Hyperbaric Medicine

Hyperbaric Medicine

Editors
Costantino Balestra
Jacek Kot

MDPI • Basel • Beijing • Wuhan • Barcelona • Belgrade • Manchester • Tokyo • Cluj • Tianjin

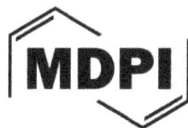

Editors
Costantino Balestra
Integrative Physiology
Haute Ecole
Bruxelles-Brabant
Brussels
Belgium

Jacek Kot
National Center for
Hyperbaric Medicine
Medical University of Gdansk
Gdynia
Poland

Editorial Office
MDPI
St. Alban-Anlage 66
4052 Basel, Switzerland

This is a reprint of articles from the Special Issue published online in the open access journal *Medicina* (ISSN 1648-9144) (available at: www.mdpi.com/journal/medicina/special_issues/hyperbaric_medicine).

For citation purposes, cite each article independently as indicated on the article page online and as indicated below:

LastName, A.A.; LastName, B.B.; LastName, C.C. Article Title. *Journal Name* **Year**, *Volume Number*, Page Range.

ISBN 978-3-0365-6467-8 (Hbk)
ISBN 978-3-0365-6466-1 (PDF)

© 2023 by the authors. Articles in this book are Open Access and distributed under the Creative Commons Attribution (CC BY) license, which allows users to download, copy and build upon published articles, as long as the author and publisher are properly credited, which ensures maximum dissemination and a wider impact of our publications.

The book as a whole is distributed by MDPI under the terms and conditions of the Creative Commons license CC BY-NC-ND.

Contents

About the Editors vii

Preface to "Hyperbaric Medicine" ix

Costantino Balestra and Jacek Kot
Oxygen: A Stimulus, Not "Only" a Drug
Reprinted from: *Medicina* **2021**, *57*, 1161, doi:10.3390/medicina57111161 1

Miguel A. Ortega, Oscar Fraile-Martinez, Cielo García-Montero, Enrique Callejón-Peláez, Miguel A. Sáez and Miguel A. Álvarez-Mon et al.
A General Overview on the Hyperbaric Oxygen Therapy: Applications, Mechanisms and Translational Opportunities
Reprinted from: *Medicina* **2021**, *57*, 864, doi:10.3390/medicina57090864 7

Katarzyna Van Damme-Ostapowicz, Mateusz Cybulski, Mariusz Kozakiewicz, Elżbieta Krajewska-Kułak, Piotr Siermontowski and Marek Sobolewski et al.
Analysis of the Increase of Vascular Cell Adhesion Molecule-1 (VCAM-1) Expression and the Effect of Exposure in a Hyperbaric Chamber on VCAM-1 in Human Blood Serum: A Cross-Sectional Study
Reprinted from: *Medicina* **2022**, *58*, 95, doi:10.3390/medicina58010095 33

Alexandru Burcea, Laurenta Lelia Mihai, Anamaria Bechir, Mircea Suciu and Edwin Sever Bechir
Clinical Assessment of the Hyperbaric Oxygen Therapy Efficacy in Mild to Moderate Periodontal Affections: A Simple Randomised Trial
Reprinted from: *Medicina* **2022**, *58*, 234, doi:10.3390/medicina58020234 47

Marie-Anne Magnan, Angèle Gayet-Ageron, Pierre Louge, Frederic Champly, Thierry Joffre and Christian Lovis et al.
Hyperbaric Oxygen Therapy with Iloprost Improves Digit Salvage in Severe Frostbite Compared to Iloprost Alone
Reprinted from: *Medicina* **2021**, *57*, 1284, doi:10.3390/medicina57111284 65

Sudhanshu Baitule, Aaran H. Patel, Narasimha Murthy, Sailesh Sankar, Ioannis Kyrou and Asad Ali et al.
A Systematic Review to Assess the Impact of Hyperbaric Oxygen Therapy on Glycaemia in People with Diabetes Mellitus
Reprinted from: *Medicina* **2021**, *57*, 1134, doi:10.3390/medicina57101134 77

Natalia D. Mankowska, Anna B. Marcinkowska, Monika Waskow, Rita I. Sharma, Jacek Kot and Pawel J. Winklewski
Critical Flicker Fusion Frequency: A Narrative Review
Reprinted from: *Medicina* **2021**, *57*, 1096, doi:10.3390/medicina57101096 89

Xavier C. E. Vrijdag, Hanna van Waart, Jamie W. Sleigh and Simon J. Mitchell
Comment on Mankowska et al. Critical Flicker Fusion Frequency: A Narrative Review. *Medicina* 2021, 57, 1096
Reprinted from: *Medicina* **2022**, *58*, 739, doi:10.3390/medicina58060739 99

Natalia D. Mankowska, Anna B. Marcinkowska, Monika Waskow, Rita I. Sharma, Jacek Kot and Pawel J. Winklewski
Reply to Vrijdag et al. Comment on "Mankowska et al. Critical Flicker Fusion Frequency: A Narrative Review. *Medicina* 2021, 57, 1096"
Reprinted from: *Medicina* **2022**, *58*, 765, doi:10.3390/medicina58060765 . . . . **101**

Laurent Deleu, Janet Catherine, Laurence Postelmans and Costantino Balestra
Effect of SCUBA Diving on Ophthalmic Parameters
Reprinted from: *Medicina* **2022**, *58*, 408, doi:10.3390/medicina58030408 . . . . **103**

Emmanuel Gouin, Costantino Balestra, Jeremy Orsat, Emmanuel Dugrenot and Erwan L'Her
Pulmonary Effects of One Week of Repeated Recreational Closed-Circuit Rebreather Dives in Cold Water
Reprinted from: *Medicina* **2022**, *59*, 81, doi:10.3390/medicina59010081 . . . . **117**

Jean-Pierre Imbert, Salih-Murat Egi and Costantino Balestra
Vascular Function Recovery Following Saturation Diving
Reprinted from: *Medicina* **2022**, *58*, 1476, doi:10.3390/medicina58101476 . . . . **131**

About the Editors

Costantino Balestra

Prof. Dr. Costantino Balestra first studied the neurophysiology of fatigue, then started studies on environmental and aging physiology issues. He teaches physiology, biostatistics, and research methodology, as well as other subjects. He is the Director of the Integrative Physiology Laboratory and a full-time professor at the Haute Ecole Bruxelles-Brabant (Brussels). He is Vice President (VP) of DAN Europe for research and education, Past President of the European Underwater and Baromedical Society (EUBS), VP of The Belgian Society of Hyperbaric and Subaquatic Medicine (SBMHS-BVOOG), and VP of the Underwater and Hyperbaric Medical Society (UHMS) (USA). His personal research interests include integrative physiology as well as challenging and extreme environments. ORCID: 0000-0001-6771-839X.

Jacek Kot

Dr. Jacek Kot is a specialist in anesthesiology and intensive care; currently he is a full-time Professor in Diving and Hyperbaric Medicine at Medical University of Gdansk, Poland, also serving as the Chief of Research and Development of the National Centre for Hyperbaric Medicine in Gdynia, Poland. The Centre is equipped with several multi-place hyperbaric chambers, a dry saturation simulator with a 'wet pot', as well as a six-bed intensive care unit within the University Hospital. Jacek Kot is the current President of the European Committee for Hyperbaric Medicine (ECHM), and from 2015 to 2018, he was President of the European Underwater and Baromedical Society (EUBS). He has been involved in international cooperation between European diving and hyperbaric centers (COST-B14, OXYNET, PHYPODE, DAN), as well as in the UHMS International Web-based Education Initiative. His professional interests mainly include HBOT in deep dives and saturation decompressions, as well as critically ill patients, especially with severe soft tissue infections. ORCID: 0000-0001-5604-8407.

Preface to "Hyperbaric Medicine"

Oxygen (both its presence and absence) acts as a potent signaling mechanism in many, if not most, cellular processes.

Oxygen has been used therapeutically mainly to alleviate or correct hypoxia, and has been administered in supra-atmospheric doses in the form of hyperbaric oxygen (a method derived from diving medicine practices, but has been used in non-diving applications since the 1960s).

Hyperbaric oxygen is, by definition, administered in an intermittent way, and in recent years, even the effects of intermittent oxygen administration at non-hyperbaric doses have been investigated and showed interesting results. Since the very beginning, because hyperbaric oxygen therapy relies on pure physics and just applying increased environmental pressure will increase partial pressure of the breathed gases (namely, oxygen), the therapeutic mechanisms involved were believed to be fully understood.

Nowadays, all reported data demonstrate how hyperoxic and hypoxic states can potentially be manipulated if oxygen is considered as a multifaceted molecule more than just a gas.

The certainties and the dogma of when hyperbaric medicine was in its adolescence are slowly being replaced.

Hyperbaric medicine is slowly moving out of its infancy. However, as in real life, with the progression away from infancy, the certainties disappear. It is now our task, as researchers, to reflect upon these uncertainties and distil out of them a coherent, balanced advice towards readers. Let us not jump to conclusions too fast, as our new "certainties"may very well prove to be "not the whole story"again. This reprint is dedicated to increase knowledge in this very interesting field, and present hyperbaric medicine in not so usual applications.

Costantino Balestra and Jacek Kot
Editors

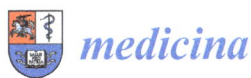

Editorial

Oxygen: A Stimulus, Not "Only" a Drug

Costantino Balestra [1] and Jacek Kot [2,*]

[1] Laboratory of Environmental and Occupational (Integrative) Physiology, Haute Ecole Bruxelles-Brabant, Auderghem, 1160 Brussels, Belgium; costantinobalestra@gmail.com
[2] National Center of Hyperbaric Medicine in Gdynia, Medical University of Gdansk, 80-210 Gdansk, Poland
* Correspondence: jacek.kot@gumed.edu.pl

Abstract: Depending on the oxygen partial pressure in a tissue, the therapeutic effect of oxygenation can vary from simple substance substitution up to hyperbaric oxygenation when breathing hyperbaric oxygen at 2.5–3.0 ATA. Surprisingly, new data showed that it is not only the oxygen supply that matters as even a minimal increase in the partial pressure of oxygen is efficient in triggering cellular reactions by eliciting the production of hypoxia-inducible factors and heat-shock proteins. Moreover, it was shown that extreme environments could also interact with the genome; in fact, epigenetics appears to play a major role in extreme environments and exercise, especially when changes in oxygen partial pressure are involved. Hyperbaric oxygen therapy is, essentially, "intermittent oxygen" exposure. We must investigate hyperbaric oxygen with a new paradigm of treating oxygen as a potent stimulus of the molecular network of reactions.

Keywords: oxygen; hyperbaric oxygen; epigenetics; normobaric oxygen paradox; hyperoxic-hypoxic paradox

1. Background

The usual path in medical sciences is typically the same: starting with understanding mechanisms; then conducting cellular tests using tissues, small animals, larger animals, then small human studies; and finally extensive clinical studies. Nevertheless, hyperbaric medicine has developed in an unusual way.

In fact, in the 1950s, a Dutch cardiac surgeon, Prof. Ite Boerema, began to use a hyperbaric chamber that was considered efficient in curing divers affected with the so-called "caissons' disease" to help his newborn patients called "blue babies". The procedure to mend cardiac septal defects needed a cardiac arrest, and the time for such a cardiac arrest was only minutes to secure a cardiovascular restart [1]. At that moment, an unacceptable number of patients were not surviving the surgery, and this surgeon wanted to find a method that would allow him to achieve better outcomes. His experiments were published in a famous paper entitled "Life without blood", and he proved that it was possible to survive critical exsanguination while remaining in a hyperbaric chamber breathing high oxygen pressures (3.0 ATA).

Increasing circulating oxygen levels in the body by increasing the barometric pressure in the operating room permits survival even after a more prolonged cardiac arrest. Of course, some years later, extracorporeal circulation became available, and the "hyperbaric operating room" was no longer needed. Hyperbaric oxygen is no longer used for maintaining general oxygenation levels, and its use has been somewhat limited for the treatment of specific diseases that are not necessarily combined with hypoxemia. Since that very moment, many hyperbaric centers have been developed, and a long list of indications and procedures have been produced.

This medical field has been so "dispersive" that reactions arose, and hyperbaric medicine was even "coined" as a "therapy in search of diseases" [2].

Significant progress has been made since the 1960s, and investigations into the mechanisms that are underlying oxygen variations were awarded a Nobel prize in 2019 [3]. This is an essential milestone in the field as, today, we have sufficient understanding to tackle two significant points that still need to be investigated in hyperbaric medicine: how much and how often. Hyperbaric medicine should be called "oxygen medicine"; an extensive range of oxygen levels may be used; and, according to these levels, repetitions of sessions must be adapted.

2. The Challenge of Oxygen Partial Pressure

Depending on the oxygen partial pressure of tissues, the therapeutic effect of oxygenation can vary from simple substance substitution, when normobaric hyperoxia is used to restore tissue oxygen levels to normal values from (120 torr in arterial blood to approx. 30–40 torr in soft tissues), up to hyperbaric oxygenation when breathing of hyperbaric oxygen at 2.5–3.0 ATA gives tissue hyperoxia well above 1000 torr.

Interestingly, the dose-effect relation is not linear but is instead "U-shaped". It is already the clinical standard that, at normobaric conditions, the arterial partial pressure must be kept in the relatively narrow range of 10–20 kPa (75–150 torr), as increased mortality was observed in critically ill patients exposed either to hypoxic or hyperoxic levels [4].

On the other hand, it is well known that exposing humans to hyperoxia induces oxygen toxicity (Paul Bert's effect on the brain and the Lorrain–Smith effect on the lungs).

3. The Challenge of Oxygen Toxicity

Today, the hyperbaric exposure dose (pressure and time) and repetitions are mainly limited by pulmonary and neurological toxicity. To remain on the safe side and not harm the patient, the OTUs (Oxygen Toxicity Units) or UTPDs (Units of Pulmonary Toxicity Dose) are calculated, even if those units are challenged in new approaches [5–8]. Permanent exposure to hyperbaric oxygen is not a clinical option. Fortunately, it seems that intermittent switching between low and high oxygen pressure is sufficiently potent to induce significant therapeutic molecular actions (Figure 1).

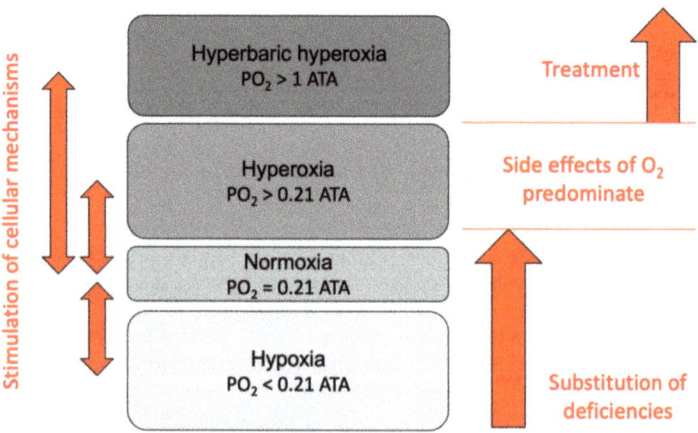

Figure 1. Oxygen levels and their therapeutic use (PO_2, partial pressure of oxygen).

4. Oxygen as a Trigger

Surprisingly, new data show that even a minimal increase in the partial pressure of oxygen efficiently triggers cellular reactions [9,10]. As we already expressed in previous works, "some decades ago, on the physiological side, the two parameters that characterize extreme environments were identified as eliciting the production of two particular elements: hypoxia-inducible factors and heat-shock proteins. The two are ubiquitous and essential for cellular life" [11,12].

These "Hypoxia-Inducible Factors can trigger several hundred genes", but it has been shown that hyperoxia, more specifically, coming back to normoxia after hyperoxic exposure (relative hypoxia), can trigger this essential factor responsible for vascular, cellular, and metabolic homeostasis and apoptosis [10,13,14]. Its beneficial actions in the fight against cancer cells have recently been advocated [12]. The second is a family of proteins acting as chaperones for other proteins and resetting impaired proteic structures triggered by many environmental stressors [15].

5. Epigenetics and the Challenge of Cellular Responses

Epigenetics seems to play a significant role in exercise and extreme environments [11]. Recently, it was shown that external stressors could indeed interact with the genome, especially when changes in the oxygen partial pressure are involved [16].

This is may not be all that surprising as we know that physical exercise can produce extensive cellular reactions, including epigenetic reactions. Physical exercise is actually an intermittent oxidative stress variation. The oxygen level is very low in the mitochondria (Figure 2) [17]. We can, therefore, understand how potent a minute variation of oxygen tension may be at that level. We may need to consider oxygen variations in the mitochondrion as the most potent homeorhetic trigger in nature.

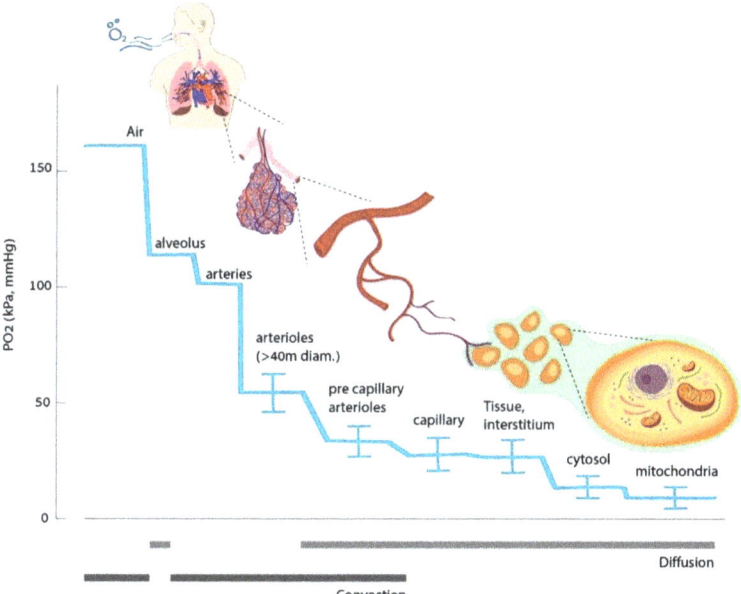

Figure 2. Oxygen cascade from ambient air down to mitochondria (figure taken from [17]).

Considering this no wonder that even variations of 10% of the inspired oxygen fraction may be effective in humans and cultured cells [9,10,18]. It is now known that genes are not always activated. They are not mandatorily expressed. They can be "turned on" or "off" by external interferences that do not change the DNA sequence. There are two major mechanisms for this: DNA methylation and histone modifications. Acute environmental changes can induce epigenetic modifications; cells constantly receive all kinds of signals informing them about their surrounding environment and adjust their activity to the situation.

Recent data showed an epigenetic change through methylation in alpinists exposed to hypoxia, demonstrating rapid changes that were even recently not considered possible in the human epigenome following acute oxygen variation [16].

Several other articles have discussed the fact that pulsed hyperoxia induces hypoxia-inducible factor 1α (HIF-1α) activation and the expression of genes involved in the response to low oxygen describing a "normobaric oxygen paradox" (NOP), i.e., that relative changes of oxygen availability, rather than steady-state hypoxic (or hyperoxic) conditions, coordinate HIF-1α transcriptional effects [14,19]. This phenomenon has different names, either "Hyperoxic–Hypoxic Paradox" [17] or "Normobaric Oxygen Paradox" [20] depending on the range of variation of PO_2 imposed. Nevertheless, a general term could be a "relative hypoxia" without reaching tissular hypoxic levels [20].

These studies investigated the activation of oxygen-sensitive transcription factors in peripheral blood mononuclear cells (PBMC) obtained from a human after breathing, increasing PO_2, generating mild, high, and very high hyperoxia (30%, 100%, and 140% O_2, respectively). The responses were followed for 24 h post exposure. It is possible that, for higher levels of hyperoxia (high and very-high), a longer time is needed to see reactive adaptations, such as the expression of nuclear factor erythroid 2-related factor 2 (NRF2) and HIF-1α. Further investigations are required with prolonged periods.

All treatments were associated with significant activation of NRF2 and HIF-1α. Conversely, the nuclear factor kappa B (NF-kB) transcription factor was significantly activated only by higher oxygen concentrations. The intracellular levels of total glutathione paralleled the nuclear transfer of NRF2 and remained elevated up to the end of the experimental observation time along with the plasmatic level of matrix metalloproteinase 9 (MMP-9). We confirmed that mild hyperoxia is sensed as hypoxic stress in vivo within the first 24 h, activating HIF-1α and NRF2, but not NF-kB.

Conversely, high hyperoxia was associated with a progressive loss of the NOP response and increased oxidative stress signals leading to NRF2 and NF-kB activation, accompanied by the synthesis of GSH. After very high hyperoxia, HIF-1α activation was absent in the first 24 h, and the oxidative stress response accompanied by NF-kB activation was prevalent. The glutathione (GSH) levels paralleled the nuclear transfer of NRF2 and remained elevated during the observation time together with the MMP-9 plasma levels. Further confirmation was published on the activation of microRNA during different oxygen exposures [21].

Interestingly, several articles have been interested in increasing hemoglobin and oxygen exposure [9,14,22–24]. To achieve such an increase in a fast way, small deltas were elicited; for a more extended response, higher oxygen variations and more distant (less frequent) variations were needed [21]. If the oxygen variations were relatively small, a repeated and frequent exposure had a fast answer (a few days) [22].

6. New Levels of Oxygen

Recent data confirmed that, in vivo, the return to normoxia after mild hyperoxia is sensed as hypoxic stress characterized by HIF-1α activation [10]. On the contrary, high hyperoxia and very high hyperoxia induce a shift toward an oxidative stress response, characterized by NRF2 and NF-κB activation in the first 24 h post-exposure.

Even though it is possible that higher levels of hyperoxia (high hyperoxia from 50% to 100%, very high hyperoxia at hyperbaric levels) may induce late responses to recover homeostasis over a longer window of time, previous studies in cultured cells [14] and in vivo [12,25] suggested that critical adaptive responses occur within shorter times. However, further investigations are needed to investigate if pulsed hyperoxia induces specific compensatory reactive adaptations at more extended periods. Future studies should focus on the two components of this paradigm: the oxygen exposure (time and PO_2) and time between sessions (intermittent exposures) [12,23].

Overall, already published data [10] suggested the occurrence of a "hormetic" adaption to high oxygen triggered by the activation of signaling cascades leading to the expression of antioxidant systems; this is in agreement with data obtained in rodents undergoing either hyperbaric or normobaric oxygen that initially induced significant oxidative stress that was eventually resolved after continued exposure [26].

To optimize applicable clinical protocols from this paradigm, future studies are expected to focus also on the "down-stream" effects of HIF-1α transcriptional activation. Depending on the therapeutic target, using mild hyperoxia (from 30% to 40–50%) may be more desirable [12,27], or, on the other hand, eliciting oxidative stress utilizing HH/VHH administration may be considered a more appropriate desirable effect.

7. Intermittent Oxygen, the Clue?

Hyperbaric oxygen therapy is, by essence, "intermittent oxygen" exposure. It is clear from previous data that we must investigate this direction with a new paradigm of treating oxygen rather as a potent stimulus of the molecular network of reactions. The vital task is answering the questions of "how much", "how long", and "how often" this stimulus should be given. The non-linearity of the dose-response curve complicates the picture. Still, to the end, we should be able to answer what oxygen dose should be given to reach a specific clinical or molecular effect.

We hope that the authors of the papers in this special issue of *Medicina* and active readers using those ideas in their research will help to shape the future of "oxygen medicine".

Author Contributions: Conceptualization, C.B. and J.K.; writing—review and editing, C.B. and J.K. All authors have read and agreed to the published version of the manuscript.

Funding: This submission received no external funding.

Institutional Review Board Statement: Not applicable.

Conflicts of Interest: The authors declare no conflict of interest.

References

1. Boerema, I.; Meyne, N.G.; Brummelkamp, W.H.; Bouma, S.; Mensch, M.H.; Kamermans, F.; Stern Hanf, M.; van Aalderen, W. Life without blood. *Ned. Tijdschr. Geneeskd.* **1960**, *104*, 949–954.
2. Phillips, T.J. Hyperbaric oxygen therapy: A therapy in search of a disease? *Dermatol. Surg.* **2000**, *26*, 1167–1169. [CrossRef]
3. Lopez-Barneo, J.; Simon, M.C. Cellular adaptation to oxygen deficiency beyond the Nobel award. *Nat. Commun.* **2020**, *11*, 607. [CrossRef]
4. De Jonge, E.; Peelen, L.; Keijzers, P.J.; Joore, H.; de Lange, D.; van der Voort, P.H.; Bosman, R.J.; de Waal, R.A.; Wesselink, R.; de Keizer, N.F. Association between administered oxygen, arterial partial oxygen pressure and mortality in mechanically ventilated intensive care unit patients. *Crit. Care* **2008**, *12*, R156. [CrossRef]
5. Wingelaar, T.T.; Brinkman, P.; Hoencamp, R.; van Ooij, P.A.; Maitland-van der Zee, A.H.; Hollmann, M.W.; van Hulst, R.A. Assessment of pulmonary oxygen toxicity in special operations forces divers under operational circumstances using exhaled breath analysis. *Diving Hyperb. Med.* **2020**, *50*, 2–7. [CrossRef]
6. Arieli, R.; Aviner, B. Acclimatization and Deacclimatization to Oxygen: Determining Exposure Limits to Avoid CNS O2 Toxicity in Active Diving. *Front. Physiol.* **2020**, *11*, 1105. [CrossRef] [PubMed]
7. Aviner, B.; Arieli, R.; Yalov, A. Power Equation for Predicting the Risk of Central Nervous System Oxygen Toxicity at Rest. *Front. Physiol.* **2020**, *11*, 1007. [CrossRef]
8. Arieli, R. Effect of an air break on the occurrence of seizures in hyperbaric oxygen therapy may be predicted by the power equation for hyperoxia at rest. *Diving Hyperb. Med. J. S. Pac. Underw. Med. Soc.* **2020**, *50*, 75–76. [CrossRef]
9. Khalife, M.; Ben Aziz, M.; Balestra, C.; Valsamis, J.; Sosnowski, M. Physiological and Clinical Impact of Repeated Inhaled Oxygen Variation on Erythropoietin Levels in Patients After Surgery. *Front. Physiol.* **2021**, *12*, 744074. [CrossRef] [PubMed]
10. Fratantonio, D.; Virgili, F.; Zucchi, A.; Lambrechts, K.; Latronico, T.; Lafere, P.; Germonpre, P.; Balestra, C. Increasing Oxygen Partial Pressures Induce a Distinct Transcriptional Response in Human PBMC: A Pilot Study on the "Normobaric Oxygen Paradox". *Int. J. Mol. Sci.* **2021**, *22*, 458. [CrossRef] [PubMed]
11. Balestra, C.; Kot, J.; Efrati, S.; Guerrero, F.; Blatteau, J.; Besnard, S. *Coping with Extreme Environments: A Physiological/Psychological Approach*; Balestra, C., Kot, J., Efrati, S., Guerrero, F., Blatteau, J., Besnard, S., Eds.; Frontiers Media SA: Lausanne, Switzerland, 2019; Volume 1.
12. De Bels, D.; Corazza, F.; Germonpre, P.; Balestra, C. The normobaric oxygen paradox: A novel way to administer oxygen as an adjuvant treatment for cancer? *Med. Hypotheses* **2011**, *76*, 467–470. [CrossRef]
13. De Bels, D.; Corazza, F.; Balestra, C. Oxygen sensing, homeostasis, and disease. *N. Engl. J. Med.* **2011**, *365*, 1845. [CrossRef]
14. Cimino, F.; Balestra, C.; Germonpre, P.; De Bels, D.; Tillmans, F.; Saija, A.; Speciale, A.; Virgili, F. Pulsed high oxygen induces a hypoxic-like response in Human Umbilical Endothelial Cells (HUVECs) and in humans. *J. Appl. Physiol.* **2012**, *113*, 1684–1689. [CrossRef]

15. Blatteau, J.E.; Gempp, E.; Balestra, C.; Mets, T.; Germonpre, P. Predive sauna and venous gas bubbles upon decompression from 400 kPa. *Aviat. Space Environ. Med.* **2008**, *79*, 1100–1105. [CrossRef] [PubMed]
16. Basang, Z.; Zhang, S.; Yang, L.; Quzong, D.; Li, Y.; Ma, Y.; Hao, M.; Pu, W.; Liu, X.; Xie, H.; et al. Correlation of DNA methylation patterns to the phenotypic features of Tibetan elite alpinists in extreme hypoxia. *J. Genet. Genom.* **2021**, *48*, 928–935. [CrossRef] [PubMed]
17. Hadanny, A.; Efrati, S. The Hyperoxic-Hypoxic Paradox. *Biomolecules* **2020**, *10*, 958. [CrossRef] [PubMed]
18. Balestra, C.; Lambrechts, K.; Mrakic-Sposta, S.; Vezzoli, A.; Levenez, M.; Germonpré, P.; Virgili, F.; Bosco, G.; Lafère, P. Hypoxic and Hyperoxic Breathing as a Complement to Low-Intensity Physical Exercise Programs: A Proof-of-Principle Study. *Int. J. Mol. Sci.* **2021**, *22*, 9200. [CrossRef] [PubMed]
19. Balestra, C.; Germonpre, P.; Poortmans, J.R.; Marroni, A. Serum erythropoietin levels in healthy humans after a short period of normobaric and hyperbaric oxygen breathing: The "normobaric oxygen paradox". *J. Appl. Physiol.* **2006**, *100*, 512–518. [CrossRef]
20. Balestra, C.; Germonpre, P. Hypoxia, a multifaceted phenomenon: The example of the "normobaric oxygen paradox". *Eur. J. Appl. Physiol.* **2012**, *112*, 4173–4175. [CrossRef]
21. Bosco, G.; Paganini, M.; Giacon, T.A.; Oppio, A.; Vezzoli, A.; Dellanoce, C.; Moro, T.; Paoli, A.; Zanotti, F.; Zavan, B.; et al. Oxidative Stress and Inflammation, MicroRNA, and Hemoglobin Variations after Administration of Oxygen at Different Pressures and Concentrations: A Randomized Trial. *Int. J. Environ. Res. Public Health* **2021**, *18*, 9755. [CrossRef]
22. Rocco, M.; D'Itri, L.; De Bels, D.; Corazza, F.; Balestra, C. The "normobaric oxygen paradox": A new tool for the anesthetist? *Minerva Anestesiol.* **2014**, *80*, 366–372. [PubMed]
23. Lafere, P.; Schubert, T.; De Bels, D.; Germonpre, P.; Balestra, C. Can the normobaric oxygen paradox (NOP) increase reticulocyte count after traumatic hip surgery? *J. Clin. Anesth.* **2013**, *25*, 129–134. [CrossRef] [PubMed]
24. De Bels, D.; Theunissen, S.; Devriendt, J.; Germonpre, P.; Lafere, P.; Valsamis, J.; Snoeck, T.; Meeus, P.; Balestra, C. The 'normobaric oxygen paradox': Does it increase haemoglobin? *Diving Hyperb. Med. J. S. Pac. Underw. Med. Soc.* **2012**, *42*, 67–71.
25. Donati, A.; Damiani, E.; Zuccari, S.; Domizi, R.; Scorcella, C.; Girardis, M.; Giulietti, A.; Vignini, A.; Adrario, E.; Romano, R.; et al. Effects of short-term hyperoxia on erythropoietin levels and microcirculation in critically Ill patients: A prospective observational pilot study. *BMC Anesthesiol.* **2017**, *17*, 49. [CrossRef] [PubMed]
26. Korpinar, S.; Uzun, H. The Effects of Hyperbaric Oxygen at Different Pressures on Oxidative Stress and Antioxidant Status in Rats. *Medicina* **2019**, *55*, 205. [CrossRef]
27. De Bels, D.; Tillmans, F.; Corazza, F.; Bizzari, M.; Germonpre, P.; Radermacher, P.; Orman, K.G.; Balestra, C. Hyperoxia Alters Ultrastructure and Induces Apoptosis in Leukemia Cell Lines. *Biomolecules* **2020**, *10*, 282. [CrossRef]

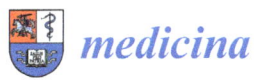

Review

A General Overview on the Hyperbaric Oxygen Therapy: Applications, Mechanisms and Translational Opportunities

Miguel A. Ortega [1,2,3,*], Oscar Fraile-Martinez [1,2,*], Cielo García-Montero [1,2], Enrique Callejón-Peláez [4], Miguel A. Sáez [1,2,5], Miguel A. Álvarez-Mon [1,2], Natalio García-Honduvilla [1,2], Jorge Monserrat [1,2], Melchor Álvarez-Mon [1,2,6], Julia Bujan [1,2] and María Luisa Canals [7]

1. Department of Medicine and Medical Specialities, Faculty of Medicine and Health Sciences, University of Alcalá, 28801 Alcala de Henares, Spain; cielo.gmontero@gmail.com (C.G.-M.); msaega1@oc.mde.es (M.A.S.); maalvarezdemon@icloud.com (M.A.Á.-M.); natalio.garcia@uah.es (N.G.-H.); jorge.monserrat@uah.es (J.M.); mademons@gmail.com (M.Á.-M.); mjulia.bujan@uah.es (J.B.)
2. Ramón y Cajal Institute of Sanitary Research (IRYCIS), 28034 Madrid, Spain
3. Cancer Registry and Pathology Department, Hospital Universitario Principe de Asturias, 28806 Alcala de Henares, Spain
4. Underwater and Hyperbaric Medicine Service, Central University Hospital of Defence—UAH Madrid, 28801 Alcala de Henares, Spain; ecalpel@fn.mde.es
5. Pathological Anatomy Service, Central University Hospital of Defence—UAH Madrid, 28801 Alcala de Henares, Spain
6. Immune System Diseases—Rheumatology, Oncology Service an Internal Medicine, University Hospital Príncipe de Asturias, (CIBEREHD), 28806 Alcala de Henares, Spain
7. ISM, IMHA Research Chair, Former of IMHA (International Maritime Health Association), 43001 Tarragona, Spain; mlcanalsp@gmail.com
* Correspondence: miguel.angel.ortega92@gmail.com (M.A.O.); oscarfra.7@hotmail.com (O.F.-M.); Tel.: +34-91-885-40-45 (M.A.O.); Fax: +34-91-885-48-85 (M.A.O.)

Abstract: Hyperbaric oxygen therapy (HBOT) consists of using of pure oxygen at increased pressure (in general, 2–3 atmospheres) leading to augmented oxygen levels in the blood (Hyperoxemia) and tissue (Hyperoxia). The increased pressure and oxygen bioavailability might be related to a plethora of applications, particularly in hypoxic regions, also exerting antimicrobial, immunomodulatory and angiogenic properties, among others. In this review, we will discuss in detail the physiological relevance of oxygen and the therapeutical basis of HBOT, collecting current indications and underlying mechanisms. Furthermore, potential areas of research will also be examined, including inflammatory and systemic maladies, COVID-19 and cancer. Finally, the adverse effects and contraindications associated with this therapy and future directions of research will be considered. Overall, we encourage further research in this field to extend the possible uses of this procedure. The inclusion of HBOT in future clinical research could be an additional support in the clinical management of multiple pathologies.

Keywords: hyperbaric oxygen therapy (HBOT); Hyperoxia; wound healing; antimicrobial properties; Coronavirus Disease-19 (COVID-19)

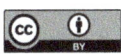

1. Introduction

Hyperbaric oxygen therapy (HBOT) is a therapeutical approach based on exposure to pure concentrations of oxygen (O_2) in an augmented atmospheric pressure. According to the Undersea and Hyperbaric Medical Society (UHMS), this pressure may equal or exceed 1.4 atmospheres (atm) [1]. However, all current UHMS-approved indications require that patients breathe near 100% oxygen while enclosed in a chamber pressurized to a minimum of 2 ATA [2].

The first documented use of hyperbaric medical therapy was in 1662 by Henshaw, a British physician who placed patients in a container with pressurized air. Interestingly, it was conducted before the formulation of the Boyle-Mariotte Law, which described the relationship between the pressure and volume of a gas, and prior to the discovery of O_2 by John Priestly over 100 years later [3]. Afterwards, the pathway of HBOT in medical care was retarded by the observation of possible O_2-derived adverse effects at 100% concentrations by Lavoisier and Seguin in 1789. Years later, in 1872 Paul Bert, considered the "father of the hyperbaric physiology", described the physiological basis of pressurized air in the human body, also defining the neurotoxic effects of O_2 in the human body, consequently named the Paul Bert effect [4], followed by the description of the pulmonary toxicity of O_2 by Lorrain Smith [5]. Simultaneously, a growing interest in the use of HBOT in the treatment of different affections was reported, including treatment for divers who suffered decompression sickness during World War II [6]. Since then, a plethora of studies were prompted, with hundreds of facilities based on HBOT being established at the beginning of the 21st century [7].

Currently, there are 14 approved indications for HBOT, including a wide variety of complications like air embolism, severe anemia, certain infectious diseases or idiopathic sensorial hearing loss. In addition, in the last European Consensus Conference on Hyperbaric Medicine highlighted the use of HBOT as a primary treatment method for certain conditions according to their moderate to high degree of evidence (e.g., after carbon monoxide (CO) poisoning), or as a potential adjuvant to consider in other conditions with a moderate amount of scientific evidence (e.g., Diabetic foot) [8]. In this work we will review in detail the basis of O_2 as a therapeutical agent and the principles of hyperbaric medicine regarding most relevant applications concerning HBOT, and potential implications for different approaches including COVID-19.

2. Physiological Role of Oxygen in the Organism

O_2 is a frequently disregarded nutrient because of its particular access inside the human body, through the lungs instead of the gastrointestinal tract, typical of all other nutrients [9]. O_2 is key for human cells to perform so-called aerobic respiration, which takes places in the mitochondria. Here, O_2 acts as an electron acceptor finally leading to ATP synthesis in a process known as oxidative phosphorylation. From an evolutionary perspective, the uptake of O_2 was the origin of eukaryotic cells, emerging as a result of an endosymbiotic relationship between prokaryotic cells (archaea and eubacteria) which were capable of using this nutrient [10]. This fact represented an adaptative advantage with regard to those cells unable to utilize it, complex organisms were coevolving with O_2, thus becoming an essential nutrient for our cells [11].

In a simple manner, O_2 is introduced in our body by two distinguished process: ventilation, in which gases are transported from the environment to the bronchial tree and diffusion, where an equilibrium in the distribution of O_2 between alveoli space and blood is reached. Given that the partial pressure of O_2 (PO_2) here is low, and rich in carbon dioxide (CO_2), gas exchange occurs [12]. Simultaneously, the difference in the pressure and volume in the chest wall and lungs are essential to permit the oxygen flow, as atmospheric pressure does not vary at all [13]. Once in the bloodstream, O_2 is mostly bound to haemoglobin (Hb) in the erythrocytes, and to a little extent in a dissolved form, being systemically distributed. Then, oxygen exchange is produced between the microcirculatory vessels—Not only capillaries, but also arterioles and venules-and the rest of the tissues, due to the different partial pressure of O_2 and the Hb oxygen saturation (SO_2), which is also dependant on other variables like temperature, PCO_2 and pH, among others [14]. If, however there is a lack of oxygen in the tissue it may appear a condition designed as hypoxia. This may be due to low O_2 content in the blood (Hypoxemia), which may be a consequence of either a disruption in the blood flow to the lungs (Perfusion), airflow to the alveoli (Ventilation) or problems in the gas diffusion in the haemato-alveolar barrier. Furthermore, low blood supply (ischaemia) or difficulties in the O_2 delivery, may also be responsible for tissue hypoxia [15]. Consequently, within cells there are specific sensors named as Hypoxia-inducible factors (HIF) that under hypoxic conditions will bind to the hypoxia response element (HRE), thereby regulating a wide variety of cellular processes [16]. Occasionally, hypoxia might provide favourable implications for health, for instance during early developmental stages [17] or in the case of intermittent exposures [18]. Nonetheless, hypoxia mostly induce a pathological stress for cells that is closely related with the appearance and progress of a broad spectrum of diseases [19]. As a result, oxygen has been proposed as a potential therapeutic agent for patients undergoing different acute or chronic conditions [20,21]. As targeting cellular hypoxia is a promising, but still an emerging approach [22], clinical management of hypoxia is directed to modulate global hypoxemia and oxygen delivery within the tissues [23]. In this context, HBOT arises as an extraordinary support in the handling of hypoxia and other hypoxia-related phenomena by increasing blood and tissue levels of oxygen [24]. Hereunder, we will describe the principles and mechanisms of action of HBOT, regarding its therapeutical basis and specific considerations of this therapy.

3. Principles of Hyperbaric Oxygen Therapy. Therapeutical Basis

As above mentioned, HBOT consist of the supply of pure oxygen under augmented pressure. This procedure is conducted in a monoplace or multiplace chamber if there are only one or various patients undergoing this procedure, respectively. In the first case, the chambers are usually compressed with O_2 whereas in the second, people breath oxygen individually through a face mask, hood, or an endotracheal tube [25]. In the case of critically ill patients, it seems that multiplace chambers allow a better monitoring of the vital functions in comparison to monoplace chambers, although the use of the latter are also safe and well tolerated by patients [26,27]. Depending on the protocol, the estimated duration of session varies from 1.5 to 2 h and may be performed from one to three times daily, being given among 20 to 60 therapeutical doses depending on the condition [28]. Frequently, this method utilizes between 2 to 3 atms of pressure. Nevertheless, it has also been obtained promising results in some studies from <2 atms (1.5 atms) for certain conditions [29,30], although according to all UHMS currently approved indications it is required a chamber pressurized to a minimum of 2 ATA [2]. Despite some protocols accept the use of 6 atms (i.e., treatment of gas embolism), little benefits are usually reported from >3 atms as it may be associated with a plethora of adverse effects [31]. Moreover, it is not possible to breath pure O_2 at higher pressures than 2.8 atm, and in those cases it is accompanied with other gases like helium, nitrogen or ozone. The alternative, normobaric oxygen therapy (NBOT), utilizes oxygen at 1 atm of pressure. In comparison with HBOT, NBOT is cheaper and easier to apply, and it could be found in almost all hospitals, as it does not require hyperbaric chambers [32]. However, some studies have reported a reduced efficacy of NBOT in comparison with HBOT [33,34], therefore showing the relevance of HBOT for certain conditions. Conversely, the use of NBOT could be critical for patients suffering from some maladies in absence of HBOT facilities.

The therapeutical basis of hyperbaric oxygenation are consequence of three main factors: (1) By breathing 100% O_2, a positive gradient is created, hence favouring diffusion for hyperoxygenated lungs to hypoxic tissues; (2) due to the high pressure, O_2 concentration in the blood raises according to Henry's Law (the amount of dissolved gas within a liquid is directly proportional to its partial pressure) and (3) it decreases the size of gas bubbles in the blood following Boyle-Mariotte Law and Henry's Law [6]. In other words, the creation of a hyperbaric environment with pure oxygen permits a significant increment of the oxygen supply to blood (Hyperoxemia) and to the tissues (Hyperoxia) even without the contribution from Hb [35]. Thus, HBOT provides multiple effects in the organism, and it could be used to correct tissue hypoxia, chronic hypoxemia and to aid in the clinical management of different pathological processes including wound healing, necrosis, or reperfusion injuries [36].

Contrary to hypoxia, the human body has not developed any specific adaptation to hyperoxia. Interestingly, the exposure to intermittent hyperoxia, share many of the mediators and cellular mechanisms which are induced by hypoxia. This is called the hyperoxic-hypoxic paradox [37]. Importantly, it does not have to be considered a negative property. As occurring with intermittent hypoxia, the submitting of short-term hyperoxia may provide favourable outcomes in the cell. The explanation resides in a crucial concept in biology, the hormesis, which correlates the type of response obtained with the dose received [38]. From a molecular perspective, high PO_2 in the tissues may have important implications in the cellular signalling, particularly through increasing the production of reactive oxygen species (ROS) and reactive nitrogen species (RNS). These changes induce multiple effects in the organism, including the synthesis of different growth factors, improving neovascularization or showing immunomodulatory properties, among others, therefore exerting its clinical efficacy [39,40]. Moreover, HBOT upregulates HIF, by ROS/RNS and Extracellular Regulated Kinases (ERK1/ERK2) pathway [37,41]. In the same manner, an excessive production of ROS and RNS due to hyperoxia may lead to the appearance of oxidative stress, DNA damage, metabolic disturbances, endothelial dysfunction, acute pulmonary injury and neurotoxicity [42]. As hyperbaric O_2 may provide both beneficial and adverse effects, it is essential to balance the different factors to clinically recommend or reject HBOT [43]. Due to the physics of HBOT, it is not easy to design adequate studies and clinical trials to fully endorse its use. Despite this, there are some predictive models that may be an additional tool to evaluate what patients may benefit the most from receiving this therapy, considering distinct therapeutical approaches if necessary [44].

In Figure 1 conditions and characteristics of hyperbaric chambers are illustrated, besides the main effect of pressurized O_2 administration. Below, main applications and translational applications of HBOT will be subsequently discussed, in order to review the actual importance of this procedure in current clinical practice and potential uses.

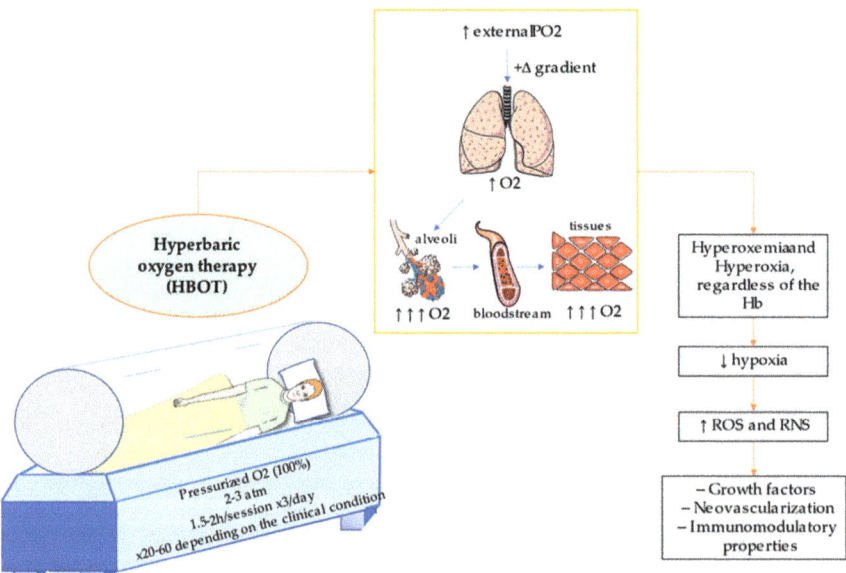

Figure 1. Illustration of a monoplace hyperbaric chamber and the effect of hyperbaric O_2. Pressurized O_2 (2–3 atm) at 100% concentration is administered normally during 1.5–2 h per session and repeated three times a day. Depending on the clinical condition sessions vary in number, from 20 to 60. The inhaled air comes from an external elevated PO_2, hence positive gradient allows higher O_2 entry, which per diffusion will be higher also in alveoli, bloodstream and therefore there will be greater arrival to tissues. This effect of "hyperoxemia" and "hyperoxia" is independent from haemoglobin (Hb), then will lessen hypoxia in tissues. This will result in a major supply of reactive oxygen species (ROS) and reactive nitrite species (RNS), with a consequent higher expression of growth factors and promotion of neovascularization and enhanced immunomodulatory properties.

4. Approved Indications for HBOT

Due to the multiple characteristics of HBOT, the possible applications of this procedure are numerous. For instance, HBOT may be used as an urgent treatment for acute pathologies but also as an additional support for chronic diseases [41]. Currently, there are 14 approved indications for HBOT are represented in Table 1. Most of these uses, can be grouped according to three main effects (a) in the wound healing acceleration and angiogenesis enhancement (b) exerting antimicrobial effects, and (c) as a medical emergency.

Table 1. Approved indications for HBOT.

Air or gas embolism
Acute thermal burn injury
Carbon monoxide poisoning
Carbon monoxide poisoning complicated by cyanide poisoning
Central retinal artery occlusion
Clostridial myositis and myonecrosis (gas gangrene)
Compromised grafts and Flaps
Crush injury, Compartment Syndrome and other acute traumatic ischemia
Decompression sickness
Delayed radiation injury (soft tissue and bony necrosis)
Enhancement of healing in selected problem wounds
Idiopathic sudden sensorineural hearing loss
Intracranial abscess
Necrotizing soft tissue infections
Refractory osteomyelitis
Severe anaemia

4.1. HBOT and Wound Healing: The Angiogenesis Enhancement

In clinical practice, it has been observed how HBOT can speed wound healing. As wounds need oxygen to regenerate tissues properly, an exposure of 100% oxygen accelerates this process. The application in this field is quite extensive, comprising microbial-infected wounds (e.g., Clostridial myonecrosis and Fournier's gangrene), traumatic wounds, thermal burns, skin grafts, radiation-induced wounds, diabetic and vascular insufficiency ulcers [45].

In the field of diabetes, there is a critical complication called "diabetic foot ulcers", an open wound at the bottom of the foot that affects 15% of patients. HBOT has been specially regarded for this injury, being implicated many inflammatory and tissue repairing parameters. For instance, there was some evidence that HBOT may improve the healing rate of wounds, by increasing nitric oxide (NO) levels and the number of endothelial progenitor cells, in the non-healing vasculitis, calcific uremic arteriolopathy (CUA), livedoid vasculopathy (LV), pyoderma gangrenosum (PG) ulcers [46]. Some trials show a prominent angiogenesis while reducing inflammation: angiogenic markers like epithelial growth factor (EGF) and VEGF become enhanced, and positively associates to Nrf2 transcription factor increase [47]. Furthermore, anaerobic infections have a lower occurrence and amputation rates immensely decrease [48,49]. Different systematic reviews support the adjuvant use of systemic but not topical HBOT in the wound healing of diabetic foot ulcers [50,51]. However, studies results are quite heterogeneous, and it is still necessary to define which group of patients may benefit most from this intervention [52]. For instance, patients with diabetic foot ulcers and peripheral arterial occlusive disease may not improve wound healing [53]. Another recent study demonstrated that the use of HBOT may be associated with improved six-year survival in patients with diabetic foots [54]. Further studies and greater samples are required to identify the most suitable candidates for HBOT.

Additionally, HBOT may be an excellent adjuvant in surgery injuries resolutions, and it is key as it may provide better outcomes if it is earlier administered. When wounds do not follow conventional treatments for healing, an extra aid can be found in HBOT.

Animal models have described the importance of this procedure in the wound healing by the acceleration of epithelialization and neovascularization [55,56]. Reported effects on these events resides in the up-regulation of host factors like tumour necrosis factor-α (TNF-α), matrix metallopeptidase 9 (MMP-9) and tissue inhibitor of metalloproteinase-1 (TIMP-1) [57]. In a rabbit model of irradiated tissue, NBOT O_2 was compared to hyperbaric demonstrating once again that O_2 is required at higher pressures to provoke an angiogenic effect [56]. More studies in vivo have alleged tension exerted by hyperbaric O_2 modulates proliferation rate of stem cells in small intestinal crypts and raises angiogenesis in chorio-allantonic membrane in *Gallus gallus* embryos [58]. In a clinical trial of patients with chronic non-healing wounds (more than 20 months without healing), HBOT was standardized for 20 sessions (five sessions/week). The results were increased levels of vascular endothelial growth factor (VEGF) and interleukine-6 (IL-6), and lower levels of endothelin-1. These facts entail an activation of host wound resolution factors, angiogenesis and vascular tone [59]. Vasculogenesis gains efficiency thanks to HBOT upregulation of nitric oxide (NO) and associates to a decrease in lesions area [60].

Multiple lines of research have also been opened to evaluate the enhanced angiogenesis and healing of tissues following HBOT. For instance, a phase 2A clinical trial demonstrated the possible benefits from HBOT in combination with steroids for patients with ulcerative colitis in terms of achieving higher rates of clinical remission, and a reduced probability of progression to second-line therapy during the hospitalization [61]. However, there are few studies in this field, and soon an updated meta-analysis and systematic review of the available evidence will be published [62]. Similar conclusions might be extrapolated to radiation-induced hemorrhagic cystitis and proctitis [63]. Osteoradionecrosis is also a frequent and worrisome condition in oncological patients after receiving radiotherapy. Frequently, this condition affects to the jaw and consists of the development aseptic, avascular necrosis which can lead to infection, tooth loss, and even pathological fracture of the jaw. Moreover, it often results in an ulceration and necrosis of the mucosa with exposed bone. HBOT plays a critical role in the treatment of this condition, improving the tissue response to surgical wounding, and even as prophylactic approach in patients with previous head and neck irradiation undergoing dental extractions or complete exodontia [64]. The enhancing angiogenesis and wound healing make HBOT an adequate adjuvant treatment in a wide variety of conditions, although future studies should be directed to evaluate the most effective dose and to identify the most suitable candidates for submitting this procedure.

4.2. HBOT and Infections: The Antimicrobial Activity

The use of HBOT as an antimicrobial adjuvant is particularly useful in healing context now that microbial infections are the most important cause of non-healing wounds: meta-analysis affirm that prevalence of bacterial biofilms in chronic wounds is 78.2% [65]. HBOT is considered a non-conventional strategy for non-healing wounds consisting in a modification of biophysical parameters in the wound microenvironment, breaking the bacterial biofilms [66]. HBOT upregulates HIF that induces the expression of Nitric Oxide Synthases (NOS) and virus killing peptides (defensins and cathelicidins such as cathelin-related antimicrobial peptide) with consequent neutrophil and monocyte phagocytosis of the microbes [67–69]. Increased cathelicidins in mice lungs provide a better response to the flu virus [70]. Cathelicidin-deficient mice show higher susceptibility to viral damage [71].

The most important applications of the antimicrobial activity of HBOT are under necrotizing soft tissue infections (NSTIs), including necrotizing fasciitis, Fournier's gangrene and gas gangrene. There is a calamitous soft tissue infection implying a wide variety of gram-positive, gram-negative, aerobic and anaerobic bacteria. It happens under conditions of trauma or minor lesions that become more complicated, normally, due to systemic problems like diabetes or vascular disfunctions [45,72]. An early and combined HBOT therapy plus current practices may be crucial as a lifesaving and cost-efficacy therapy, particularly in the most critical patients [73]. Clinical practice agrees on the necessity of HBOT in the event of an anaerobic infection, as anaerobic bacteria are killed by a much higher amount of pressurized O_2 [74,75]. For instance, the use of HBOT in the anaerobic *Clostridium perfringens* bacteria is specially recommended [76]. This bacterium produces more than 20 recognized toxins. However, two toxins, alpha and theta are the main mediators of the infection caused by this agent. *Clostridium perfringens* growth is restricted at O_2 tensions up to 70 mm Hg, and alpha-toxin production is halted at tensions of 250 mm Hg, also achieving bacteriostasis and other antimicrobial effects. Thus, recommended treatment is O_2 at 3 ATA for 90 min three times in the first 24 h and twice a day for the next 2 to 5 days, always in combination with proper antibiotic use [77]. The anti-inflammatory potential of HBOT also aids to lessen tissue damage and infection expansion [72], also explained by a decrease in neutrophil activation, eviting rolling and accumulation of white blood cells (WBCs), hence limiting the production of ROS by neutrophils and avoiding reperfusion injury [45]. Moreover, this is observed in In vitro studies, having been demonstrated the biofilm shrinkage ability with the significant decreases in cellular load of anaerobic bacteria and fungi after HBOT [75]. A sepsis mouse model showed a significant increase in survival rate, >50%, with early HBOT compared to a control group that did not receive the treatment and was associated with lower expression of TNF-α, IL-6 and IL-10 [78]. Translation to clinical experience reports that the improvements in oxygenation follow the neovascularization, which avoid undesired events like amputation [28]. This is the case, for example, of Fournier's gangrene, where bacteremia and sepsis are top factors of fatality, which can be avoided by adjuvant HBOT, providing much higher survival rates in clinical trials [79]. Sometimes unwanted events are underestimated until it is late and polymicrobial infection has bursted into surgical bone and joint lesions [80]. For that reason, molecular assessments of bacterial identification like mass spectrometry, are every time more accomplished to consider if HBOT is worthy for patients' better recovering.

On the other hand, the use of HBOT might provide a central therapeutical option in the intracranial abscess (ICA). ICA presentation includes cerebral abscess, subdural empyema, and epidural empyema, and it is caused by an encapsulated infection in which the proper inflammatory response may damage the surrounding brain parenchyma [81]. The etiological agent might be bacteria, fungi, or a parasite, and it might appear as a consequence of a dissemination of previous infections like sinusitis, otitis, mastoiditis, dental infection; hematogenous seeding or cranial trauma [82]. Due to the high morbidity and mortality, along with the urgency of a non-invasive and effective method, HBOT has been proposed as a well-accepted adjunctive therapy for ICA, being regarded as a safe and tolerated method [83]. The main mechanisms by which HBOT represent an additional tool in the management of ICA resides on the impairment of the acidotic and hypoxic environment in ICAs due to the proper infection and the use of antibiotics [84]. Similarly, osteomyelitis is a chronic infection in the bone marrow frequently caused by bacteria or mycobacteria. It is a difficult condition to treat, as many antimicrobials do not penetrate in the bone properly. When this condition does not respond to the treatment or reemerge after receiving the therapy it is designed refractory osteomyelitis [85]. HBOT is a potential indication of refractory osteomyelitis as it provides synergist antibiotic activity, while enhancing angiogenesis, leukocyte oxidative killing and osteogenesis process [86]. A recent systematic review [87] reported that adjuvant HBOT provided almost a 75% of therapeutic success in patients with chronic refractory osteomyelitis, hence showing the importance of this treatment in bacterial infections. Malignant otitis externa, another infection, a necrotizing infection of the soft tissue of the external auditory canal which may rapidly cause skull base osteomyelitis may also benefit from the use of HBOT, although further studies are needed to conclude its effects [88].

Finally, some authors have also proposed a potential clinical use of HBOT as a medical emergency treatment of mucormycosis, a fungal infection [89]. Despite there still being few studies supporting its use, a compelling evidence show its potential use in a similar manner than necrotizing fasciitis, although further research is needed in this area.

4.3. HBOT in Medical Emergencies

Apart from the previously discussed applications, there has been further conditions in which HBOT may be considered. Some of them are designed as medical emergencies, in which the use of HBOT is an urgent indication for these patients. These are the cases of some infections above mentioned, decompression sickness, air or gas embolism, acute arterial insufficiencies such as central retinal arterial occlusion (CRAO), crush injury, compartment syndrome and acute traumatic ischemia, along with CO/Cyanide poisoning [89]. In this context, the central role of HBOT is derived from the rapid and effective response of the tissues under certain conditions that may be severe and even life-threatening [90].

A. Decompression sickness is a condition occurring due to the formation of bubbles caused by a reduction in ambient pressure that introduced dissolved gases within the body accidents. In turn, these bubbles drive to mechanical disruption of tissues, blood flow occlusion, endothelial dysfunction, platelet activation and capillary leakage. [91]. However, the term decompression sickness has been abandoned by the ECHM to be replaced by "Decompression illness" (DCI) [92], so in this article we will refer this malady as DCI. Clinical manifestations are at least one of more of the following: generalized fatigue or rash, joint pain, hypesthesia and in serious cases motor weakness, ataxia, pulmonary edema, shock and death [71]. DCI can occur in aviators, divers, astronauts, compressed air workers and, in some cases, it may appear due to iatrogenic causes [93]. HBOT/recompression therapy tables (US Navy Treatment Table 6 or helium/oxygen (Heliox Comex Cx30 or equivalent) are recommended for the initial treatment of DCI (Type 1 recommendation, Level C evidence). US Navy Treatment Table 5 can be used as the first recompression schedule for selected mild cases [94]. Therapies at higher pressure could be administered in exceptional cases, but it entails higher difficulties and risks. To maximize its efficacy, different adjunctive therapies are used in combination with HBOT including fluid administration, non-steroidal anti-inflammatory drugs and prophylactic agents to prevent venous thromboembolism events, particularly in paralyzed patients [93,95]. Overall, because of the high pressure, HBOT provide the opposite effects of the pathological mechanisms of DCIs, therefore exerting its therapeutical efficacy.

B. Air embolism. Apart from DCI, bubble formation of large arterial air embolism during operations are unusual occurrences but also ruinous and life-threatening. For bubble gas formation in veins from lung biopsy, arterial catheterization, cardiopulmonary bypass, HBOT is strictly necessary as there are no better alternatives in time. It provides tissue oxygenation by promoting gas reabsorption, and hence reduces ischemic injuries [96]. In this context, retrograde cerebral air embolism is a worrisome condition that may appear in major procedures (neurosurgery and cardiovascular operations, endoscopy), or during minor interventions (peripheral or central venous access), being particularly lethal when presented with encephalopathy [97]. The therapeutic basis of air embolism is similar to DCS, with HBOT as first-line therapy [98]. Some reports have emphasized the importance of an early HBOT, in the first 6 h since diagnosis, for this complication to obtain better outcomes, less sequelae or death rate [99]. However, there is some evidence of late benefits from its use, up to 60 h after the onset [100]. Even when there is no gas seen in on image test, patients may benefit from the use of HBOT [101]. On the other hand, recent data indicates that less cases appears to be treated by HBOT probably by the lack of belief of some physicians in HBOT, particularly in UK [102]. However, available evidence supports the use of this therapy to prevent and improve the outcome of such a dangerous condition.

C. CRAO is an ophthalmological complication caused by a permanent occlusion of the central retinal artery, mostly due to a embolus at its narrowest part that is typically associated with a sudden, massive loss of vision in the affected eye [103]. Prognosis for visual recovery is poor, as the retinal tissue is not tolerant to hypoxia, and it presents the highest oxygen consumption rate in the body at 13 mL/100 g per min [104]. As a result, HBOT is a robust indication for patients with CRAO and many studies have reported encouraging results from its use, minimum at eight sessions, with some advantages presented in comparison to other lines of treatment such as being a non-invasive method with low adverse effects [104–107]. However, and despite these benefits, HBOT is rarely offered for patients with CRAO [108], probably due to the lack of facilities in the hospital services.

D. Another approved indication for HBOT is crush injury and acute ischemia occurred as result of a trauma. Presentations of these damage vary from mild contusions to limb threatening damage, involving multiple tissues, from skin to muscles and bones. A severe consequence of trauma is the skeletal muscle-compartment syndrome (SMCS), a condition affecting both muscle and nerves [1]. Subsequently to trauma, the affected tissue will suffer from hypoxia, edema and ischemia. Here, the efficacy of angiogenesis has been also proved to be boosted by HBOT in animal models for ischemic limbs when combined with bone marrow derived mononuclear cells transplantation [109]. Some translational studies of multicenter randomized trials did not show a significant complete progress of healing [110], but in contrast, other trials showed the advantage of HBOT as adjunct for ischemic limbs when reconstructive surgery was not possible [111]. Evaluating skin peripheral circulation as well, the outcomes showed significant improvements in revascularization [112], therefore demonstrating the important role of HBOT in this condition.

E. CO poisoning is a problem that happens when household devices which use gas or coal produce CO due to an uncomplete combustion. Inhalation of this gas can be lethal and cause long-term problems particularly cognitive and brain deficits, presented up to a 40% of the patients and approximately one in three people develop cardiac dysfunction, like arrhythmia, left ventricular systolic dysfunction, and myocardial infarction [113]. To address these problems, HBOT has been applied [114] being associated to neurological sequelae reduction [115] and when applied in the first 24 h can reduce the risk of cognitive sequelae months later more efficiently [116]. In general, NBOT is immediately used after CO poisoning until HBOT is available [117]. Evidence indicates that HBOT should be considered for all cases of serious acute CO poisoning, loss of consciousness, ischemic cardiac changes, neurological deficits, significant metabolic acidosis, or COHb greater than 25% [113]. Another kind of poisoning in which HBOT has its application is cyanide toxicity. This issue appears with uncomplete combustion, this time, of materials like plastics, vinyl, acrylics, nylon, etc. HBOT is the primary treatment, but it exceeds when is combined with the antidote hydroxycobalamin, ameliorating mitochondrial oxidative phosphorylation function [118,119]. Potential uses of HBOT in a wide range of urgent conditions at least might be considered as an important tool in medical emergencies.

F. Severe anemias and idiopathic sudden sensorineural hearing loss. Despite not being considered a medical emergency, the use of HBOT is also indicated for these conditions [89]. In the first case, as Hb levels critically drops, O_2 delivery to the tissues may be impaired. In this line, the use of 100%, hyperbaric O_2 might solve this issue, simultaneously exerting a wide range of favorable effects in the hematological profile [120]. This could be especially important in patients who cannot be transfused for religion, immunologic reasons, or blood availability problems. Idiopathic sudden sensorineural hearing loss or acute acoustic trauma (AAT) are also important conditions in which HBOT could be a valuable tool. In fact, a recent systematic review and meta-analysis conducted by Rhee et al. [121] showed that the addition of HBOT to standard medical therapy is a valuable treatment option particularly for patients with severe to profound hearing loss and in those patients which received, at least 1200 min of HBOT. Apart from the regulation of ROS and inflammatory response, previous research has demonstrated the protective role of HBOT in the hair cell stereocilia, probably through hormetic mechanisms [122].

G. Finally HBOT can significantly improve symptoms and quality of life of patients affected by femoral head necrosis (ECHM recommendation type II level of evidence B) [123] as well as the previously mentioned NSTI, gas gangrene and urgent HBO alpha toxin neutralized

5. Translational and Potential Applications of HBOT

Besides approved indications, further lines of research have demonstrated the potential applications and translation of HBOT in the field of inflammatory and systemic conditions, cancer, COVID-19 and other conditions are summarized.

5.1. HBOT and Inflammation: Immunomodulatory Properties

HBOT might also be applicated in the regulation of inflammatory responses and its derived complications. Among the most important immunomodulatory effects, HBOT drives an alteration in CD4+:CD8+ ratio, a reduced proliferation of lymphocytes, and an activation of neutrophils with migration to hyperoxic regions [124]. Thus, HBOT might be used in a wide variety of conditions presenting an altered immune system as part of its pathogenesis. In this sense, it has been proposed the role of HBOT in the management of autoimmune diseases (ADs). A study conducted by Xu et al. [125] observed the overall effect of HBOT in general immune populations and particular Th1 and B lymphocytes subsets, proving its promising role in certain ADs. Furthermore, long-term exposure to HBOT was proven to supress the development of autoimmune symptoms, including proteinuria, facial erythema and lymphadenopathy [126]. In the same manner, the use of HBOT in early and middle stage of disease mice also show a significant increase in survival with a decrease in inflammatory cells, anti-dsDNA antibody titers, and amelioration of immune-complex deposition in comparison to later stage of disease [127] The use of HBOT has also proven its efficacy on rheumatoid arthritis, particularly due to the polarization of Th17 cells to T reg, with a significative reduction of cell hypoxia [128].

Similarly, these results could be extrapolated to other inflammatory conditions. For instance, HBOT provides an anti-inflammatory response in DSS-induced colitis. Through direct effects on HIF, HBOT induces antioxidant expression and the downregulation of proinflammatory cytokines like IL-6, therefore reducing colonic inflammation [129]. In vitro studies with lymphocytes from type 1 diabetes mellitus have proved effects of HBOT on inducible NOS expression, observing lower activity with a consequent decreased levels of NFkB [130]. Additionally, HBOT comprises another potential approach regarding musculoskeletal dysfunctions. Fibromyalgia represents an incapacitant disorder characterized by a widespread muscle and joint pain, frequently accompanied by systemic symptoms including cognitive dysfunction, mood disorders, fatigue, and insomnia [131]. HBOT exerts direct effects on brain activity, chronic pain and immune dysregulation, therefore improving quality of life of affected patients [132]. Interestingly, Woo et al. [133] also observed that HBOT could be considered an interesting alternative to attenuate exercise-induced inflammation and muscle damage.

Overall, previous research has indicated the favourable effects of HBOT in the immune system and also on the whole body.

5.2. Role of HBOT in the COVID-19 Pandemic

COVID-19 pandemic has challenged healthcare systems worldwide, overloading them with a huge burden in economy and our normalcy [134,135]. The urge of conducting massive vaccination programs besides finding better therapies for clinical management, have been the focus these months. In this context, HBOT has been proposed as an adjuvant for clinical practice in severe patients, and also for recovery after SARS-CoV-2 infection. Results from clinical trials have already demonstrated the potential uses of this treatment to redirect O_2 diffusion avoided by hypoxemia, and its ability to eliminate inflammatory cytokines.

Nevertheless, not only hyperbaric O_2 may be worthy for severe patients, but also for treating the named "silent" hypoxemia in those patients that do not have a bad clinical course yet [136]. This silent hypoxemia is not characterized by typical respiratory distress in critically ill patients, but it may be dangerous if it is not sooner detected as a prompt deterioration can occur without noticing [137]. In fact, previous studies have demonstrated the association between hypoxemia with fatal outcomes in patients with COVID-19 [138].

In the same manner, physicians observed that patients exhibit hypoxemia without dyspnea, being crucial to find care solutions to anticipate a problem with more patients at important risk [139]. Some cases of people with mild or even without symptoms, that contracted multi-organ failure and then died, have emphasized the importance of self-monitoring of pulse oximetry, which typically presents reduced readings in these patients [140]. Collected data from patients that did not present problems of breathing at admission, agreed with the suggestion of utilizing pulse oximetry to predict the outcome of hypoxemia/hypocapnia syndrome that defines asymptomatic hypoxia [141]. Steps forward in the understanding of our complex respiratory system have also launched reviews about the higher oxygenation rate in prone position, concerning variables like gravity, lung structure and the higher expression of nitric oxide (NO) in dorsal lung vessels than in ventral ones [142]. It has been demonstrated that HBOT increases the production of NO and ROS/RNS, inhibiting SARS-CoV-2 replication in previous In vitro models [41].

Moreover, all these facts have shed a light on finding better treatments to prevent fast hypoxia, fatality or even the need for mechanical ventilation [143,144] being HBOT a suggested adjuvant for its promising outcomes from previous animal models and clinical cases of sepsis and inflammatory diseases [145]. Preliminary comparisons of HBOT applications in COVID-19 to other maladies, like livedoid vasculopathy, have exposed the possible mechanisms that may occur: anti-inflammatory actions (decreased ICAM-1, proinflammatory cytokines and neutrophil rolling), anticoagulant actions (boosted fibrinolysis and increased plasminogen activator) and tissue healing actions (increased fibroblasts and stem cells) [146].

First studies in a severe patient affirmed that, compared to normobaric oxygen supply, the better empiric outcome agreed with the theoretic expectance of the potential uses of HBOT in COVID-19 [147]. Although it is still being evaluated scientifically, positive results are arising for COVID-19 treatment, finding an attenuation of the innate immune system, and increasing hypoxia tolerance [148]. In every report, this therapy has been rated as a potential support in the relieving of cytokine storm [149]. Now that mechanical ventilation may be long lasting and, preferably, avoided, in a controlled trial, safety and efficacy of HBOT for COVID-19 patients was successfully evaluated [150]. Another preliminary study showed rapid alleviation of hypoxemia from the beginning of the treatment in patients with COVID-19 pneumonia [151].

Anatomically, pathologic examinations of lung with early-phase COVID-19 have shown edema, proteinaceous exudate, inflammatory cellular infiltration, and interstitial thickening that entails a disproportional gas exchange. This is due to CO_2 diffuses through tissues much faster than O_2, about 20 times, what leads to hypocapnia [152]. Alveolar structure is altered in the COVID-19 patient, there is also hyaline membrane formation, there is thickness in alveolar membrane and the space for the diffusion of oxygen generates a lot of exudate and inflammation. Hence, diffusion from the alveolus through the haematoalveolar membrane does not occur correctly, the concentration of oxygen in the blood and in the tissues begins to fall and the exchange of the dioxide also becomes difficult. Due to possible viral interactions with Hb [153] and a hypoxemia-induced shift in the oxyhemoglobin dissociation curve to the left, there is O_2 saturation but low arterial blood pressure [154].

Clinical evidence from few studies about COVID-19 patients undergoing HBOT, notes that this therapy may make possible to contribute to reverse hypoxemia and ameliorating the pulmonary capillary circulation diffusion despite the thickness in alveolar membrane in disease. According to Henry's Law, HBOT allows to increase pressure of O_2 in the alveoli above ambient pressure. In this way, there will be a large increase of O_2 diffusion into the pulmonary capillary circulation, more than 10 times, for its arrival in the plasma and reach the tissues independently of Hb. There will be a gain of O_2 supply to the tissues mediated by the increase in pressure. Experimentally, hematological, biochemical and inflammatory parameters were significantly improved after HBOT. In first trials the observation of lymphocyte count was increased, whereas lactate and fibrinogen were decreased [147,151].

However, during this procedure patients may suffer from desaturation reflexes. Despite the etiology of this reflex is unclear, it might be probably caused by a vasoconstriction affecting the pulmonary arteries, due to the oxidative stress as well as direct damage in type II pneumocytes and thrombus associated with COVID-19 [124].

Notwithstanding the ongoing clinical trials and the efforts of standardize better protocols for safety, COVID-19 is not yet an accepted indication for HBOT, but this may be recommended for post-viral sequelae [155]. In order to guarantee its beneficial effects, there is still a need of more controlled trials to measure different inflammatory and hematological parameters that demonstrate that exudate and inflammation are reduced besides the improvements in alveolar circulation diffusion. This would confirm the potential of this adjuvant, also for considering the financial investment in hyperbaric chambers in hospitals.

5.3. HBOT and Cancer

Cancer is a complex entity which encompasses a broad spectrum of unique pathologies that share the following hallmarks: Immune system evasion, tumor-promoting inflammation, genome instability, enabling replicative immortality, activating invasion and metastasis sustaining proliferative signaling, evading growth suppressors, resisting cell death, inducing angiogenesis, and metabolic reprogramming [156]. Tumor-hypoxia plays a central role in many of these carcinogenic features, promoting an aggressive phenotype besides limit the effectiveness of radiotherapy, chemotherapy, and immunotherapy thereby worsening prognosis in the oncological patients [157]. Thus, targeting tumoral hypoxia and its downstream effectors have been proposed as a potential therapeutical approach in cancer management [158–160]. In this line, accumulating evidence supports the role of HBOT in the inhibition of tumor growth and therapy success, by three main mechanisms: (1) By limiting cancer-associated hypoxia, (2) through the generation of ROS and RNS and (3) restoring immune function [161]. Actual investigations show the promising role of HBOT in a wide variety of malignancies, including breast cancer, prostate cancer, head and neck cancer, colorectal cancer, leukemia, brain tumors, cervical cancer and bladder cancer [162]. Main applications derived from HBOT in oncology may be (a) As part of the treatment (b) as a radiotherapy adjuvant and (c) as a chemotherapy adjuvant [163].

The use of HBOT as part of the cancer therapy is not currently an approved indication, although some promising results have arisen recently. In this context, Thews & Vaupel [164] compared the efficacy of NBOT (1 atm) versus HBOT (2 atm) oxygenation reporting broader reductions of hypoxia under hyperbaric conditions. However, even at high pressure oxygenation, tumor hypoxia was not completely removed, hence showing that HBOT alone efficacy is limited. Importantly, as previously described HBOT was associated with increased angiogenesis, these effects are not significative in tumour cells, so its use could be important in the cancer management [165]. Conversely, a study conducted by Pande et al. [166] revealed that notwithstanding HBOT-treated mice initially induced a decrease in tumor progression, a tumorigenic effect was observed post-therapy, probably due to impaired DNA repair, mutagenicity and chromosomic aneuploidies together with an altered blood supply and nutrients. On the other hand, some authors suggest that the lack of therapeutical efficacy of HBOT might be due to the difficulty on creating a hyperoxic environment in the tumor and that, by combining HBOT with other methods it could act a as a potential cure in certain types of cancer. In this line, Lu et al. [167] proposed a combined use in prostate cancer patients of HBOT with ultrasound guided transrectal prostate puncture, in order to create a hyperoxic environment within the tumor, which may lead to DNA damage and a detention in the G2/M cycle, hence establishing the basis for future research. Similarly, tumor hypoxia is associated with the metabolic reprogramming of tumour cells, also known as the aerobic glycolysis or "Warburg effect". This consists of a glycolytic switch of cancer cells, which refrain from performing oxidative phosphorylation [168]. In this sense, Poff et al. [169] described the combined effects of HBOT in combination with ketogenic diet in a murine model, preventing tumoral metastasis while expanding overall survival. Furthermore, HBOT alone or combined with low glucose and ketone supplementation also exert multiple benefits against late-stage metastatic cancers, by increasing the production of ROS and oxidative stress [170]. Despite the encouraging results, further research is required to establish the efficacy of HBOT in the different types of cancer, also searching for the most adequate use of this therapy in a global context.

Radiotherapy (RT) is a central component in cancer management, with approximately 50% of patients receiving this therapy contributing up to a 40% of curative success for cancer [171]. Through ionizing radiation, it creates a ROS and RNS overproduction, leading to double strand breaks, chromosomal aberrations and rearrangements with subsequent cell death or dysfunction, thus exerting its anti-tumoral effects. The effect of HBOT on human glioblastoma (GBM) was investigated, in laboratory, on patient-derived cells and on microglia cell biology (CHME-5). The results obtained from the combination of HBO and RT clearly showed a radiosensitising effect of HBO on GBM cells grown [172]. Hypofractionated stereotactic radiotherapy (HSRT) after HBO (HBO-RT) appears to be effective for the treatment of recurrent high-grade glioma (rHGG), as pointed out on a cohort of 9 adult rHGG patients. It could represent an alternative, with low toxicity, to systemic therapies for patients who cannot or refuse to undergo such treatments [173]. However, although non-tumour cells are less sensitive, radiation could also affect them, altering multiple cellular signaling pathways or inducing apoptosis, hence explaining its multiple adverse effects [174] One of the most severe consequences resulted from irradiation is the appearance of post-radiation injuries, a process starting during radiotherapy that involves the dysregulation of multiple bioactive compounds, particularly fibrogenic cytokines like TGF-β [175]. Similarly, almost all tissues with delayed irradiation injury present a histological feature named as obliterative endarteritis, finally leading to a tissue damage characterized by hypoxia, hypovascularity and hypocellularity [176]. In this line, HBOT has consistently demonstrated its therapeutical effectivity against radiation-induced injury also approved by the UHMS [177] and the ECHM [8]. Last 2016 Cochrane review [178] evidenced that the use of HBOT in head, neck, anus and rectum injured tissues were associated with improved outcomes and, at some extent with osteoradionecrosis following tooth extraction in an irradiated field. According to ECHM recommendation the use of HBOT is recommended in the treatment of radiation proctitis (Type 1 recommendation, Level A evidence), mandibular osteoradionecrosis and haemorrhagic radiation cystitis (Type 1 recommendation, Level B evidence) and suggested in the treatment of osteoradionecrosis of other bone than the mandible, for preventing loss of osseointegrated implants in irradiated bone and in the treatment of soft-tissue radionecrosis (other than cystitis and proctitis), in particular in the head and neck area (Type 2 recommendation, Level C evidence). Furthermore, it would be reasonable to use HBOT for treating or preventing radio-induced lesions of the larynx, in the treatment of radio-induced lesions of the central nervous system (Type 3 recommendation, Level C evidence) [8]

Finally, the combined use of HBOT plus chemotherapy have reported certain benefits. In this line, a recent study conducted by Brewer et al. [179] demonstrated the effectiveness of using HBOT to prevent chemotherapy-induced neuropathy In vivo. This fact appears to be due to the various implications of HBOT in the neuronal activity and signaling [180–182] Kawasoe et al. also observed [183] that an integrative strategy of carboplatin plus HBOT significantly reduced mortality in C3H mice with inoculated osteosarcoma cells Similar results were obtained with HBOT and chemotherapy in lung cancer cultures and animal models [184]. In particular, the combination of paclitaxel and carboplatin plus HBOT and hyperthermia show promising results for treating patients with non-small cell lung cancer and multiple metastasis [185]. Despite these results, the use of HBOT and chemotherapy may also represent a contraindication for the patients. For instance, the combination of HBOT with doxorubicin, bleomycin, or cisplatin may exert synergic cardiotoxicity, pulmonary toxicity or impaired wound healing, respectively [186]. This is an important issue to address in the oncologic patient. In these cases, it is important to separate chemotherapy from the use of necessary HBOT, to avoid undesired effects. In addition, further strategies could be considered targeting tumour hypoxia and functioning as therapeutic adjuvants like physical activity [187]. Overall, the benefits of HBOT in cancer management is a potential field to keep on exploring.

5.4. Other Applications

In the same manner, other novel lines of research are exploring potential uses of HBOT in a plethora of conditions. For instance, some studies related to microvascular or macrovascular insufficiencies causing erectile dysfunction (ED) have hypothesized the effects of HBOT in patients with this problem. Empirical data suggests that it can induce penile angiogenesis and improve erectile function in men suffering from ED. This is due to vasodilatation relies on proper blood vessels in corpora cavernosa. Then, being a major concentration of oxygen in tissues, there is an increased angiogenesis by VEGF and endothelial cells differentiation [188]. This application has not provided significant data on rehabilitation after prostatectomy [189] but it has obtained good symptoms resolution for other clinical manifestations like ED in diabetes mellitus [190] or in recovery after urethral reconstruction [191].

Equally, the use of HBOT for ischemic stroke and brain injury is an interesting point of study. For instance, different studies have demonstrated the importance of this procedure as a prophylactic approach for sequestration of inflammation inherent in stroke and traumatic brain injury, preventing neuronal death [192]. Other uses such as brain preconditioning before stem cells transplantation have also been explored [193]. However, the efficacy and safety of HBOT in these conditions remains to be fully elucidated, although some basic and clinical research have shown encouraging results [194].

Finally, the use of HBOT could be potentially extended to novel fields like aging. Hachmo et al. [195] reported the effect of hyperbaric oxygen in the prevention of telomere shortening and immunosenescence by the clearance of senescent immune cells. In this line, other studies have reported the same results in the aging skin, through the acceleration of epidermal basal cells proliferation [196], in the endothelial cells, where it induces antioxidants expression [197] and also in the brain, where HBOT appears to improve the cerebral blood flow [198], restoring cognitive parameters, hippocampal functions and even improved insulin resistance in both normal-weigh and obese aging rats [199].

As summarized in Figure 2, the main consequences of HBOT and its related hyperoxemia and hyperoxia in the human body could be related with the angiogenesis enhancement, antimicrobial properties and immunomodulatory effects. Approved indications for this therapy could also be grouped according to its emergency.

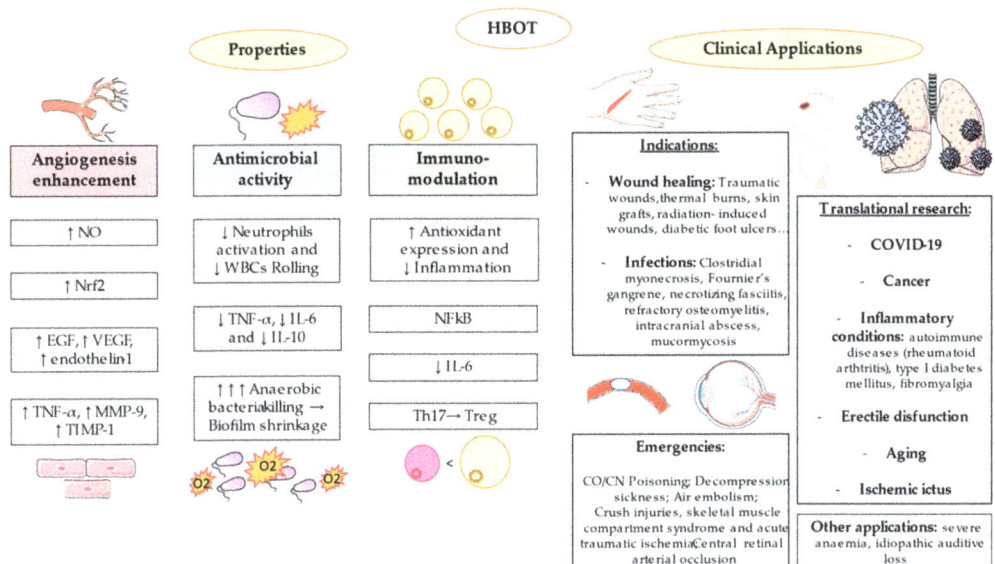

Figure 2. Summary of top properties of HBOT and its clinical applications. Firstly, it can provide an angiogenesis enhancement, observed by the prime production of NO which subsequently brings an upregulation of Nrf2 and growth factors like epidermal growth factor (EGF), vascular endothelial growth factor (VEGF) and endothelin-1. TNF-α, matrix metallopeptidase 9 (MMP-9) and tissue inhibitor of metalloproteinase-1 (TIMP-1) will be boosted too. Secondly, the antimicrobial activity is visible due to bacterial killing by O_2, removing biofilm and lessening white blood cells (WBCs) rolling and neutrophils recruitment, hence promoting a downregulation of proinflammatory cytokines (TNF-α, IL-6 and IL-10). The immunomodulation properties are observed by a downregulation of transcriptional factor NFkB, involving a proinflammatory response switch off (IL-6) and a polarization from Th17 lymphocytes to Treg. Summarized applications include: indications for which HBOT is approved (mostly wound healing and infections), primary emergencies (like CO/CN poisoning or air embolism), and translational research (comprising COVID-19, cancer, inflammatory conditions or aging among others).

6. Adverse Effects and Contraindications

Notwithstanding the multiple benefits and applications of HBOT, there are important adverse effects that may appear during this procedure. As a result of the hyperoxia and the hyperbaric environment, there are some issues when using this therapy. The two most common complications during HBOT are claustrophobia and barotrauma. Both occur during monoplace or multiplace chamber compression [200]. In the case of barotrauma, it could be defined as an injury caused by an inability to equalize pressure from an air-containing space and the surrounding environment. Ear barotrauma is the most frequent condition affecting the middle ear, although sinus/paranasal, dental or pulmonary barotrauma could also be reported [201]. Despite the incidence of this complication being extremely rare [202], its seriousness should be taken into account, considering clinical history of patients at risk of suffering from these complications while implementing different strategies to prevent this complication, such as anti-epileptic therapy, prolonged air brakes or controlling treatment pressure [203]. The last event is associated with the appearance of the Paul Bert effect because of the formation of seizures that may bring transient but negative consequences for cognitive functioning and behavioural patterns [204]. These effects are primarily due to the toxic properties of oxygen at high concentrations. However, to date, no threshold has been described to precisely assess the pathological levels of oxygen, which could be an important issue for critical patients [205]. Pulmonary toxicity is not associated with the use of repeated hyperbaric oxygen following current protocols [206]. Ocular manifestations from HBOT may also be described, particularly hyperbaric myopia, transitory in most cases. Other ophthalmological complications less frequent observed are cataracts, keratoconus or retinopathy of prematurity, in the case of pregnant women exposed to HBOT [207,208]. All these adverse effects may be ameliorated prominently by an adequate screening, through the use of certain devices and the adjustment of the treatment protocols [200,201]

On the other hand, there are certain conditions in which HBOT might be absolutely contraindicated or relatively contraindicated. The first case is exclusively represented by untreated pneumothorax, as it could be a life-threatening procedure [209]. The rest of contraindications are relative, its indication will depend on the real necessity of this therapy. Aside from the chemotherapheutic agents previously described other treatments like sulfamylon (Mafenide), could also share the same action than cisplatin impeding wound healing effects derived from HBOT, and it should also be interrupted before this therapy [45]. If patient has a pacemaker or any type of implantable devices, it is necessary to verify its safety with increased pressure or with pure concentrations of oxygen. Hereditary spherocytosis may also be a contraindication, as hyperbaric oxygen could cause severe haemolysis [43]. Pregnancy is another potential contraindication for this therapy in exception of CO poisoning [210]. Although rare in non-diabetic individuals, patients may also suffer from hypoglycaemia during this procedure, and it is important to evaluate their blood glucose levels before HBOT, as it could aggravate their hypoglycaemic profile [211]. Similarly, patients with underlying respiratory pathologies like chronic obstructive pulmonary disease (COPD), asthma and even upper respiratory infections might be also possible contraindications from receiving HBOT, as it could increase the risk of hypercapnia, pulmonary barotrauma and sinus or middle ear barotrauma, respectively [209]. An additional effect derived from HBOT is the increment of blood pressure [212]. Hyperbaric oxygen may also induce pulmonary oedema and cardiovascular difficulties in patients with heart failure or in patients with reduced cardiac ejection fractions [213]. Finally, the history of epilepsy, hypoglycaemia, hyperthyroidism, current fever, and certain drugs such as penicillin and disulfiram are also thought to lower the seizure threshold during this therapy [214]. Diabetic patients may be warned from regulating its doses of HBOT in order to prevent the hypoglycaemic effect of this therapy.

To summarize, despite the multiple applications of HBOT it is equally important to consider its potential adverse effects and underlying conditions in which this therapy is not going to exert its efficacy, also representing a potential risk for these patients.

7. Conclusions and Future Directions

HBOT is an effective method to increase blood and tissue oxygen levels, independently from Hb transportation. Its therapeutic basis could be understood from three different perspectives: Physical (Hyperbaric 100% oxygen), physiological (Hyperoxia and hyperoxemia) and cellular/molecular effects. All these effects provide HBOT its efficacy in the management of hypoxia derived conditions and hypoxemia, respectively, also exerting direct effects in infectious agents and immune cells, modulating a wide variety of cellular signaling pathways, cytokine production and tissue processes such as angiogenesis. Herein, the use of HBOT might be extended to a broad spectrum of pathologies, from infections and inflammatory/systemic maladies to wound healing and vascular complications, also reporting its efficacy in the management of medical emergencies like air embolism or gas poisoning. Although respiratory infections and diseases have been mentioned as contraindications for HBOT, the case of SARS-CoV-2 is an exception. Nowadays, the potential use of HBOT in the COVID-19 has been specially regarded, exposing results in numerous controlled clinical trials. Moreover, the use of this procedure in different types of malignancies represents an important support in the delayed radiation injury. In the same manner, the use of HBOT as a therapeutical agent have shown promising results in trials as an adjunctive substance with other approved treatments like chemotherapy and even, recent research have also reported significant improvements in nanomedicine approaches when combined with HBOT [215].

Despite its benefits, there are still certain challenges which need to be overcome to improve the current and potential applications of HBOT. In this line, a worrisome issue would be to develop sophisticated strategies to address tissue hypoxia, as for certain conditions like tumoral cells, the HBOT induced hyperoxia does not completely eliminate tumour hypoxia. An adequate combination of HBOT with another procedure might be interesting to targeting this problem [167]. On the other hand, it is equally important to determine and quantify potential adverse effects derived from HBOT, as well as potential contraindications from receiving this therapy. Future research should be destinated on developing accurate systems to determine potential benefits and risks for patients before submitting HBOT. In this line, the development of predictive models as previously mentioned or novel strategies could be interesting approaches in these fields.

Currently, there are only 14 approved indications for this therapeutical approach. We encourage further studies to extend the possible uses of this procedure, always considering individual benefits and risks from receiving this therapy. The inclusion of HBOT in future clinical research could be an additional support in the clinical management of multiple pathologies.

Author Contributions: Conceptualization, M.A.O., O.F.-M., C.G.-M., M.Á.-M., J.B., M.L.C.; Methodology, M.A.O., O.F.-M., C.G.-M.; Formal Analysis, M.A.O., O.F.-M., C.G.-M.; Investigation, M.A.O., O.F.-M., C.G.-M., E.C.-P., M.A.S., M.A.Á.-M., N.G.-H., J.M., M.Á.-M., J.B., M.L.C.; Data Curation, M.A.O., O.F.-M., C.G.-M.; Writing-Original Draft Preparation, M.A.O., O.F.-M., C.G.-M., E.C.-P., M.A.S., M.A.Á.-M., N.G.-H., J.M., M.Á.-M., J.B., M.L.C.; Writing-Review & Editing, M.A.O., O.F.-M., C.G.-M., E.C.-P., M.A.S., M.A.Á.-M., N.G.-H., J.M., M.Á.-M., J.B., M.L.C.; Supervision, M.Á.-M., J.B., M.L.C.; Project Administration, M.Á.-M., J.B.; Funding Acquisition, M.Á.-M., J.B. All authors have read and agreed to the published version of the manuscript.

Funding: The study was supported by the Comunidad de Madrid (B2017/BMD-3804 MITIC-CM), Univer-sidad de Alcalá (32/2013, 22/2014, 26/2015) and Halekulani S.L.

Institutional Review Board Statement: Not applicable.

Informed Consent Statement: Not applicable.

Data Availability Statement: The data used to support the findings of the present study are available from the corresponding author upon request.

Acknowledgments: Oscar Fraile-Martinez had a predoctoral fellowship from the University of Alcalá during the course of this work.

Conflicts of Interest: The authors declare no conflict of interest.

References

1. HBO Indications—Undersea & Hyperbaric Medical Society. Available online: https://www.uhms.org/resources/hbo-indications.html# (accessed on 3 April 2021).
2. UHMS Position Statement: Low-Pressure Fabric Hyperbaric Chambers Title: Low-Pressure Fabric Hyperbaric Chambers. 2017. Available online: https://www.uhms.org/images/Position-Statements/UHMS_Position_Statement_LP_chambers_revised.pdf (accessed on 23 May 2021).
3. Edwards, M.L. Hyperbaric Oxygen Therapy. Part 1: History and Principles. *J. Vet. Emergy Crit. Care* **2010**, *20*, 284–288. [CrossRef] [PubMed]
4. Dejours, P.; Dejours, S. The Effects of Barometric Pressure According to Paul Bert: The Question Today. *Int. J. Sports Med.* **1992**, *13*, S1–S5. [CrossRef] [PubMed]
5. Hedley-Whyte, J. Pulmonary Oxygen Toxicity: Investigation and Mentoring. *Ulst. Med. J.* **2008**, *77*, 39–42.
6. Jones, M.W.; Wyatt, H.A. *Hyperbaric, Physics*; StatPearls Publishing: Treasure Island, FL, USA, 2019.
7. Moon, R.E.; Camporesi, E.M. Hyperbaric Oxygen Therapy: From the Nineteenth to the Twenty-First Century. *Respir. Care Clin. N. Am.* **1999**, *5*, 1–5.
8. Mathieu, D.; Marroni, A.; Kot, J. Tenth European Consensus Conference on Hyperbaric Medicine: Recommendations for Accepted and Non-Accepted Clinical Indications and Practice of Hyperbaric Oxygen Treatment. *Diving Hyperb. Med.* **2017**, *47*, 24–31. [CrossRef]
9. Trayhurn, P. Oxygen—The Forgotten Nutrient. *J. Nutr. Sci.* **2017**, *6*, e47. [CrossRef]

10. Martin, W.F.; Garg, S.; Zimorski, V. Endosymbiotic Theories for Eukaryote Origin. *Philos. Trans. R. Soc. B Biol. Sci.* **2015**, *370*, 20140330. [CrossRef]
11. Trayhurn, P. Oxygen—A Critical, but Overlooked, Nutrient. *Front. Nutr.* **2019**, *6*, 10. [CrossRef]
12. Butler, J.P.; Tsuda, A. Transport of Gases between the Environment and Alveoli-Theoretical Foundations. *Compr. Physiol.* **2011**, *1*, 1301–1316. [CrossRef]
13. Harris, R.S. Pressure-Volume Curves of the Respiratory System. *Respir. Care* **2005**, *50*, 78–99.
14. Pittman, R.N. Oxygen Gradients in the Microcirculation. *Acta Physiol.* **2011**, *202*, 311–322. [CrossRef]
15. Gossman, W.; Alghoula, F.; Berim, I. *Anoxia (Hypoxic Hypoxia)*; StatPearls Publishing: Treasure Island, FL, USA, 2019.
16. Choudhry, H.; Harris, A.L. Advances in Hypoxia-Inducible Factor Biology. *Cell Metab.* **2018**, *27*, 281–298. [CrossRef]
17. Soares, M.J.; Iqbal, K.; Kozai, K. Hypoxia and Placental Development. *Birth Defects Res.* **2017**, *109*, 1309–1329. [CrossRef]
18. Navarrete-Opazo, A.; Mitchell, G.S. Therapeutic Potential of Intermittent Hypoxia: A Matter of Dose. *Am. J. Physiol. Regul. Integr. Comp. Physiol.* **2014**, *307*, R1181–R1197. [CrossRef]
19. Chen, P.S.; Chiu, W.T.; Hsu, P.L.; Lin, S.C.; Peng, I.C.; Wang, C.Y.; Tsai, S.J. Pathophysiological Implications of Hypoxia in Human Diseases. *J. Biomed. Sci.* **2020**, *27*, 63. [CrossRef]
20. Horner, D.; O'Driscoll, R. Oxygen Therapy for Medical Patients. *BMJ* **2018**, *363*. [CrossRef]
21. Daste, T. The Oxygen Therapy. *Prat. Vet* **2013**, *20*, 30–32. [CrossRef]
22. Lee, J.W.; Ko, J.; Ju, C.; Eltzschig, H.K. Hypoxia Signaling in Human Diseases and Therapeutic Targets. *Exp. Mol. Med.* **2019**, *51*, 1–13. [CrossRef]
23. Macintyre, N.R. Tissue Hypoxia: Implications for the Respiratory Clinician. *Respir. Care* **2014**, *59*, 1590–1596. [CrossRef]
24. Choudhury, R. Hypoxia and Hyperbaric Oxygen Therapy: A Review. *Int. J. Gen. Med.* **2018**, *11*, 431–442. [CrossRef]
25. Kirby, J.P.; Snyder, J.; Schuerer, D.J.E.; Peters, J.S.; Bochicchio, G. V Essentials of Hyperbaric Oxygen Therapy: 2019 Review. *Mol. Med.* **2019**, *116*, 176–179.
26. Lind, F. A pro/Con Review Comparing the Use of Mono- and Multiplace Hyperbaric Chambers for Critical Care. *Diving Hyperb. Med.* **2015**, *45*, 56–60.
27. Weaver, L.K. Monoplace Hyperbaric Chamber Use of U.S. Navy Table 6: A 20-Year Experience. *Undersea Hyperb. Med.* **2006**, *33*, 85.
28. Lam, G.; Fontaine, R.; Ross, F.L.; Chiu, E.S. Hyperbaric Oxygen Therapy: Exploring the Clinical Evidence. *Adv. Ski. Wound Care* **2017**, *30*, 181–190. [CrossRef]
29. Harch, P.G.; Andrews, S.R.; Fogarty, E.F.; Amen, D.; Pezzullo, J.C.; Lucarini, J.; Aubrey, C.; Taylor, D.V.; Staab, P.K.; Van Meter, K.W. A Phase I Study of Low-Pressure Hyperbaric Oxygen Therapy for Blast-Induced Post-Concussion Syndrome and Post-Traumatic Stress Disorder. *J. Neurotrauma* **2012**, *29*, 168–185. [CrossRef]
30. Izquierdo-Alventosa, R.; Inglés, M.; Cortés-Amador, S.; Gimeno-Mallench, L.; Sempere-Rubio, N.; Chirivella, J.; Serra-Añó, P. Comparative Study of the Effectiveness of a Low-Pressure Hyperbaric Oxygen Treatment and Physical Exercise in Women with Fibromyalgia: Randomized Clinical Trial. *Ther. Adv. Musculoskelet. Dis.* **2020**, *12*, 1759720X20930493. [CrossRef]
31. Camporesi, E.M.; Mascia, M.F.; Thom, S.R. Physiological Principles of Hyperbaric Oxygenation. In *Handbook on Hyperbaric Medicine*; Springer: Milan, Italy, 1996; pp. 35–58.
32. Bennett, M.H.; French, C.; Schnabel, A.; Wasiak, J.; Kranke, P.; Weibel, S. Normobaric and Hyperbaric Oxygen Therapy for the Treatment and Prevention of Migraine and Cluster Headache. *Cochrane Database Syst. Rev.* **2015**, *2015*, CD005219. [CrossRef]
33. Lin, C.-H.; Su, W.-H.; Chen, Y.-C.; Feng, P.-H.; Shen, W.-C.; Ong, J.-R.; Wu, M.-Y.; Wong, C.S. Treatment with Normobaric or Hyperbaric Oxygen and Its Effect on Neuropsychometric Dysfunction after Carbon Monoxide Poisoning. *Medicine* **2018**, *97*, e12456. [CrossRef]
34. Casillas, S.; Galindo, A.; Camarillo-Reyes, L.A.; Varon, J.; Surani, S.R. Effectiveness of Hyperbaric Oxygenation Versus Normobaric Oxygenation Therapy in Carbon Monoxide Poisoning: A Systematic Review. *Cureus* **2019**, *11*, e5916. [CrossRef]
35. Leach, R.M.; Rees, P.J.; Wilmshurst, P. ABC of Oxygen: Hyperbaric Oxygen Therapy. *Br. Med. J.* **1998**, *317*, 1140–1143. [CrossRef]
36. Brugniaux, J.V.; Coombs, G.B.; Barak, O.F.; Dujic, Z.; Sekhon, M.S.; Ainslie, P.N. Highs and Lows of Hyperoxia: Physiological, Performance, and Clinical Aspects. *Am. J. Physiol. Regul. Integr. Comp. Physiol.* **2018**, *315*, R1–R27. [CrossRef] [PubMed]
37. Amir, H.; Shai, E. The Hyperoxic-hypoxic Paradox. *Biomolecules* **2020**, *10*, 958.
38. Calabrese, E.J. Hormesis: Path and Progression to Significance. *Int. J. Mol. Sci.* **2018**, *19*, 2871. [CrossRef] [PubMed]
39. Thom, S.R. Hyperbaric Oxygen: Its Mechanisms and Efficacy. *Plast. Reconstr. Surg.* **2011**, *127*, 131S–141S. [CrossRef]
40. Camporesi, E.M.; Bosco, G. Mechanisms of Action of Hyperbaric Oxygen Therapy. *Undersea Hyperb. Med.* **2014**, *41*, 247–252.
41. Longobardi, P.; Hoxha, K.; Perreca, F. Is Hyperbaric Oxygen an Effective Treatment for the Prevention of Complications in SARS-CoV-2 Asymptomatic Patients? *Infect. Microbes Dis.* **2021**, *3*, 109–111. [CrossRef]
42. Chen, W.; Liang, X.; Nong, Z.; Li, Y.; Pan, X.; Chen, C.; Huang, L. The Multiple Applications and Possible Mechanisms of the Hyperbaric Oxygenation Therapy. *Med. Chem.* **2019**, *15*, 459–471. [CrossRef]
43. DuBose, K.J.; Cooper, J.S. *Hyperbaric Patient Selection*; StatPearls Publishing: Treasure Island, FL, USA, 2018.
44. Fife, C.E.; Eckert, K.A.; Carter, M.J. An Update on the Appropriate Role for Hyperbaric Oxygen: Indications and Evidence. *Plast. Reconstr. Surg.* **2016**, *138*, 107S–116S. [CrossRef]
45. Bhutani, S.; Vishwanath, G. Hyperbaric Oxygen and Wound Healing. *Indian J. Plast. Surg.* **2012**, *45*, 316–324. [CrossRef]

46. Longobardi, P.; Hoxha, K.; Bennett, M.H. Is There a Role for Hyperbaric Oxygen Therapy in the Treatment of Refractory Wounds of Rare Etiology? *Diving Hyperb. Med.* **2019**, *49*, 216–224. [CrossRef]
47. Dhamodharan, U.; Karan, A.; Sireesh, D.; Vaishnavi, A.; Somasundar, A.; Rajesh, K.; Ramkumar, K.M. Tissue-Specific Role of Nrf2 in the Treatment of Diabetic Foot Ulcers during Hyperbaric Oxygen Therapy. *Free Radic. Biol. Med.* **2019**, *138*, 53–62. [CrossRef]
48. Löndahl, M.; Katzman, P.; Nilsson, A.; Hammarlund, C. Hyperbaric Oxygen Therapy Facilitates Healing of Chronic Foot Ulcers in Patients with Diabetes. *Diabetes Care* **2010**, *33*, 998–1003. [CrossRef]
49. Salama, S.E.; Eldeeb, A.E.; Elbarbary, A.H.; Abdelghany, S.E. Adjuvant Hyperbaric Oxygen Therapy Enhances Healing of Nonischemic Diabetic Foot Ulcers Compared With Standard Wound Care Alone. *Int. J. Low. Extrem. Wounds* **2019**, *18*, 75–80. [CrossRef]
50. Sharma, R.; Sharma, S.K.; Mudgal, S.K.; Jelly, P.; Thakur, K. Efficacy of Hyperbaric Oxygen Therapy for Diabetic Foot Ulcer, a Systematic Review and Meta-Analysis of Controlled Clinical Trials. *Sci. Rep.* **2021**, *11*, 2189. [CrossRef]
51. Game, F.L.; Apelqvist, J.; Attinger, C.; Hartemann, A.; Hinchliffe, R.J.; Löndahl, M.; Price, P.E.; Jeffcoate, W.J. Effectiveness of Interventions to Enhance Healing of Chronic Ulcers of the Foot in Diabetes: A Systematic Review. *Diabetes Metab. Res. Rev.* **2016**, *32* (Suppl. 1), 154–168. [CrossRef]
52. Lalieu, R.C.; Brouwer, R.J.; Ubbink, D.T.; Hoencamp, R.; Raap, R.B.; Van Hulst, R.A. Hyperbaric Oxygen Therapy for Nonischemic Diabetic Ulcers: A Systematic Review. *Wound Repair Regen. Off. Publ. Wound Health Soc. Eur. Tissue Repair Soc.* **2020**, *28*, 266–275. [CrossRef]
53. Brouwer, R.J.; Lalieu, R.; Hoencamp, R.; van Hulst, R.A.; Ubbink, D.T. A Systematic Review and Meta-Analysis of Hyperbaric Oxygen Therapy for Diabetic Foot Ulcers with Arterial Insufficiency. *J. Vasc. Surg.* **2020**, *71*, 682–692. [CrossRef]
54. Londahl, M.; Fagher, K.; Nilson, A.; Katzman, P. Hyperbaric Oxygen Therapy Is Associated with Improved Six-Year Survival in People with Chronic Diabetic Foot Ulcers. *Diabetes* **2018**, *67*, 2225. [CrossRef]
55. Edwards, M.L. Hyperbaric Oxygen Therapy. Part 2: Application in Disease. *J. Vet. Emerg. Crit. Care* **2010**, *20*, 289–297. [CrossRef]
56. Marx, R.E.; Ehler, W.J.; Tayapongsak, P.; Pierce, L.W. Relationship of Oxygen Dose to Angiogenesis Induction in Irradiated Tissue. *Am. J. Surg.* **1990**, *160*, 519–524. [CrossRef]
57. Sander, A.L.; Henrich, D.; Muth, C.M.; Marzi, I.; Barker, J.H.; Frank, J.M. In Vivo Effect of Hyperbaric Oxygen on Wound Angiogenesis and Epithelialization. *Wound Repair Regen.* **2009**, *17*, 179–184. [CrossRef]
58. Peña-Villalobos, I.; Casanova-Maldonado, I.; Lois, P.; Prieto, C.; Pizarro, C.; Lattus, J.; Osorio, G.; Palma, V. Hyperbaric Oxygen Increases Stem Cell Proliferation, Angiogenesis and Wound-Healing Ability of WJ-MSCs in Diabetic Mice. *Front. Physiol.* **2018**, *9*, 995. [CrossRef]
59. Sureda, A.; Batle, J.M.; Martorell, M.; Capó, X.; Tejada, S.; Tur, J.A.; Pons, A. Antioxidant Response of Chronic Wounds to Hyperbaric Oxygen Therapy. *PLoS ONE* **2016**, *11*, e0163371. [CrossRef]
60. Boykin, J.V.; Baylis, C. Hyperbaric Oxygen Therapy Mediates Increased Nitric Oxide Production Associated with Wound Healing. *Adv. Ski. Wound Care* **2007**, *20*, 382–389. [CrossRef]
61. Dulai, P.S.; Buckey, J.C.; Raffals, L.E.; Swoger, J.M.; Claus, P.L.; O'Toole, K.; Ptak, J.A.; Gleeson, M.W.; Widjaja, C.E.; Chang, J.; et al. Hyperbaric Oxygen Therapy Is Well Tolerated and Effective for Ulcerative Colitis Patients Hospitalized for Moderate-Severe Flares: A Phase 2A Pilot Multi-Center, Randomized, Double-Blind, Sham-Controlled Trial. *Am. J. Gastroenterol.* **2018**, *113*, 1516–1523. [CrossRef]
62. Wang, W.; He, Y.; Wen, D.; Jiang, S.; Zhao, X. Efficacy and Safety Evaluation of Hyperbaric Oxygen Therapy for Patients with Ulcerative Colitis: A Protocol of Systematic Review and Meta-Analysis. *Medicine* **2021**, *100*, e23966. [CrossRef]
63. Oliai, C.; Fisher, B.; Jani, A.; Wong, M.; Poli, J.; Brady, L.W.; Komarnicky, L.T. Hyperbaric Oxygen Therapy for Radiation-Induced Cystitis and Proctitis. *Int. J. Radiat. Oncol. Biol. Phys.* **2012**, *84*, 733–740. [CrossRef]
64. Davis, D.D.; Hanley, M.E.; Cooper, J.S. Osteoradionecrosis. *Curr. Otorhinolaryngol. Rep.* **2021**, *6*, 285–291.
65. Malone, M.; Bjarnsholt, T.; McBain, A.J.; James, G.A.; Stoodley, P.; Leaper, D.; Tachi, M.; Schultz, G.; Swanson, T.; Wolcott, R.D. The Prevalence of Biofilms in Chronic Wounds: A Systematic Review and Meta-Analysis of Published Data. *J. Wound Care* **2017**, *26*, 20–25. [CrossRef]
66. Kadam, S.; Shai, S.; Shahane, A.; Kaushik, K.S. Recent Advances in Non-Conventional Antimicrobial Approaches for Chronic Wound Biofilms: Have We Found the "Chink in the Armor"? *Biomedicines* **2019**, *7*, 35. [CrossRef]
67. Kościuczuk, E.M.; Lisowski, P.; Jarczak, J.; Strzałkowska, N.; Jóźwik, A.; Horbańczuk, J.; Krzyżewski, J.; Zwierzchowski, L.; Bagnicka, E. Cathelicidins: Family of Antimicrobial Peptides. A Review. *Mol. Biol. Rep.* **2012**, *39*, 10957–10970. [CrossRef] [PubMed]
68. Peyssonnaux, C.; Datta, V.; Cramer, T.; Doedens, A.; Theodorakis, E.A.; Gallo, R.L.; Hurtado-Ziola, N.; Nizet, V.; Johnson, R.S. HIF-1α Expression Regulates the Bactericidal Capacity of Phagocytes. *J. Clin. Investig.* **2005**, *115*, 1806–1815. [CrossRef] [PubMed]
69. Zarember, K.A.; Malech, H.L. HIF-1alpha: A Master Regulator of Innate Host Defenses? *J. Clin. Investig.* **2005**, *115*, 1702–1704. [CrossRef] [PubMed]
70. Tecle, T.; Tripathi, S.; Hartshorn, K. Review: Defensins and Cathelicidins in Lung Immunity. *Innate Immun.* **2010**, *16*, 151–159. [CrossRef]
71. Gaudreault, É.; Gosselin, J. Leukotriene B4 Induces Release of Antimicrobial Peptides in Lungs of Virally Infected Mice. *J. Immunol.* **2008**, *180*, 6211–6221. [CrossRef]

72. Memar, M.Y.; Yekani, M.; Alizadeh, N.; Baghi, H.B. Hyperbaric Oxygen Therapy: Antimicrobial Mechanisms and Clinical Application for Infections. *Biomed. Pharmacother.* **2019**, *109*, 440–447. [CrossRef]
73. Shaw, J.J.; Psoinos, C.M.; Emhoff, T.A.; Shah, S.A.; Santry, H. Not Just Full of Hot Air: Hyperbaric Oxygen Therapy Increases Survival in Cases of Necrotizing Soft Tissue Infections. *Surg. Infect.* **2014**, *15*, 328–335. [CrossRef]
74. Nedrebø, T.; Bruun, T.; Skjåstad, R.; Holmaas, G.; Skrede, S. Hyperbaric Oxygen Treatment in Three Cases of Necrotizing Infection of the Neck. *Infect. Dis. Rep.* **2012**, *4*, 73–76. [CrossRef]
75. Sanford, N.E.; Wilkinson, J.E.; Nguyen, H.; Diaz, G.; Wolcott, R. Efficacy of Hyperbaric Oxygen Therapy in Bacterial Biofilm Eradication. *J. Wound Care* **2018**, *27*, S20–S28. [CrossRef]
76. Gibson, A.; Davis, F.M. Hyperbaric Oxygen Therapy in the Management of Clostridium Perfringens Infections. *N. Z. Med. J.* **1986**, *99*, 617–620.
77. Sison-Martinez, J.; Hendriksen, S.; Cooper, J.S. Hyperbaric Treatment Of Clostridial Myositis And Myonecrosis. 2021. Available online: https://europepmc.org/article/nbk/nbk500002 (accessed on 13 May 2021).
78. Halbach, J.L.; Prieto, J.M.; Wang, A.W.; Hawisher, D.; Cauvi, D.M.; Reyes, T.; Okerblom, J.; Ramirez-Sanchez, I.; Villarreal, F.; Patel, H.H.; et al. Early Hyperbaric Oxygen Therapy Improves Survival in a Model of Severe Sepsis. *Am. J. Physiol.-Regul. Integr. Comp. Physiol.* **2019**, *317*, R160–R168. [CrossRef]
79. Hung, M.C.; Chou, C.L.; Cheng, L.C.; Ho, C.H.; Niu, K.C.; Chen, H.L.; Tian, Y.F.; Liu, C.L. The Role of Hyperbaric Oxygen Therapy in Treating Extensive Fournier's Gangrene. *Urol. Sci.* **2016**, *27*, 148–153. [CrossRef]
80. Walter, G.; Vernier, M.; Pinelli, P.O.; Million, M.; Coulange, M.; Seng, P.; Stein, A. Bone and Joint Infections Due to Anaerobic Bacteria: An Analysis of 61 Cases and Review of the Literature. *Eur. J. Clin. Microbiol. Infect. Dis.* **2014**, *33*, 1355–1364. [CrossRef]
81. Muzumdar, D.; Jhawar, S.; Goel, A. Brain Abscess: An Overview. *Int. J. Surg.* **2011**, *9*, 136–144. [CrossRef]
82. Tomoye, E.O.; Moon, R.E. Hyperbaric Oxygen for Intracranial Abscess. *Undersea Hyperb. Med.* **2021**, *48*, 97–102. [CrossRef]
83. Bartek, J.; Jakola, A.S.; Skyrman, S.; Förander, P.; Alpkvist, P.; Schechtmann, G.; Glimåker, M.; Larsson, A.; Lind, F.; Mathiesen, T. Hyperbaric Oxygen Therapy in Spontaneous Brain Abscess Patients: A Population-Based Comparative Cohort Study. *Acta Neurochir.* **2016**, *158*, 1259–1267. [CrossRef]
84. M Das, J.; Tommeraasen, M.A.; Cooper, J.S. *Hyperbaric Evaluation and Treatment of Intracranial Abscess*; StatPearls Publishing: Treasure Island, FL, USA, 2020.
85. Hanley, M.E.; Hendriksen, S.; Cooper, J.S. *Hyperbaric Treatment of Chronic Refractory Osteomyelitis*; StatPearls Publishing: Treasure Island, FL, USA, 2021.
86. Rose, D. Hyperbaric Oxygen Therapy for Chronic Refractory Osteomyelitis. *Am. Fam. Physician* **2012**, *86*, 888–893.
87. Savvidou, O.D.; Kaspiris, A.; Bolia, I.K.; Chloros, G.D.; Goumenos, S.D.; Papagelopoulos, P.J.; Tsiodras, S. Effectiveness of Hyperbaric Oxygen Therapy for the Management of Chronic Osteomyelitis: A Systematic Review of the Literature. *Orthopedics* **2018**, *41*, 193–199. [CrossRef]
88. Byun, J.; Patel, J.; Nguyen, S.A.; Lambert, P.R. Hyperbaric Oxygen Therapy in Malignant Otitis Externa: A Systematic Review of the Literature. *World J. Otorhinolaryngol. Head Neck Surg.* **2020**. [CrossRef]
89. Kirby, J.P. Hyperbaric Oxygen Therapy Emergencies. *Mol. Med.* **2019**, *116*, 180–183.
90. Leung, J.K.S.; Lam, R.P.K. Hyperbaric Oxygen Therapy: Its Use in Medical Emergencies and Its Development in Hong Kong. *Hong Kong Med. J.* **2018**, *24*, 191–199. [CrossRef]
91. Cooper, J.S.; Hanson, K.C. *Decompression Sickness (DCS, Bends, Caisson Disease)*; StatPearls Publishing: Treasure Island, FL, USA, 2019.
92. Pollock, N.W.; Buteau, D. Updates in Decompression Illness. *Emerg. Med. Clin. N. Am.* **2017**, *35*, 301–319. [CrossRef]
93. Vann, R.D.; Butler, F.K.; Mitchell, S.J.; Moon, R.E. Decompression Illness. *Lancet* **2011**, *377*, 153–164. [CrossRef]
94. Moon, R.E. Hyperbaric Oxygen Treatment for Decompression Sickness. *Undersea Hyperb. Med.* **2014**, *41*, 151–157.
95. Moon, R.E. Adjunctive Therapy for Decompression Illness: A Review and Update. *Diving Hyperb. Med.* **2009**, *39*, 81–87.
96. Malik, N.; Claus, P.L.; Illman, J.E.; Kligerman, S.J.; Moynagh, M.R.; Levin, D.L.; Woodrum, D.A.; Arani, A.; Arunachalam, S.P.; Araoz, P.A. Air Embolism: Diagnosis and Management. *Future Cardiol.* **2017**, *13*, 365–378. [CrossRef]
97. Yesilaras, M.; Atılla, O.D.; Aksay, E.; Kilic, T.Y.; Atilla, O.D. Retrograde Cerebral Air Embolism. *Am. J. Emerg. Med.* **2014**, *32*, 1562.e1–1562.e2. [CrossRef]
98. Moon, R.E. Hyperbaric Treatment of Air or Gas Embolism: Current Recommendations. *Undersea Hyperb. Med.* **2019**, *46*, 673–683. [CrossRef]
99. Blanc, P.; Boussuges, A.; Henriette, K.; Sainty, J.; Deleflie, M. Iatrogenic Cerebral Air Embolism: Importance of an Early Hyperbaric Oxygenation. *Intensive Care Med.* **2002**, *28*, 559–563. [CrossRef]
100. Bitterman, H.; Melamed, Y. Delayed Hyperbaric Treatment of Cerebral Air Embolism. *Isr. J. Med. Sci.* **1993**, *29*, 22–26.
101. Schlimp, C.J.; Bothma, P.A.; Brodbeck, A.E. Cerebral Venous Air Embolism: What Is It and Do We Know How to Deal With It Properly? *JAMA Neurol.* **2014**, *71*, 243. [CrossRef] [PubMed]
102. Bothma, P.A.; Schlimp, C.J., II. Retrograde Cerebral Venous Gas Embolism: Are We Missing Too Many Cases? *Br. J. Anaesth.* **2014**, *112*, 401–404. [CrossRef] [PubMed]
103. Hayreh, S.S. Central Retinal Artery Occlusion. *Indian J. Ophthalmol.* **2018**, *66*, 1684–1694. [CrossRef] [PubMed]
104. Hanley, M.E.; Cooper, J.S. *Hyperbaric, Central Retinal Artery Occlusion*; StatPearls Publishing: Treasure Island, FL, USA, 2018.

105. Bağlı, B.S.; Çevik, S.G.; Çevik, M.T. Effect of Hyperbaric Oxygen Treatment in Central Retinal Artery Occlusion. *Undersea Hyperb. Med.* **2018**, *45*, 421–425. [CrossRef]
106. Olson, E.A.; Lentz, K. Central Retinal Artery Occlusion: A Literature Review and the Rationale for Hyperbaric Oxygen Therapy. *Mol. Med.* **2016**, *113*, 53–57.
107. Kim, S.H.; Cha, Y.S.; Lee, Y.; Kim, H.; Yoon, I.N. Successful Treatment of Central Retinal Artery Occlusion Using Hyperbaric Oxygen Therapy. *Clin. Exp. Emerg. Med.* **2018**, *5*, 278–281. [CrossRef]
108. Youn, T.S.; Lavin, P.; Patrylo, M.; Schindler, J.; Kirshner, H.; Greer, D.M.; Schrag, M. Current Treatment of Central Retinal Artery Occlusion: A National Survey. *J. Neurol.* **2018**, *265*, 330–335. [CrossRef]
109. Yu, M.; Yuan, H.S.; Li, Q.; Li, Q.; Teng, Y.F. Combination of Cells-Based Therapy with Apelin-13 and Hyperbaric Oxygen Efficiently Promote Neovascularization in Ischemic Animal Model. *Eur. Rev. Med. Pharmacol. Sci.* **2019**, *23*, 2630–2639. [CrossRef]
110. Santema, K.T.B.; Stoekenbroek, R.M.; Koelemay, M.J.W.; Reekers, J.A.; Van Dortmont, L.M.C.; Oomen, A.; Smeets, L.; Wever, J.J.; Legemate, D.A.; Ubbink, D.T. Hyperbaric Oxygen Therapy in the Treatment of Ischemic Lower-Extremity Ulcers in Patients with Diabetes: Results of the DAMO2CLES Multicenter Randomized Clinical Trial. *Diabetes Care* **2018**, *41*, 112–119. [CrossRef]
111. Abidia, A.; Laden, G.; Kuhan, G.; Johnson, B.F.; Wilkinson, A.R.; Renwick, P.M.; Masson, E.A.; McCollum, P.T. The Role of Hyperbaric Oxygen Therapy in Ischaemic Diabetic Lower Extremity Ulcers: A Double-Blind Randomized-Controlled Trial. *Eur. J. Vasc. Endovasc. Surg.* **2003**, *25*, 513–518. [CrossRef]
112. Nakamura, H.; Makiguchi, T.; Atomura, D.; Yamatsu, Y.; Shirabe, K.; Yokoo, S. Changes in Skin Perfusion Pressure After Hyperbaric Oxygen Therapy Following Revascularization in Patients With Critical Limb Ischemia: A Preliminary Study. *Int. J. Low. Extrem. Wounds* **2020**, *19*, 57–62. [CrossRef]
113. Rose, J.J.; Wang, L.; Xu, Q.; McTiernan, C.F.; Shiva, S.; Tejero, J.; Gladwin, M.T. Carbon Monoxide Poisoning: Pathogenesis, Management, and Future Directions of Therapy. *Am. J. Respir. Crit. Care Med.* **2017**, *195*, 596–606. [CrossRef]
114. Martani, L.; Cantadori, L.; Paganini, M.; Camporesi, E.M.; Bosco, G. Carbon Monoxide Intoxication: Prehospital Diagnosis and Direct Transfer to the Hyperbaric Chamber. *Minerva Anestesiol.* **2019**, *85*, 920–922. [CrossRef]
115. Rose, J.J.; Nouraie, M.; Gauthier, M.C.; Pizon, A.F.; Saul, M.I.; Donahoe, M.P.; Gladwin, M.T. Clinical Outcomes and Mortality Impact of Hyperbaric Oxygen Therapy in Patients With Carbon Monoxide Poisoning. *Crit. Care Med.* **2018**, *46*, e649–e655. [CrossRef]
116. Weaver, L.K.; Hopkins, R.O.; Chan, K.J.; Churchill, S.; Elliott, C.G.; Clemmer, T.P.; Orme, J.F.; Thomas, F.O.; Morris, A.H. Hyperbaric Oxygen for Acute Carbon Monoxide Poisoning. *N. Engl. J. Med.* **2002**, *347*, 1057–1067. [CrossRef]
117. Hampson, N.B.; Piantadosi, C.A.; Thom, S.R.; Weaver, L.K. Practice Recommendations in the Diagnosis, Management, and Prevention of Carbon Monoxide Poisoning. *Am. J. Respir. Crit. Care Med.* **2012**, *186*, 1095–1101. [CrossRef]
118. Hanley, M.E.; Murphy-Lavoie, H.M. *Hyperbaric, Cyanide Toxicity*; StatPearls Publishing: Treasure Island, FL, USA, 2019.
119. Lawson-Smith, P.; Jansen, E.C.; Hilsted, L.; Johnsen, A.H.; Hyldegaard, O. Effect of Acute and Delayed Hyperbaric Oxygen Therapy on Cyanide Whole Blood Levels during Acute Cyanide Intoxication. *Undersea Hyperb. Med.* **2011**, *38*, 17–26.
120. Van Meter, K.W. The Effect of Hyperbaric Oxygen on Severe Anemia. *Undersea Hyperb. Med.* **2012**, *39*, 937–942.
121. Rhee, T.M.; Hwang, D.; Lee, J.S.; Park, J.; Lee, J.M. Addition of Hyperbaric Oxygen Therapy vs. Medical Therapy Alone for Idiopathic Sudden Sensorineural Hearing Loss: A Systematic Review and Meta-Analysis. *JAMA Otolaryngol. Head Neck Surg.* **2018**, *144*, 1153–1161. [CrossRef]
122. Bayoumy, A.B.; de Ru, J.A. The Use of Hyperbaric Oxygen Therapy in Acute Hearing Loss: A Narrative Review. *Eur. Arch. Oto-Rhino-Laryngol.* **2019**, *276*, 1859–1880. [CrossRef]
123. Paderno, E.; Zanon, V.; Vezzani, G.; Giacon, T.; Bernasek, T.; Camporesi, E.; Bosco, G. Evidence-Supported HBO Therapy in Femoral Head Necrosis: A Systematic Review and Meta-Analysis. *Int. J. Environ. Res. Public Health* **2021**, *18*, 2888. [CrossRef]
124. Brenner, I.; Shephard, R.J.; Shek, P.N. Immune Function in Hyperbaric Environments, Diving, and Decompression. *Undersea Hyperb. Med.* **1999**, *26*, 27–39.
125. Xu, X.; Yi, H.; Kato, M.; Suzuki, H.; Kobayashi, S.; Takahashi, H.; Nakashima, I. Differential Sensitivities to Hyperbaric Oxygen of Lymphocyte Subpopulations of Normal and Autoimmune Mice. *Immunol. Lett.* **1997**, *59*, 79–84. [CrossRef]
126. Saito, K.; Tanaka, Y.; Ota, T.; Eto, S.; Yamashita, U. Suppressive Effect of Hyperbaric Oxygenation on Immune Responses of Normal and Autoimmune Mice. *Clin. Exp. Immunol.* **1991**, *86*, 322–327. [CrossRef]
127. Chen, S.Y.; Chen, Y.C.; Wang, J.K.; Hsu, H.P.; Ho, P.S.; Chen, Y.C.; Sytwu, H.K. Early Hyperbaric Oxygen Therapy Attenuates Disease Severity in Lupus-Prone Autoimmune (NZB × NZW) F1 Mice. *Clin. Immunol.* **2003**, *108*, 103–110. [CrossRef]
128. Harnanik, T.; Soeroso, J.; Suryokusumo, M.G.; Juliandhy, T. Effects of Hyperbaric Oxygen on t Helper 17/Regulatory t Polarization in Antigen and Collagen-Induced Arthritis: Hypoxia-Inducible Factor-1α as a Target. *Oman Med. J.* **2020**, *35*, e90. [CrossRef] [PubMed]
129. Novak, S.; Drenjancevic, I.; Vukovic, R.; Kellermayer, Z.; Cosic, A.; Tolusic Levak, M.; Balogh, P.; Culo, F.; Mihalj, M. Anti-Inflammatory Effects of Hyperbaric Oxygenation during DSS-Induced Colitis in BALB/c Mice Include Changes in Gene Expression of HIF-1 α, Proinflamatory Cytokines, and Antioxidative Enzymes. *Mediat. Inflamm.* **2016**, *2016*, 7141430. [CrossRef] [PubMed]
130. Resanovic, I.; Gluvic, Z.; Zaric, B.; Sudar-Milovanovic, E.; Jovanovic, A.; Milacic, D.; Isakovic, R.; Isenovic, E.R. Early Effects of Hyperbaric Oxygen on Inducible Nitric Oxide Synthase Activity/Expression in Lymphocytes of Type 1 Diabetes Patients: A Prospective Pilot Study. *Int. J. Endocrinol.* **2019**, *2019*, 2328505. [CrossRef] [PubMed]

131. Bellato, E.; Marini, E.; Castoldi, F.; Barbasetti, N.; Mattei, L.; Bonasia, D.E.; Blonna, D. Fibromyalgia Syndrome: Etiology, Pathogenesis, Diagnosis, and Treatment. *Pain Res. Treat.* **2012**, *2012*, 17. [CrossRef]
132. Guggino, G.; Schinocca, C.; Lo Pizzo, M.; Di Liberto, D.; Garbo, D.; Raimondo, S.; Alessandro, R.; Brighina, F.; Ruscitti, P.; Giacomelli, R.; et al. T Helper 1 Response Is Correlated with Widespread Pain, Fatigue, Sleeping Disorders and the Quality of Life in Patients with Fibromyalgia and Is Modulated by Hyperbaric Oxygen Therapy. *Clin. Exp. Rheumatol.* **2019**, *37* (Suppl. 116), 81–89.
133. Woo, J.; Min, J.H.; Lee, Y.H.; Roh, H.T. Effects of Hyperbaric Oxygen Therapy on Inflammation, Oxidative/Antioxidant Balance, and Muscle Damage after Acute Exercise in Normobaric, Normoxic and Hypobaric, Hypoxic Environments: A Pilot Study. *Int. J. Environ. Res. Public Health* **2020**, *17*, 7377. [CrossRef]
134. Ortega, M.A.; Fraile-Martínez, O.; García-Montero, C.; García-Gallego, S.; Sánchez-Trujillo, L.; Torres-Carranza, D.; Álvarez-Mon, M.Á.; Pekarek, L.; García-Honduvilla, N.; Bujan, J.; et al. An Integrative Look at SARS-CoV-2 (Review). *Int. J. Mol. Med.* **2021**, *47*, 415–434. [CrossRef]
135. del Barco, A.A.; Ortega, M.A. Epidemiology and Public Health in the COVID-19 Epidemic. *Medicine* **2020**, *13*, 1297–1304. [CrossRef]
136. Chandra, A.; Chakraborty, U.; Pal, J.; Karmakar, P. Silent Hypoxia: A Frequently Overlooked Clinical Entity in Patients with COVID-19. *BMJ Case Rep.* **2020**, *13*, 237207. [CrossRef]
137. Dhont, S.; Derom, E.; Van Braeckel, E.; Depuydt, P.; Lambrecht, B.N. The Pathophysiology of "happy" Hypoxemia in COVID-19. *Respir. Res.* **2020**, *21*, 198. [CrossRef]
138. Álvarez-Mon, M.; Ortega, M.A.; Gasulla, Ó.; Fortuny-Profitós, J.; Mazaira-Font, F.A.; Saurina, P.; Monserrat, J.; Plana, M.N.; Troncoso, D.; Moreno, J.S.; et al. A Predictive Model and Risk Factors for Case Fatality of Covid-19. *J. Pers. Med.* **2021**, *11*, 36. [CrossRef]
139. Tobin, M.J.; Laghi, F.; Jubran, A. Why COVID-19 Silent Hypoxemia Is Baffling to Physicians. *Am. J. Respir. Crit. Care Med.* **2020**, *202*, 356–360. [CrossRef]
140. Wilkerson, R.G.; Adler, J.D.; Shah, N.G.; Brown, R. Silent Hypoxia: A Harbinger of Clinical Deterioration in Patients with COVID-19. *Am. J. Emerg. Med.* **2020**, *38*, 2243.e5–2243.e6. [CrossRef]
141. Brouqui, P.; Amrane, S.; Million, M.; Cortaredona, S.; Parola, P.; Lagier, J.C.; Raoult, D. Asymptomatic Hypoxia in COVID-19 Is Associated with Poor Outcome. *Int. J. Infect. Dis.* **2021**, *102*, 233–238. [CrossRef]
142. Lindahl, S.G.E. Using the Prone Position Could Help to Combat the Development of Fast Hypoxia in Some Patients with COVID-19. *Acta Paediatr. Int. J. Paediatr.* **2020**, *109*, 1539–1544. [CrossRef]
143. Oliaei, S.; SeyedAlinaghi, S.; Mehrtak, M.; Karimi, A.; Noori, T.; Mirzapour, P.; Shojaei, A.; Mohsseni Pour, M.; Mirghaderi, S.P.; Alilou, S.; et al. The effects of hyperbaric oxygen therapy (HBOT) on coronavirus disease-2019 (COVID-19): A systematic review. *Eur. J. Med. Res.* **2021**, *26*, 96. [CrossRef] [PubMed]
144. Paganini, M.; Bosco, G.; Perozzo, F.A.G.; Kohlscheen, E.; Sonda, R.; Bassetto, F.; Garetto, G.; Camporesi, E.M.; Thom, S.R. The Role of Hyperbaric Oxygen Treatment for COVID-19: A Review. *Adv. Exp. Med. Biol.* **2021**, *1289*, 27–35. [CrossRef] [PubMed]
145. De Maio, A.; Hightower, L.E. COVID-19, Acute Respiratory Distress Syndrome (ARDS), and Hyperbaric Oxygen Therapy (HBOT): What Is the Link? *Cell Stress Chaperones* **2020**, *25*, 717–720. [CrossRef] [PubMed]
146. Criado, P.R.; Miot, H.A.; Pincelli, T.P.H.; Fabro, A.T. From Dermatological Conditions to COVID-19: Reasoning for Anticoagulation, Suppression of Inflammation, and Hyperbaric Oxygen Therapy. *Dermatol. Ther.* **2021**, *34*, e14565. [CrossRef]
147. Xiaoling, Z.; Xiaolan, T.; Yanchao, T.; Ruiyong, C. The Outcomes of Hyperbaric Oxygen Therapy to Retrieve Hypoxemia of Severe Novel Coronavirus Pneumonia: First Case Report. *Chin. J. Naut. Med. Hyperb. Med.* **2020**, *27*, E001. [CrossRef]
148. Kjellberg, A.; De Maio, A.; Lindholm, P. Can Hyperbaric Oxygen Safely Serve as an Anti-Inflammatory Treatment for COVID-19? *Med. Hypotheses* **2020**, *144*, 110224. [CrossRef]
149. Senniappan, K.; Jeyabalan, S.; Rangappa, P.; Kanchi, M. Hyperbaric Oxygen Therapy: Can It Be a Novel Supportive Therapy in COVID-19? *Indian J. Anaesth.* **2020**, *64*, 835–841.
150. Thibodeaux, K.; Speyrer, M.; Raza, A.; Yaakov, R.; Serena, T.E. Hyperbaric Oxygen Therapy in Preventing Mechanical Ventilation in COVID-19 Patients: A Retrospective Case Series. *J. Wound Care* **2020**, *29*, S4–S8. [CrossRef]
151. Guo, D.; Pan, S.; Wang, M.; Guo, Y. Hyperbaric Oxygen Therapy May Be Effective to Improve Hypoxemia in Patients with Severe COVID-2019 Pneumonia: Two Case Reports. *Undersea Hyperb. Med. J. Undersea Hyperb. Med. Soc. Inc.* **2020**, *47*, 181–187. [CrossRef]
152. Tian, S.; Hu, W.; Niu, L.; Liu, H.; Xu, H.; Xiao, S.Y. Pulmonary Pathology of Early-Phase 2019 Novel Coronavirus (COVID-19) Pneumonia in Two Patients With Lung Cancer. *J. Thorac. Oncol.* **2020**, *15*, 700–704. [CrossRef]
153. Cavezzi, A.; Troiani, E.; Corrao, S. COVID-19: Hemoglobin, Iron, and Hypoxia beyond Inflammation. A Narrative Review. *Clin. Pract.* **2020**, *10*, 24–30. [CrossRef]
154. Allali, G.; Marti, C.; Grosgurin, O.; Morélot-Panzini, C.; Similowski, T.; Adler, D. Dyspnea: The vanished warning symptom of COVID-19 pneumonia. *J. Med. Virol.* **2020**, *92*, 2272–2273. [CrossRef]
155. El Hawa, A.A.A.; Charipova, K.; Bekeny, J.C.; Johnson-Arbor, K.K. The Evolving Use of Hyperbaric Oxygen Therapy during the COVID-19 Pandemic. *J. Wound Care* **2021**, *30*, S8–S11. [CrossRef]
156. Hanahan, D.; Weinberg, R.A. Hallmarks of Cancer: The next Generation. *Cell* **2011**, *144*, 646–674. [CrossRef]

157. Muz, B.; de la Puente, P.; Azab, F.; Azab, A.K. The Role of Hypoxia in Cancer Progression, Angiogenesis, Metastasis, and Resistance to Therapy. *Hypoxia* **2015**, *3*, 83. [CrossRef]
158. Ortega, M.A.; Fraile-Martínez, O.; Asúnsolo, Á.; Buján, J.; García-Honduvilla, N.; Coca, S. Signal Transduction Pathways in Breast Cancer: The Important Role of PI3K/Akt/MTOR. *J. Oncol.* **2020**, *2020*, 9258396. [CrossRef]
159. Jing, X.; Yang, F.; Shao, C.; Wei, K.; Xie, M.; Shen, H.; Shu, Y. Role of Hypoxia in Cancer Therapy by Regulating the Tumor Microenvironment. *Mol. Cancer* **2019**, *18*, 157. [CrossRef]
160. Dhani, N.; Fyles, A.; Hedley, D.; Milosevic, M. The Clinical Significance of Hypoxia in Human Cancers. *Semin. Nucl. Med.* **2015**, *45*, 110–121. [CrossRef]
161. Kim, S.W.; Kim, I.K.; Lee, S.H. Role of Hyperoxic Treatment in Cancer. *Exp. Biol. Med.* **2020**, *245*, 851–860. [CrossRef]
162. Moen, I.; Stuhr, L.E.B. Hyperbaric Oxygen Therapy and Cancer—A Review. *Target. Oncol.* **2012**, *7*, 233–242. [CrossRef]
163. Stępień, K.; Ostrowski, R.P.; Matyja, E. Hyperbaric Oxygen as an Adjunctive Therapy in Treatment of Malignancies, Including Brain Tumours. *Med. Oncol.* **2016**, *33*, 101. [CrossRef] [PubMed]
164. Thews, O.; Vaupel, P. Spatial Oxygenation Profiles in Tumors during Normo- and Hyperbaric Hyperoxia. *Strahlenther Onkol.* **2015**, *191*, 875–882. [CrossRef] [PubMed]
165. Feldmeier, J.; Carl, U.; Hartmann, K.; Sminia, P. Hyperbaric Oxygen: Does It Promote Growth or Recurrence of Malignancy? *Undersea Hyperb. Med.* **2003**, *30*, 1–18. [PubMed]
166. Pande, S.; Sengupta, A.; Srivastava, A.; Gude, R.P.; Ingle, A. Re-Evaluate the Effect of Hyperbaric Oxygen Therapy in Cancer—A Preclinical Therapeutic Small Animal Model Study. *PLoS ONE* **2012**, *7*, e48432. [CrossRef]
167. Lu, Q.Z.; Li, X.; Ouyang, J.; Li, J.Q.; Chen, G. Further Application of Hyperbaric Oxygen in Prostate Cancer. *Med. Gas Res.* **2018**, *8*, 167–171.
168. Batra, S.; Adekola, K.; Rosen, S.; Shanmugam, M. Cancer Metabolism as a Therapeutic Target. *Oncology* **2013**, *27*, 460–467.
169. Poff, A.M.; Ari, C.; Seyfried, T.N.; D'Agostino, D.P. The Ketogenic Diet and Hyperbaric Oxygen Therapy Prolong Survival in Mice with Systemic Metastatic Cancer. *PLoS ONE* **2013**, *8*, e65522. [CrossRef]
170. Poff, A.M.; Ward, N.; Seyfried, T.N.; Arnold, P.; D'Agostino, D.P. Non-Toxic Metabolic Management of Metastatic Cancer in VM Mice: Novel Combination of Ketogenic Diet, Ketone Supplementation, and Hyperbaric Oxygen Therapy. *PLoS ONE* **2015**, *10*, e0127407. [CrossRef]
171. Baskar, R.; Lee, K.A.; Yeo, R.; Yeoh, K.W. Cancer and Radiation Therapy: Current Advances and Future Directions. *Int. J. Med. Sci.* **2012**, *9*, 193–199. [CrossRef]
172. Arienti, C.; Pignatta, S.; Zanoni, M.; Zamagni, A.; Cortesi, M.; Sarnelli, A.; Romeo, A.; Arpa, D.; Longobardi, P.; Bartolini, D.; et al. High-Pressure Oxygen Rewires Glucose Metabolism of Patient-Derived Glioblastoma Cells and Fuels Inflammasome Response. *Cancer Lett.* **2021**, *506*, 152–166. [CrossRef]
173. Arpa, D.; Parisi, E.; Ghigi, G.; Cortesi, A.; Longobardi, P.; Cenni, P.; Pieri, M.; Tontini, L.; Neri, E.; Micheletti, S.; et al. Role of Hyperbaric Oxygenation Plus Hypofractionated Stereotactic Radiotherapy in Recurrent High-Grade Glioma. *Front. Oncol.* **2021**, *11*, 964. [CrossRef]
174. Majeed, H.; Gupta, V. *Adverse Effects of Radiation Therapy*; StatPearls Publishing: Treasure Island, FL, USA, 2020.
175. Brush, J.; Lipnick, S.L.; Phillips, T.; Sitko, J.; McDonald, J.T.; McBride, W.H. Molecular Mechanisms of Late Normal Tissue Injury. *Semin. Radiat. Oncol.* **2007**, *17*, 121–130. [CrossRef]
176. Cooper, J.S.; Hanley, M.E.; Hendriksen, S.; Robins, M. *Hyperbaric Treatment of Delayed Radiation Injury*; StatPearls Publishing: Treasure Island, FL, USA, 2020.
177. Feldmeier, J.J. Hyperbaric Oxygen Therapy and Delayed Radiation Injuries (Soft Tissue and Bony Necrosis): 2012 Update. *Undersea Hyperb. Med.* **2012**, *39*, 1121–1139.
178. Bennett, M.H.; Feldmeier, J.; Hampson, N.B.; Smee, R.; Milross, C. Hyperbaric Oxygen Therapy for Late Radiation Tissue Injury. *Cochrane Database Syst. Rev.* **2016**, *2016*, CD005005. [CrossRef]
179. Brewer, A.L.; Shirachi, D.Y.; Quock, R.M.; Craft, R.M. Effect of Hyperbaric Oxygen on Chemotherapy-Induced Neuropathy in Male and Female Rats. *Behav. Pharmacol.* **2020**, *31*, 61–72. [CrossRef]
180. Fu, H.; Li, F.; Thomas, S.; Yang, Z. Hyperbaric Oxygenation Alleviates Chronic Constriction Injury (CCI)-Induced Neuropathic Pain and Inhibits GABAergic Neuron Apoptosis in the Spinal Cord. *Scand. J. Pain* **2017**, *17*, 330–338. [CrossRef]
181. Zhang, Y.; Brewer, A.L.; Nelson, J.T.; Smith, P.T.; Shirachi, D.Y.; Quock, R.M. Hyperbaric Oxygen Produces a Nitric Oxide Synthase-Regulated Anti-Allodynic Effect in Rats with Paclitaxel-Induced Neuropathic Pain. *Brain Res.* **2019**, *1711*, 41–47. [CrossRef]
182. Gibbons, C.R.; Liu, S.; Zhang, Y.; Sayre, C.L.; Levitch, B.R.; Moehlmann, S.B.; Shirachi, D.Y.; Quock, R.M. Involvement of Brain Opioid Receptors in the Anti-Allodynic Effect of Hyperbaric Oxygen in Rats with Sciatic Nerve Crush-Induced Neuropathic Pain. *Brain Res.* **2013**, *1537*, 111–116. [CrossRef]
183. Kawasoe, Y.; Yokouchi, M.; Ueno, Y.; Iwaya, H.; Yoshida, H.; Komiya, S. Hyperbaric Oxygen as a Chemotherapy Adjuvant in the Treatment of Osteosarcoma. *Oncol. Rep.* **2009**, *22*, 1045–1050. [CrossRef]
184. Petre, P.M.; Baciewicz, F.A.; Tigan, S.; Spears, J.R.; Patterson, G.A.; Swisher, S.G.; Harpole, D.H.; Goldstraw, P. Hyperbaric Oxygen as a Chemotherapy Adjuvant in the Treatment of Metastatic Lung Tumors in a Rat Model. *J. Thorac. Cardiovasc. Surg.* **2003**, *125*, 85–95. [CrossRef]

185. Ohguri, T.; Imada, H.; Narisada, H.; Yahara, K.; Morioka, T.; Nakano, K.; Miyaguni, Y.; Korogi, Y. Systemic Chemotherapy Using Paclitaxel and Carboplatin plus Regional Hyperthermia and Hyperbaric Oxygen Treatment for Non-Small Cell Lung Cancer with Multiple Pulmonary Metastases: Preliminary Results. *Int. J. Hyperth.* **2009**, *25*, 160–167. [CrossRef]
186. Baude, J.; Cooper, J.S. *Hyperbaric Contraindicated Chemotherapeutic Agents*; StatPearls Publishing: Treasure Island, FL, USA, 2020.
187. Ortega, M.A.; Fraile-Martínez, O.; García-Montero, C.; Pekarek, L.; Guijarro, L.G.; Castellanos, A.J.; Sanchez-Trujillo, L.; García-Honduvilla, N.; Álvarez-Mon, M.; Buján, J.; et al. Physical Activity as an Imperative Support in Breast Cancer Management. *Cancers* **2021**, *13*, 55. [CrossRef]
188. Hadanny, A.; Lang, E.; Copel, L.; Meir, O.; Bechor, Y.; Fishlev, G.; Bergan, J.; Friedman, M.; Zisman, A.; Efrati, S. Hyperbaric Oxygen Can Induce Angiogenesis and Recover Erectile Function. *Int. J. Impot. Res.* **2018**, *30*, 292–299. [CrossRef]
189. Chiles, K.A.; Staff, I.; Johnson-Arbor, K.; Champagne, A.; McLaughlin, T.; Graydon, R.J. A Double-Blind, Randomized Trial on the Efficacy and Safety of Hyperbaric Oxygenation Therapy in the Preservation of Erectile Function after Radical Prostatectomy. *J. Urol.* **2018**, *199*, 805–811. [CrossRef]
190. Cormier, J.; Theriot, M. Patient Diagnosed with Chronic Erectile Dysfunction Refractory to PDE 5 Inhibitor Therapy Reports Improvement in Function after Hyperbaric Oxygen Therapy. *Undersea Hyperb. Med.* **2016**, *43*, 463–465.
191. Yuan, J.-B.; Yang, L.Y.; Wang, Y.H.; Ding, T.; Chen, T.D.; Lu, Q. Hyperbaric Oxygen Therapy for Recovery of Erectile Function after Posterior Urethral Reconstruction. *Int. Urol. Nephrol.* **2011**, *43*, 755–761. [CrossRef]
192. Lippert, T.; Borlongan, C.V. Prophylactic Treatment of Hyperbaric Oxygen Mitigates Inflammatory Response via Mitochondria Transfer. *CNS Neurosci. Ther.* **2019**, *25*, 815–823. [CrossRef]
193. Liska, G.M.; Lippert, T.; Russo, E.; Nieves, N.; Borlongan, C. V A Dual Role for Hyperbaric Oxygen in Stroke Neuroprotection: Preconditioning of the Brain and Stem Cells. *Cond. Med.* **2018**, *1*, 151–166.
194. Ding, Z.; Tong, W.C.; Lu, X.-X.; Peng, H.-P. Hyperbaric Oxygen Therapy in Acute Ischemic Stroke: A Review. *Interv. Neurol.* **2014**, *2*, 201–211. [CrossRef]
195. Hachmo, Y.; Hadanny, A.; Abu Hamed, R.; Daniel-Kotovsky, M.; Catalogna, M.; Fishlev, G.; Lang, E.; Polak, N.; Doenyas, K.; Friedman, M.; et al. Hyperbaric Oxygen Therapy Increases Telomere Length and Decreases Immunosenescence in Isolated Blood Cells: A Prospective Trial. *Aging* **2020**, *12*, 22445–22456. [CrossRef]
196. Nishizaka, T.; Nomura, T.; Higuchi, K.; Takemura, A.; Ishihara, A. Mild Hyperbaric Oxygen Activates the Proliferation of Epidermal Basal Cells in Aged Mice. *J. Dermatol.* **2018**, *45*, 1141–1144. [CrossRef] [PubMed]
197. Godman, C.A.; Joshi, R.; Giardina, C.; Perdrizet, G.; Hightower, L.E. Hyperbaric Oxygen Treatment Induces Antioxidant Gene Expression. *Ann. N. Y. Acad. Sci.* **2010**, *1197*, 178–183. [CrossRef] [PubMed]
198. Amir, H.; Malka, D.K.; Gil, S.; Rahav, B.G.; Merav, C.; Kobi, D.; Yafit, H.; Ramzia, A.H.; Efrat, S.; Gregory, F.; et al. Cognitive Enhancement of Healthy Older Adults Using Hyperbaric Oxygen: A Randomized Controlled Trial. *Aging* **2020**, *12*, 13740–13761. [CrossRef] [PubMed]
199. Shwe, T.; Bo-Htay, C.; Ongnok, B.; Chunchai, T.; Jaiwongkam, T.; Kerdphoo, S.; Kumfu, S.; Pratchayasakul, W.; Pattarasakulchai, T.; Chattipakorn, N.; et al. Hyperbaric Oxygen Therapy Restores Cognitive Function and Hippocampal Pathologies in Both Aging and Aging-Obese Rats. *Mech. Ageing Dev.* **2021**, *195*, 111465. [CrossRef]
200. Camporesi, E.M. Side Effects of Hyperbaric Oxygen Therapy. *Undersea Hyperb. Med.* **2014**, *41*, 253–257.
201. Heyboer, M.; Sharma, D.; Santiago, W.; McCulloch, N. Hyperbaric Oxygen Therapy: Side Effects Defined and Quantified. *Adv. Wound Care* **2017**, *6*, 210–224. [CrossRef]
202. Hadanny, A.; Meir, O.; Bechor, G.; Fishlev, J.; Efrati, S. Seizures during Hyperbaric Oxygen Therapy: Retrospective Analysis of 62,614 Treatment Sessions. *Undersea Hyperb. Med.* **2016**, *43*, 21–28.
203. Cooper, J.S.; Phuyal, P.; Shah, N. *Oxygen Toxicity*; StatPearls Publishing: Treasure Island, FL, USA, 2021. Available online: https://www.ncbi.nlm.nih.gov/books/NBK430743/ (accessed on 28 March 2021).
204. Domachevsky, L.; Rachmany, L.; Barak, Y.; Rubovitch, V.; Abramovich, A.; Pick, C.G. Hyperbaric Oxygen-Induced Seizures Cause a Transient Decrement in Cognitive Function. *Neuroscience* **2013**, *247*, 328–334. [CrossRef]
205. Nakane, M. Biological Effects of the Oxygen Molecule in Critically Ill Patients. *J. Intensive Care* **2020**, *8*, 95. [CrossRef]
206. Hadanny, A.; Zubari, T.; Tamir-Adler, L.; Bechor, Y.; Fishlev, G.; Lang, E.; Polak, N.; Bergan, J.; Friedman, M.; Efrati, S. Hyperbaric Oxygen Therapy Effects on Pulmonary Functions: A Prospective Cohort Study. *BMC Pulm. Med.* **2019**, *19*, 148. [CrossRef]
207. Mcmonnies, C.W. Hyperbaric Oxygen Therapy and the Possibility of Ocular Complications or Contraindications. *Clin. Exp. Optom.* **2015**, *98*, 122–125. [CrossRef]
208. Sola, A.; Chow, L.; Rogido, M. Retinopathy of Prematurity and Oxygen Therapy: A Changing Relationship. *An. Pediatr.* **2005**, *62*, 48–63. [CrossRef]
209. Gawdi, R.; Cooper, J.S. *Hyperbaric Contraindications*; StatPearls Publishing: Treasure Island, FL, USA, 2020.
210. Arslan, A. Hyperbaric Oxygen Therapy in Carbon Monoxide Poisoning in Pregnancy: Maternal and Fetal Outcome. *Am. J. Emerg. Med.* **2021**, *43*, 41–45. [CrossRef]
211. Stevens, S.L.; Narr, A.J.; Claus, P.L.; Millman, M.P.; Steinkraus, L.W.; Shields, R.C.; Buchta, W.G.; Haddon, R.; Wang, Z.; Murad, M.H. The Incidence of Hypoglycemia during HBO_2 Therapy: A Retrospective Review. *Undersea Hyperb. Med.* **2015**, *42*, 191–196.
212. Al-Waili, N.S.; Butler, G.J.; Beale, J.; Abdullah, M.S.; Finkelstein, M.; Merrow, M.; Rivera, R.; Petrillo, R.; Carrey, Z.; Lee, B.; et al. Influences of Hyperbaric Oxygen on Blood Pressure, Heart Rate and Blood Glucose Levels in Patients with Diabetes Mellitus and Hypertension. *Arch. Med. Res.* **2006**, *37*, 991–997. [CrossRef]

213. Weaver, L.K.; Churchill, S. Pulmonary Edema Associated with Hyperbaric Oxygen Therapy. *Chest* **2001**, *120*, 1407–1409. [CrossRef]
214. Kahle, A.C.; Cooper, J.S. *Hyperbaric Physiological And Pharmacological Effects Gases*; StatPearls Publishing: Treasure Island, FL, USA, 2019.
215. Wang, X.; Li, S.; Liu, X.; Wu, X.; Ye, N.; Yang, X.; Li, Z. Boosting Nanomedicine Efficacy with Hyperbaric Oxygen Therapy. In *Advances in Experimental Medicine and Biology*; Springer: Berlin/Heidelberg, Germany, 2021; Volume 1295, pp. 77–95.

Article

Analysis of the Increase of Vascular Cell Adhesion Molecule-1 (VCAM-1) Expression and the Effect of Exposure in a Hyperbaric Chamber on VCAM-1 in Human Blood Serum: A Cross-Sectional Study

Katarzyna Van Damme-Ostapowicz [1,*], Mateusz Cybulski [2], Mariusz Kozakiewicz [3], Elżbieta Krajewska-Kułak [2], Piotr Siermontowski [4], Marek Sobolewski [5] and Dorota Kaczerska [6]

[1] Department of Health and Caring Sciences, Faculty of Health and Social Sciences, Western Norway University of Applied Sciences, Svanehaugvegen 1 Str., 6812 Førde, Norway

[2] Department of Integrated Medical Care, Faculty of Health Sciences, Medical University of Białystok, Skłodowskiej-Curie 7A Str., 15-096 Białystok, Poland; mateusz.cybulski@umb.edu.pl (M.C.); elzbieta.krajewska-kulak@umb.edu.pl (E.K.-K.)

[3] Division of Biochemistry and Biogerontology, Department of Geriatrics, Nicolaus Copernicus University in Toruń, L. Rydygier Collegium Medicum in Bydgoszcz, Dębowa 3 Str., 85-626 Bydgoszcz, Poland; markoz@cm.umk.pl

[4] Department of Submarine Work Technology, Faculty of Mechanical and Electrical Engineering, Polish Naval Academy, Śmidowicza 69 Str., 81-127 Gdynia, Poland; p.siermontowski@amw.gdynia.pl

[5] Department of Quantitative Methods, Faculty of Management, Rzeszów University of Technology, Powstańców Warszawy 8 Str., 35-959 Rzeszów, Poland; msobolew@prz.edu.pl

[6] Department of Physiotherapy and Health Sciences, Faculty of Dietetics, Gdańsk College of Health, Pelplińska 7 Str., 80-335 Gdańsk, Poland; dorotakaczerska@tlen.pl

* Correspondence: katarzyna.van-damme-ostapowicz@hvl.no; Tel.: +47-57-72-25-31

Abstract: *Background and Objectives:* Vascular cell adhesion molecule-1 (VCAM-1) was identified as a cell adhesion molecule that helps to regulate inflammation-associated vascular adhesion and the transendothelial migration of leukocytes, such as macrophages and T cells. VCAM-1 is expressed by the vascular system and can be induced by reactive oxygen species, interleukin 1 beta (IL-1β) or tumor necrosis factor alpha (TNFα), which are produced by many cell types. The newest data suggest that VCAM-1 is associated with the progression of numerous immunological disorders, such as rheumatoid arthritis, asthma, transplant rejection and cancer. The aim of this study was to analyze the increase in VCAM-1 expression and the impact of exposure in a hyperbaric chamber to VCAM-1 levels in human blood serum. *Materials and Methods:* The study included 92 volunteers. Blood for the tests was taken in the morning, from the basilic vein of fasting individuals, in accordance with the applicable procedure for blood collection for morphological tests. In both groups of volunteers, blood was collected before and after exposure, in heparinized tubes to obtain plasma and hemolysate, and in clot tubes to obtain serum. The level of VCAM-1 was determined using the immunoenzymatic ELISA method. *Results:* The study showed that the difference between the distribution of VCAM-1 before and after exposure corresponding to diving at a depth of 30 m was at the limit of statistical significance in the divers group and that, in most people, VCAM-1 was higher after exposure. Diving to a greater depth had a much more pronounced impact on changes in VCAM-1 values, as the changes observed in the VCAM-1 level as a result of diving to a depth of 60 m were statistically highly significant (p = 0.0002). The study showed an increase in VCAM-1 in relation to the baseline value, which reached as much as 80%, i.e., VCAM-1 after diving was almost twice as high in some people. There were statistically significant differences between the results obtained after exposure to diving conditions at a depth of 60 m and the values measured for the non-divers group. The leukocyte level increased statistically after exposure to 60 m. In contrast, hemoglobin levels decreased in most divers after exposure to diving at a depth of 30 m (p = 0.0098). *Conclusions:* Exposure in the hyperbaric chamber had an effect on serum VCAM-1 in the divers group and non-divers group. There is a correlation between the tested morphological parameters and the VCAM-1 level before and after exposure in the divers group and the non-divers group. Exposure may result in activation of the endothelium.

Keywords: atmosphere exposure chambers; diving physiology; decompression

1. Introduction

Vascular cell adhesion molecule-1 (VCAM-1) is an endothelial cell adhesion factor. It is expressed on endothelium activated by cytokines, but may also occur in a soluble form in serum [1]. VCAM-1 was identified as a cell adhesion molecule that helps regulate inflammation-associated vascular adhesion and the transendothelial migration of leukocytes, such as macrophages and T cells. VCAM-1 is expressed by the vascular system and can be induced by reactive oxygen species, interleukin 1 beta (IL-1β) or tumor necrosis factor alpha (TNFα), which are produced by many cell types. The newest data suggests that VCAM-1 is associated with the progression of numerous immunological disorders, such as rheumatoid arthritis, asthma, transplant rejection and cancer [1]. Homeostasis is a necessary condition for health and the proper functioning of the body, and hence, diseases result from disturbances in mechanisms that maintain homeostasis [2]. Commercial saturation divers work in high-pressure environments, in which their bodies must acclimatize to a variety of physiological stress factors [3].

Research shows that intercellular adhesion molecule-1 (ICAM-1) and VCAM-1 adhesive molecules are potential markers of changes in the endothelium [4]. These molecules are of great interest both in order to understand the mechanisms of their action and their usefulness in the diagnosis and treatment of diseases [4,5]. Brubakk et al. [6], in their studies on vesicle formation and endothelial function in human and animal models, showed a decrease in the arterial endothelial function after a single dive using air.

The researchers [7–9] indicated that the endothelium was sensitive to oxidative stress and the shear rate, leading to vascular remodeling and a release of micro molecules. According to Freyssinet [9], endothelial microparticles are constantly shed into the circulation of healthy individuals and have been shown to be elevated in many diseases, most notably those characterized by endothelial dysfunction. This was supported by Horstman et al. [10].

It would be interesting to deepen the knowledge of the role of the VCAM-1 biomarker in the human body during decompression. The aim of this study was to analyze the increase in VCAM-1 expression and the impact of exposure in a hyperbaric chamber to the VCAM-1 level in human blood serum.

The research problem was to answer the following questions:

1. Does exposure in the hyperbaric chamber affect the VCAM-1 level in the divers group and non-divers group (a group who stayed in the same chamber for the same time period and breathed in the same pattern with the same breathing mix to best reflect the effect of the same pressure during exposure and decompression)?
2. Is there a correlation between the blood cell counts (BCC) and VCAM-1, before and after exposure in the chamber, in the divers group?

The following hypotheses were formulated:

1. Exposure in a hyperbaric chamber has an effect on the serum VCAM-1 level in the divers group and the non-divers group.
2. There is a correlation between tested BCC and VCAM-1 before and after exposure in the chamber in the divers group.

2. Materials and Methods

2.1. Design of the Study

The cross-sectional study involved four exposures. Short-term simulated hyperbaric air exposures corresponding to diving at a depth of 30 and 60 m were carried out. The exposure corresponding to a 60 m dive was chosen because it was the maximum allowable depth for a dive using air as a breathing mixture, and 30 m as half the maximum depth. Air was used for breathing in the hyperbaric chamber during dives. This was an experimental chamber complex DGKN 120 belonging to the Department of Underwater Works Technology of the Naval Academy in Gdynia. It consists of 3 chambers located at the same level: dry, wet and transient. In a dry chamber, where the study was carried out on short-term exposures, there may be 7 people, with longer ones—4, and with saturated ones—2. The maximum working pressure is 120 m of water column, i.e., 12 at or 13 ata. Additional inhalers (beeps) allow you to breathe, e.g., oxygen in a different atmosphere in the chamber. Pressure unit converters were the following: 760 mmHg = 760 tracks ~ 1 atm. = 1.033227 at. = 1.01325 N/m^2 = 1.01325 Pa = 14.69 psi.

Exposures were based on the Naval Table for the decompression and recompression of divers (Table 1). Exposures were carried out by compressing the subjects in a hyperbaric chamber to a pressure of 400 kPa, corresponding to a dive at a depth of 30 m, and to a pressure of 700 kPa, corresponding to a dive at a depth of 60 m. This pressure was maintained for 30 min. The entire time of exposure to 4 atm was 1 h, and to 7 atm—2 h. The plateau of both exposures was 30 min. The pressure exposure profiles are shown on Figures 1 and 2. Exposures were performed at the Department of Underwater Works Technology of the Naval Academy in cooperation with the Department of Maritime and Hyperbaric Medicine of the Military Medical Institute in Gdynia. Exposures were carried out by a qualified physician and a technical employee of the Department of Underwater Works Technology of the Naval Academy in Gdynia.

Table 1. 3 MW decompression tables.

Exposition	Depth	Bottom Time	Time to First Stop	Decompression Stops (mH$_2$O)														Total Ascent Time			
				42	39	36	33	30	27	24	21	18	15	12	9	6	3	Air		Oxygen	
				Time on the Stops (min)														(h)	(min)	(h)	(min)
	(mH$_2$O)	(min)	(min)	Air								Air or (Oxygen)									
30 m	33	35	3												6(3)	10(5)	16(8)		35		19
60 m	63	35	6						9	13	16	18(9)	22(11)	32(16)	47(24)	58(29)		3	41	2	13

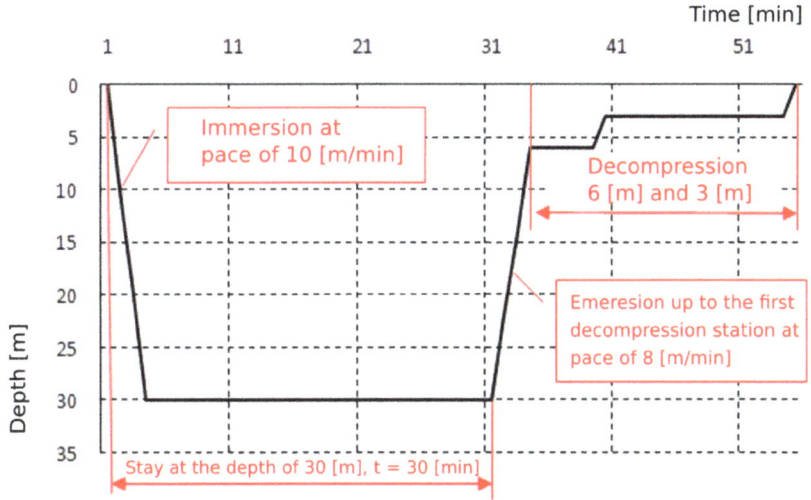

Figure 1. Pressure exposure profile 30 m/30 min.

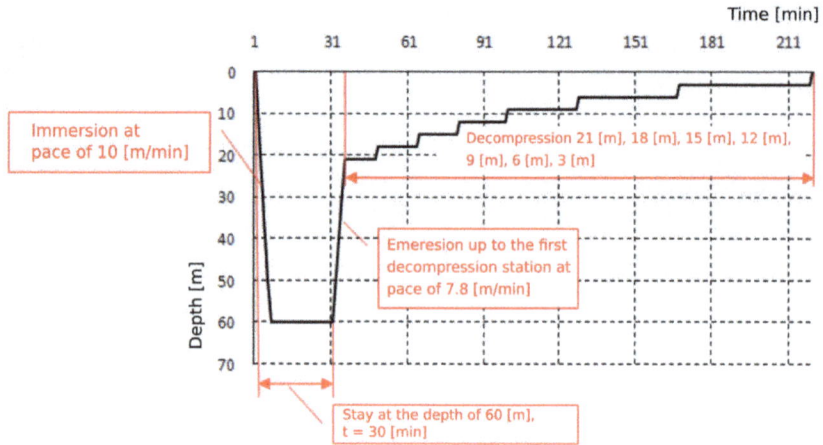

Figure 2. Pressure exposure profile 60 m/30 min.

2.2. Characteristics of Subject Population

Volunteers also completed a questionnaire, providing information concerning their age, sex, place of residence, education, seniority, type of work, type of physical exertion, smoking status, coffee consumption and a self-assessment of their physical condition. A total of 45 professional divers volunteered to participate in the study. They were subjected to hyperbaric exposure in a pressure chamber. A total of 47 volunteers—non-divers who had never been subjected to hyperbaric exposure—were also included. The non-divers group stayed in the same chamber for the same time period and breathed in the same pattern with the same (identical) breathing mixture to best reflect the effect of the same pressure during exposure and decompression. The non-divers group, who were not exposed, sat in the in the same chamber, with the same temperature and lighting conditions and breathed the same breathing mixture.

Criteria for inclusion in the divers group were professionally active diver, mentally and physically healthy and aged from 24 to 55 years. Exclusion criteria were respiratory tract infection, age under 24 and over 55 years, using intoxicating drugs, using any other medications and resignation from participation in the study. Ultimately, 18 people participated in the study. Inclusion criteria for the non-divers group were non-divers, who had never been subjected to hyperbaric exposure before, mentally and physically healthy and aged 24 to 55 years. Exclusion criteria were respiratory tract infection, aged under 24 and over 55, using intoxicating drugs, using any other medications and resignation from participation in the study Ultimately, 14 people participated in the study.

All the people who participated in the study breathed air and were not subjected to physical exertion.

Basic information about the divers group (N = 18) and the non-divers group (N = 14) is presented in Table 2. There were statistically significant differences between the sex (p = 0.0391), type of work (p = 0.0436) and physical effort (p = 0.0043) between the groups. In the divers group, manual workers predominated. The descriptive statistics presented below show that both groups were completely comparable in terms of age and occupational seniority.

Table 2. Demographic and occupational status of subjects.

Demographic and Occupational Status	Group				p
	Divers (N = 18)		Non-Divers (N = 14)		
	N	%	N	%	
Sex					
female	0	0.0%	3	21.4%	0.0391 *
male	18	100.0%	11	78.6%	
Age (years)	33.9 ± 6.6		33.0 ± 8.4		0.5521
Place of residence					
Rural	5	29.4%	0	0.0%	
municipality up to 50,000 inhabitants	8	47.1%	5	35.7%	0.0515
municipality 50,000–100,000 inhabitants	1	5.9%	1	7.1%	
municipality over 100,000 inhabitants	3	17.6%	8	57.1%	
Education					
Secondary	8	44.4%	3	21.4%	0.1739
Higher	10	55.6%	11	78.6%	
Occupational seniority (years)	10.4 ± 7.3		10.6 ± 7.8		0.9254
Type of work					
physical	15	83.3%	7	50.0%	0.0436 *
mental	3	16.7%	7	50.0%	
Type of physical effort					
Intensive	3	17.0%	2	14.3%	
Moderate	4	22.0%	2	14.3%	0.0043 **
Variable	3	17.0%	0	0.0%	
Aerobic	0	0.0%	8	57.1%	
None	8	44.0%	2	14.3%	

Abbreviations: *—$p < 0.05$; **—$p < 0.01$.

2.3. Methods

Blood for the tests was taken in the morning, from the basilic vein of fasting individuals, in accordance with the applicable procedure for blood collection for morphological tests. Tests were performed by a certified medical analytical laboratory. VCAM-1 measurements were performed with serum and BCC with plasma.

In both groups, blood was collected at the same time, before and after exposure, to heparin anticoagulant tubes to obtain plasma and hemolysate and to clot tubes to obtain serum. The level of VCAM-1 was determined using the immunoenzymatic ELISA method, with the DIACLONE kit.

2.4. Procedural and Ethical Considerations

The study was performed from September 2018 to June 2019 and the study obtained ethical approval from the Bioethics Committee of the Medical University in Bialystok, Poland (R-I-002/237/2015). Members of the research team provided oral and written information about the study. Subjects gave their informed consent for participation in the study. Each participant received written and oral information about the possibility of withdrawing from the study at any time and without any consequences. The research conformed with the Good Clinical Practice guidelines, and the procedures were in accordance with the principles of the 1975 Declaration of Helsinki, as revised in 2000, and with the ethical standards of the institutional committee on human experimentation.

2.5. Statistical Analysis

To present listings as elements of the description of both groups, summary tables contain numbers and percentages, and for age and occupational seniority—means (M) ± standard deviations (SD); the p-value was calculated using the chi-square test of independence (for comparison of percentage structure) or the Mann–Whitney U test (for comparison of numerical values—age and occupational seniority of the subjects).

Selected numerical characteristics of the examined parameters were determined: arithmetic mean (M), median (Me), the highest (maximum) and the lowest (minimum) value and standard deviation (SD).

A test of the statistical significance of the relationship under study was performed. For all statistical analyses, the significance level was set at $p < 0.05$.

Additionally, information on the 95% confidence interval for the average VCAM-1 level measured in the four tested situations is presented. The normality of VCAM-1 level distribution in various tested situations was assessed using the Shapiro–Wilk test. The statistical significance of differences in the distribution of VCAM-1 before and after exposure was analyzed. As the measurements were made on the same group of divers, the Wilcoxon test was used for the analysis. Results were graphically illustrated using scatter plots. The Mann–Whitney U test was used to compare the distribution of VCAM-1 among non-divers (in various tested situations). The difference between the results obtained in both groups was assessed using the Mann–Whitney U test. The Wilcoxon test was also used to examine the significance of changes between tests performed before and after exposure.

Spearman's rank correlation coefficient (r_S) was used to assess the strength of relationships between the BCC and VCAM-1.

3. Results

There were no significant differences between the divers and non-divers groups in terms of coffee consumption, smoking status or self-assessment of physical condition.

The *p*-value calculated for "coffee consumption" was $p = 0.3365$, for "smoking status" —$p = 0.7876$ and for "self-assessment of physical condition"—$p = 0.0842$ (Table 3).

Table 3. Subject lifestyle.

Lifestyle	Group				*p*
	Divers (N = 18)		Non-Divers (N = 14)		
	N	%	N	%	
Drinking coffee					
None	6	33.3%	4	28.6%	
Once a day	4	22.2%	3	21.4%	0.3365
Twice a day	6	33.3%	2	14.3%	
More	2	11.1%	5	35.7%	
Tobacco smoking					
Yes	2	11.1%	2	14.3%	0.7876
No	16	88.9%	12	85.7%	
Self-assessment of physical condition					
Ideal	1	5.6%	4	28.6%	
Good	17	94.4%	8	57.1%	0.0842
Intermediate	0	0.0%	1	7.1%	
Hard to tell	0	0.0%	1	7.1%	

The table below (Table 4) provides information on the 95% confidence intervals for the average level of VCAM-1 in the four tested situations.

Table 4. 95% confidence intervals for the average level of VCAM-1 parameter measured in four tested situations in the divers group.

VCAM-1 (ng/mL)	95% CI
Before exposure—30 m	(10.7; 20.5)
After exposure—30 m	(12.3; 21.9)
Before exposure—60 m	(9.2; 16.4)
After exposure—60 m	(12.8; 24.6)

Abbreviations: CI—confidence interval; VCAM-1—vascular cell adhesion molecule-1.

The difference between the VCAM-1 distribution before and after the exposure with a diving depth of 30 m was on the limit of statistical significance ($p = 0.0582$). In most people, VCAM-1 after exposure was higher, on average, by about 1.5 ng/mL (but a decrease in the VCAM-1 level was also noted in some people). Diving to a greater depth had a much more pronounced impact on the changes in the VCAM-1 value. In all the subjects, VCAM-1 increased after exposure by at least 0.8, and at most by 24.2 ng/mL. On average, the change was about 5.9 ng/mL, although the average was somewhat overestimated by the quite outlying peak value of VCAM-1 growth of 24.2. Therefore, a median of 4.2 ng/mL may be a better measure of the average level of VCAM-1 changes after a dive (Table 5).

Table 5. Distribution of VCAM-1 before and after the exposure corresponding to a 30 m and 60 m dive in the divers group.

		M	Me	SD	Min.	Max.
VCAM-1 [ng/mL] 30	Before dive	15.6	14.6	9.9	5.6	46.1
	After dive	17.1	16.6	9.6	6.7	41.5
	Change ($p = 0.0582$)	1.5	1.1	2.8	−4.6	6.6
VCAM-1 [ng/mL] 60	Before dive	12.8	12.4	7.2	5.0	31.1
	After dive	18.7	17.5	11.8	6.7	55.3
	Change ($p = 0.0002$ ***)	5.9	4.2	5.3	0.8	24.2

Abbreviations: M—mean; Me—median; SD—standard deviation; Min.—minimum; Max.—maximum; ***—$p < 0.001$.

The changes in VCAM-1 as a result of diving to a depth of 60 m were highly statistically significant (the p-value determined using the Wilcoxon test was 0.0002).

As seen in the chart below, the relative increase in VCAM-1 in some people was as high as 60% of the initial value (Figure 3).

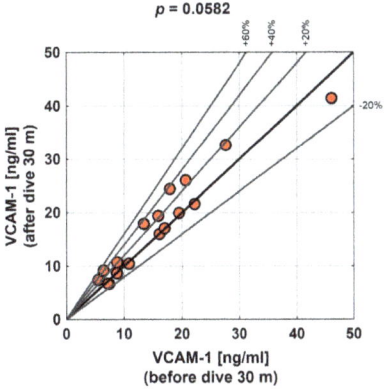

Figure 3. Distribution of VCAM-1 before and after exposure to a 30 m dive in the study group.

As presented in the graph below (Figure 4), the relative increase in VCAM-1 over the baseline was as high as 80% (i.e., in some subjects, VCAM-1 was almost twice as high after diving).

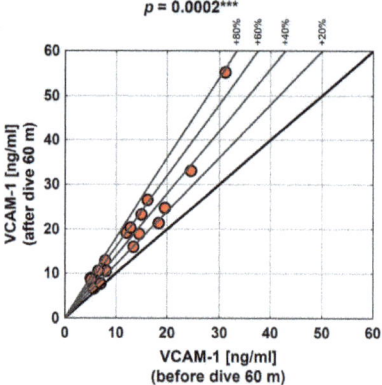

Figure 4. VCAM-1 values with diving to 60 m in the study group. Abbreviations: ***—$p < 0.001$.

The distribution of results obtained before and after exposure to the conditions corresponding to diving at a depth of 30 m did not differ in a statistically significant way from the distribution of results in the non-divers group.

Statistically significant differences existed between the results obtained after exposure to diving conditions at a depth of 60 m and the values measured for the non-divers group ($p = 0.0494$; Table 6).

Table 6. Values of descriptive statistics characterizing the distribution of VCAM-1 in the compared groups.

VCAM-1 (ng/mL)	Group										p
	Divers (N = 18)					Non-Divers (N = 14)					
	$\bar{x}$	Me	s	Min	Max	$\bar{x}$	Me	s	Min	Max	
before exposure—30 m	15.6	14.6	9.9	5.6	46.1	11.1	9.9	4.5	7.2	25.0	0.2666
after exposure—30 m	17.1	16.6	9.6	6.7	41.5						0.1251
before exposure—60 m	12.8	12.4	7.2	5.0	31.1						0.8662
after exposure—60 m	18.7	17.5	11.8	6.7	55.3						0.0494 *

Abbreviations: *—$p < 0.05$.

The graph (Figure 5) shows the values of position statistics of the VCAM-1 distribution in the compared groups and test series.

The leukocyte count increased in a statistically significant manner after exposure to a 60 m dive. However, exposure to the conditions corresponding to diving at a depth of 30 m did not affect the unequivocally directed change in the leukocyte count. Longer exposure results in greater tissue saturation with gases (among others with nitrogen) during decompression, which lasts significantly longer; in this case, many more microbubbles are formed, which activate the immune system. The hemoglobin level decreased in most divers after exposure to a 30 m dive ($p = 0.0098$). Detailed data presenting the distribution of leukocytes and hemoglobin counts in individual tests, showing the significance of changes between the tests completed before and after exposure, are presented in Table 7.

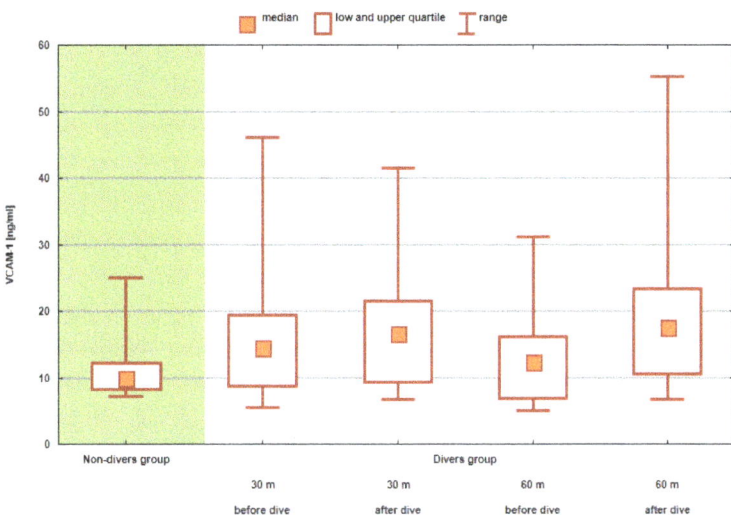

Figure 5. Values of position statistics of VCAM-1 distribution in the compared groups and test series.

Table 7. Descriptive statistics characterizing the distribution of leukocytes and hemoglobin counts in individual tests, showing the significance of changes between tests completed before and after exposure.

		M	Me	SD	Min.	Max.
Leukocytes [G/L]	Before dive 30 m	6.20	6.19	1.05	4.23	9.03
	After dive 30 m	6.43	6.22	1.23	4.42	8.87
	Change ($p = 0.2485$)	0.23	0.18	0.74	−0.76	1.56
	Before dive 60 m	5.95	6.01	0.96	3.70	7.56
	After dive 60 m	7.10	7.26	1.28	4.55	9.33
	Change ($p = 0.0004$ ***)	1.17	0.94	0.85	0.12	3.20
Hemoglobin [g/dL]	Before dive 30 m	15.2	15.3	0.8	14.0	16.8
	After dive 30 m	15.0	15.0	0.9	13.4	16.8
	Change ($p = 0.0098$ **)	−0.2	−0.2	0.3	−1.0	0.4
	Before dive 60 m	15.2	15.2	0.8	13.8	16.4
	After dive 60 m	15.0	15.1	0.8	13.8	16.3
	Change ($p = 0.1673$)	−0.1	0.0	0.3	−0.9	0.3

Abbreviations: G/L—billion per liter; M—mean; Me—median; SD—standard deviation; Min.—minimum; Max.—maximum; **—$p < 0.01$; ***—$p < 0.001$.

The results of BCC after the exposure of the subjects in the divers group to conditions corresponding to a 30 m dive were not correlated with the VCAM-1 values. All the correlation coefficients were statistically insignificant ($p > 0.05$). Those few correlations that were close to the level of statistical significance, and also in a single case that was statistically significant, occurred between BCC and VCAM-1 after exposure to conditions corresponding to a 60 m dive.

These relationships were as follows:

- Relationships between the neutrophil count and VCAM-1—the higher the level of neutrophils was, the lower the value of VCAM-1 was ($p = 0.0456$, R = −0.51);
- A similar relationship existed between the leukocyte count and VCAM-1 (it was slightly weaker and only close to the level of statistical significance);
- VCAM-1 was higher in subjects with a higher lymphocyte ratio (R = 0.44)—this correlation was close to the level of statistical significance ($p = 0.0848$).

Changes in the BCC and VCAM-1 level after exposure to conditions corresponding to a 30 m dive were not statistically significantly correlated with each other.

More statistically significant relationships existed between the changes in BCC and the changes in VCAM-1 after exposure to the conditions corresponding to a 60 m dive.

There were the following relationships:

- Higher increases in VCAM-1 were associated with a greater increase (in some cases, a smaller decrease) in the mean corpuscular hemoglobin (MCH) and the mean corpuscular hemoglobin concentration (MCHC)—these were relationships of average strength and statistical significance;
- Quite a strong correlation occurred between the changes in the neutrophil counts and the changes in VCAM-1—the greater the increase in the number of neutrophils was, the smaller the increase in VCAM-1 was;
- In turn, the increase in the lymphocyte count after exposure to the conditions corresponding to a 60 m dive was correlated with the increase in VCAM-1 (R = 0.54; p = 0.0304);
- Similar correlations (i.e., positive) were found for VCAM-1 and the lymphocyte and monocyte ratio (although the latter relationship was no longer statistically significant—p = 0.1156).

4. Discussion

The aim of this study was to analyze the increase in VCAM-1 expression and the impact of exposure in a hyperbaric chamber on VCAM-1 in human blood serum. We believe that the results that have been obtained will allow for a better understanding of the biological changes that take place in our body during pressure changes at various depths, a deeper knowledge about the role of the VCAM-1 biomarker in our body and the possible impact of exposure in a hyperbaric chamber on human blood serum.

Madden and Laden [11], in their study, suggested that endothelial microparticles (MP) can be used as a decompression sickness (DCI) stress marker by assessing the antigenic markers of circulating MP that not only allow a specific origin, but also reflect endothelial integrity. According to these researchers, after endothelial disruption, the expression of adhesion molecules was expressed in accordance with the adopted configuration, and one such molecule, the VCAM-1 molecule, is an attractive marker due to the fact that it was only expressed on the activated endothelium, which was achieved after vascular trauma and is therefore a prognostic marker of a pro-inflammatory endothelium.

In this study, the statistical significance of differences in the distribution of VCAM-1 before and after exposure was analyzed. The difference between the VCAM-1 distribution before and after the exposure corresponding to a 30 m dive was on the limit of statistical significance (p = 0.0582). For most people, VCAM-1 was higher after exposure; on average, it was around 1.5 ng/mL, but there were also subjects who experienced a decrease in VCAM-1. The relative increase in VCAM-1 in some subjects was as high as 60% of the baseline value. Vince et al. [12] reported a significant increase in VCAM-1 positive microparticles (VCAM + MP), observed 1 h after diving using air compared to the non-divers group (p = 0.013), which was not observed after oxygen diving (p = 0.095).

The discussed study showed that diving at a greater depth had a much more pronounced effect on changes in VCAM-1 values. In all the subjects, VCAM-1 increased after exposure—at least by 0.8, and at most by 24.2 ng/mL. The average change was about 5.9 ng/mL. The changes in VCAM-1, as a result of diving to a depth of 60 m, were highly statistically significant. A study by Bao et al. [13] found that diving caused significantly reduced VCAM-1 levels.

Our research showed that the relative increase in VCAM-1 compared to the baseline value was as high as 80%, i.e., VCAM-1 after diving almost doubled in some subjects. A study performed by Zhang et al. [14] showed that VCAM-1 levels increased post-decompression in DCI rats.

In the presented study, a comparison of VCAM-1 distribution among divers before and after exposure to a 30 m and 60 m dive and the non-divers group was performed.

The distribution of the results obtained before and after exposure to the conditions corresponding to a 30 m dive did not statistically significantly differ from the distribution of results in the non-divers group. The research showed that there were statistically significant differences between the results obtained after exposure to conditions of a 60 m dive and the values measured for the non-divers group ($p = 0.0494$). VCAM-1 is expressed exclusively on the activated endothelium following vascular insult, and therefore, is a marker of a proinflammatory endothelium, as a study by Bao et al. [13] showed.

Research by Vince et al. [12] in which the VCAM + MP was quantified before diving (09:00 a.m. and 1:00 p/m.) and after diving (+1, +3 and +15 h), showed that both for diving with air and oxygen, and compared to control samples collected from the same subjects, VCAM + MP showed a similar trend in all the experiments. However, both dives resulted in a change in endothelial status as measured by VCAM + MP. A significant increase in VCAM + MP was observed 1 h after diving using air compared to the controls ($p = 0.013$), which was not observed after oxygen diving ($p = 0.095$). The researchers [12] observed an increase in the circulating VCAM + MP population after simulated diving with both compressed air and oxygen, compared to their non-dive controls taken at the same time of day. Due to its expression only on the activated endothelium, VCAM + MP can be used as a sensitive marker of endothelial function/dysfunction. Researchers hypothesized that the increase in circulating VCAM + MP could reflect changes in the state of the endothelium and could be potentially used as a biomarker of sensitivity to, for example, decompression sickness, when vascular mechanisms are involved [12].

This research showed that the results of BCC after the exposure of the subjects in the divers and non-divers group to conditions corresponding to a 30 m dive were not correlated with values of VCAM-1. However, the leukocyte count increased in a statistically significant manner after exposure to a 60 m dive, and exposure to conditions corresponding to a 30 m dive did not affect the unequivocally targeted change in the leukocyte count, which could be explained by an insufficient number of subjects in the divers group. A study performed by Glavas et al. [15] showed that the microbubbles produced during the decompression process induce endothelial damage and affect leukocyte mobilization.

In our study, the hemoglobin level decreased in most divers after exposure to diving conditions at a depth of 30 m and this effect should be considered as not accidental ($p = 0.0098$), and after a stronger exposure—to conditions corresponding to a depth of 60 m—such effects were not observed. The scale of the decrease in hemoglobin levels was small—only 0.2 g/dL on average; therefore, it was not a change affecting the health of the divers. Several studies have reported an altered hematological status and hemoglobin reduction after saturation diving [16–19].

A decrease in the number of neutrophils in the blood in our study is unlikely to indicate inflammation. Most likely, these results decrease from the fact that microbubbles are treated as hostile pathogens by neutrophils; as a result of the so-called oxygen burst (respiratory burst), microbubbles are eliminated, and thus the neutrophil cells are destroyed. This would confirm the increased generation of reactive oxygen species and the intensification of oxidative stress (we also observed an increase in oxidative stress in our volunteers).

More statistically significant relationships existed between the changes in the BCC parameters and the changes in VCAM-1 after exposure to conditions corresponding to a 60 m dive in the non-divers group. The relationships that occurred were as follows: higher increments of VCAM-1 were associated with a greater increase (in some cases a smaller decrease) in MCH and MCHC—these were relationships of average strength and statistically significant; quite a strong correlation was found between changes in neutrophils count and changes in VCAM-1—the greater the increase in the number of neutrophils is, the smaller the increase in VCAM-1 is.

Our study showed that the number of blood platelets decreased in a statistically significant ($p = 0.0382$) manner after exposure to the conditions corresponding to a dive to a depth of 60 m, and the level of neutrophils increased in a statistically significant manner after exposure to conditions corresponding to a dive to a depth of 60 m. Olszański et al. [20] demonstrated in his study that the diving technology employed did not generate substantial changes in the examined parameters of blood in divers, and the increase in neutrophils, blood platelets and the fibrinogen concentration in the blood plasma immediately after diving is of a temporary character, being a typical reaction observed during diving.

In turn, the increase in the number of lymphocytes after exposure to conditions corresponding to a 60 m dive correlated with the increase in VCAM-1 ($R = 0.54$; $p = 0.0304$); similar (i.e., positive) correlations apply to VCAM-1 and the lymphocyte ratio. This research also showed that those few correlations that were close to the level of statistical significance, and in one case statistically significant, occurred between BCC and VCAM-1 after exposure to conditions corresponding to a 60 m dive in the divers group. The relationships were as follows: there was a relationship between the neutrophils count and VCAM-1—the higher the number of neutrophils was, the lower the value of VCAM-1 was (this correlation was statistically significant—$p = 0.0456$; its strength was average—$R = -0.51$); a similar relationship was found between the number of leukocytes and VCAM-1 (it was slightly weaker and only close to the level of statistical significance); VCAM-1 was higher in the subjects with a higher lymphocyte ratio ($R = 0.44$)—this correlation was close to the level of statistical significance ($p = 0.0848$). In a study performed by Bao et al. [13], deep heliox diving caused a significant decrease in red blood cells (RBC) but had no significant effect on hemoglobin (HGB) levels. These changes can be explained by the oxidative damage-induced fragility of the RBC membrane. A study by Perovic et al. [21] showed that neutrophils increased, and monocytes decreased immediately after 30 m-depth compressed-diving using air. Since the number of intermediate cells in humans is small, the reduction in the percentage of intermediate cells may be a transient response to external stimuli. Obad at al. [22] have shown in their study that this may be caused by trans-endothelial migration due to altered vascular/endothelial function after diving. Sureda et al. [23] has shown in his study that scuba diving at 50 m deep for a total time of 35 min was enough to induce a post-diving neutrophil mobilization in normobaria, suggesting the initiation of an immune-like response, similar to that which occurs after an infection or an acute bout of exercise. Exactly these results could be expected, because VCAM-1 is a key cell adhesion molecule involved in inflammation that is closely implicated in various immunological disorders [24,25]. The VCAM-1 protein mediates the adhesion of neutrophils, monocytes, eosinophils and basophils to the vascular endothelium [14,26]. It is also active in the signal transduction of leukocytes and endothelial cells [24,27–29]. A study by Glavas et al. [15] showed that the absolute number of monocytes was slightly, but not significantly, increased after a dive, and this study suggests that biochemical changes induced by scuba diving primarily activate existing monocytes rather than increase the number of monocytes at a time of acute arterial endothelial dysfunction.

Strengths and Limitations of the Study

A strength of this study was the well-matched divers and non-divers groups.

The limitations of the present study should be noted. Due to the small sample size, the present study has limited power. We believe that further research with a larger population is required and warranted. In searching for the relationship between the BCC results of blood counts and the values of VCAM-1 in the test group (conditions corresponding to a 30 m dive), the lack of a relationship with white blood cells can also be explained by the group of respondents being too small.

5. Conclusions

1. The results confirm our hypothesis that exposure to a hyperbaric chamber has an effect on VCAM-1 in blood serum in the divers group.
2. There is a correlation between the tested BCC and VCAM-1 before and after exposure in the chamber in the divers group.

3. We believe that exposure in a hyperbaric chamber may result in the activation of the endothelium.

Author Contributions: Conceptualization, K.V.D.-O., M.C., M.K., E.K.-K., P.S. and D.K.; data curation, K.V.D.-O., M.C., M.K., P.S. and D.K.; formal analysis, K.V.D.-O., M.C., M.K., P.S. and M.S.; funding acquisition, K.V.D.-O.; investigation, K.V.D.-O., M.C., M.K., P.S. and M.S.; methodology, K.V.D.-O., M.K., P.S. and D.K.; project administration, K.V.D.-O.; supervision, M.C., M.K., E.K.-K., P.S. and D.K.; writing—original draft, K.V.D.-O., M.K., P.S., M.S. and D.K.; writing—review and editing, K.V.D.-O., M.C., M.K.,E.K.-K., P.S. and M.S. All authors have read and agreed to the published version of the manuscript.

Funding: The research was funded with grant no. N/ST/ZB/15/001/3310 from the Ministry of Science and Higher Education in Poland. The funders had no role in the study design, data collection and analysis, preparation of the manuscript or decision about its publication.

Institutional Review Board Statement: The study was conducted according to the guidelines of the Declaration of Helsinki and approved by the Ethics Committee of the Medical University of Białystok, Poland (no. R-I-002/237/2015; approval date: 25 June 2015).

Informed Consent Statement: Informed consent was obtained from all subjects involved in the study.

Data Availability Statement: Data are available upon reasonable request.

Conflicts of Interest: The authors declare no conflict of interest.

References

1. Kong, D.H.; Kim, Y.K.; Kim, M.R.; Jang, J.H.; Lee, S. Emerging roles of Vascular Cell Adhesion Molecule-1 (VCAM-1) in immunological disorders and cancer. *Int. J. Mol. Sci.* **2018**, *19*, 1057. [CrossRef]
2. Gunes, A.E.; Celik, H.; Yilmaz, O.; Erbas, C.; Gumus, E. Acute and chronic effects of pressure on dynamic Thiol-Disulphide homoeostasis in divers. *Fresenius Environ. Bull.* **2019**, *28*, 2949–2956.
3. Łuczyński, D.; Lautridou, J.; Hjelde, A.; Monnoyer, R.; Eftedal, I. Hemoglobin during and following a 4-week commercial saturation dive to 200 m. *Front. Physiol.* **2019**, *10*, 1494. [CrossRef]
4. Ridker, P.M. Intercellular adhesion molecule (ICAM-1) and the risk of developing atherosclerotic disease. *Eur. Heart J.* **1998**, *19*, 1119–1121.
5. Morisaki, N.; Saito, I.; Tamura, K.; Tashiro, J.; Masuda, M.; Kanzaki, T.; Watanabe, S.; Masuda, Y.; Saito, Y. New indicates of ischemic heart disease and aging: Studies on the serum levels of soluble intercellular adhesion molecule-1 (ICAM-1) and soluble vascular cell adhesion molecul-1 (VCAM-1) in patients with hypercholesterolemia and ischemic heart disease. *Atherosclerosis* **1997**, *131*, 43–48. [CrossRef]
6. Brubakk, A.O.; Duplancic, D.; Valic, Z.; Palada, I.; Obad, A.; Bakovic, D.; Wisloff, U.; Dujic, Z. A single air dive reduces arterial endothelial function in man. *J. Physiol.* **2005**, *566 Pt 3*, 901–906. [CrossRef]
7. Lehoux, S.; Castier, Y.; Tedgui, A. Molecular mechanisms of the vascular responses to haemodynamic forces. *J. Intern. Med.* **2006**, *259*, 381–392. [CrossRef]
8. Ungvari, Z.; Wolin, M.S.; Csiszar, A. Mechanosensitive production of reactive oxygen species in endothelial and smooth muscle cells: Role in microvascular remodeling? *Antioxid. Redox Signal* **2006**, *8*, 1121–1129. [CrossRef] [PubMed]
9. Freyssinet, J.M. Cellular microparticles: What are they bad or good for? *J. Thromb. Haemost.* **2003**, *1*, 1655–1662. [CrossRef]
10. Horstman, L.L.; Jy, W.; Jimenez, J.J.; Ahn, Y.S. Endothelial microparticles as markers of endothelial dysfunction. *Front. Biosci.* **2004**, *9*, 1118–1135. [CrossRef] [PubMed]
11. Madden, L.A.; Laden, G. Endothelial microparticles in vascular disease and as a potential marker of decompression illness. *EJUHM* **2007**, *8*, 6–10.
12. Vince, R.V.; McNaughton, L.R.; Taylor, L.; Midgley, A.W.; Laden, G.; Madden, L.A. Release of VCAM-1 associated endothelial microparticles following simulated SCUBA dives. *Eur. J. Appl. Physiol.* **2009**, *105*, 507–513. [CrossRef]
13. Bao, X.C.; Shen, Q.; Fang, Y.Q.; Wu, J.G. Human Physiological Responses to a Single Deep Helium-Oxygen Diving. *Front. Physiol.* **2021**, *12*, 735986. [CrossRef] [PubMed]
14. Zhang, K.; Wang, D.; Jiang, Z.; Ning, X.; Buzzacott, P.; Xu, W. Endothelial dysfunction correlates with decompression bubbles in rats. *Sci. Rep.* **2016**, *6*, 33390. [CrossRef]
15. Glavas, D.; Markotic, A.; Valic, Z.; Kovacic, N.; Palada, I.; Martinic, R.; Breskovic, T.; Bakovic, D.; Brubakk, A.O.; Dujic, Z. Expression of endothelial selectin ligands on human leukocytes following dive. *Exp. Biol. Med.* **2008**, *233*, 1181–1188. [CrossRef] [PubMed]
16. Thorsen, E.; Haave, H.; Hofso, D.; Ulvik, R.J. Exposure to hyperoxia in diving and hyperbaric medicine—Effects on blood cell counts and serum ferritin. *Undersea Hyperb. Med.* **2001**, *28*, 57–62.

17. Smith, S.M.; Davis-Street, J.E.; Fesperman, J.V.; Smith, M.D.; Rice, B.L.; Zwart, S.R. Nutritional status changes in humans during a 14-day saturation dive: The NASA extreme environment mission operations V project. *J. Nutr.* **2004**, *134*, 1765–1771. [CrossRef] [PubMed]
18. Deb, S.; Burgess, K.; Swinton, P.; Dolan, E. Physiological responses to prolonged saturation diving: A field-based pilot study. *Undersea Hyperb. Med.* **2017**, *44*, 581–587. [CrossRef]
19. Kiboub, F.Z.; Balestra, C.; Loennechen, O.; Eftedal, I. Hemoglobin and erythropoietin after commercial saturation diving. *Front. Physiol.* **2018**, *9*, 1176. [CrossRef]
20. Olszański, R.; Konarski, M.; Kierznikowicz, B. Changes of selected morphotic parameters and blood plasma proteins in blood of divers after a single short-time operational heliox exposure. *Int. Marit. Health* **2002**, *53*, 111–121.
21. Perovic, A.; Nikolac, N.; Braticevic, M.N.; Milcic, A.; Sobocanec, S.; Balog, T.; Dabelic, S.; Dumic, J. Does recreational scuba diving have clinically significant effect on routine haematological parameters? *Biochem. Med.* **2017**, *27*, 325–331. [CrossRef] [PubMed]
22. Obad, A.; Palada, I.; Valic, Z.; Ivancev, V.; Baković, D.; Wisløff, U.; Brubakk, A.O.; Dujić, Z. The effects of acute oral antioxidants on diving-induced alterations in human cardiovascular function. *J. Physiol.* **2007**, *578 Pt 3*, 859–870. [CrossRef]
23. Sureda, A.; Batle, J.M.; Capo, X.; Martorell, M.; Córdova, A.; Tur, J.A.; Pons, A. Scuba diving induces nitric oxide synthesis and the expression of inflammatory and regulatory genes of the immune response in neutrophils. *Physiol. Genom.* **2014**, *46*, 647–654. [CrossRef] [PubMed]
24. Yuan, M.L.; Tong, Z.H.; Jin, X.G.; Zhang, J.C.; Wang, X.J.; Ma, W.L.; Yin, W.; Zhou, Q.; Ye, H.; Shi, H.Z. Regulation of $CD4^+$ T Cells by Pleural Mesothelial Cells via Adhesion Molecule-Dependent Mechanisms in Tuberculous Pleurisy. *PLoS ONE* **2013**, *8*, e74624.
25. Miyamoto, Y.; Torii, T.; Tanoue, A.; Yamauchi, J. VCAM1 acts in parallel with CD69 and is required for the initiation of oligodendrocyte myelination. *Nat. Commun.* **2016**, *7*, 13478. [CrossRef]
26. Brett, K.D.; Nugent, N.Z.; Fraser, N.K.; Bhopale, V.M.; Yang, M.; Thom, S.R. Microparticle and interleukin-1β production with human simulated compressed air diving. *Sci. Rep.* **2019**, *9*, 13320. [CrossRef]
27. Leitner, J.; Grabmeier-Pfistershammer, K.; Steinberger, P. Receptors and ligands implicated in human T cell costimulatory processes. *Immunol. Lett.* **2010**, *128*, 89–97. [CrossRef]
28. Nasreen, N.; Mohammed, K.A.; Ward, M.J.; Antony, V.B. Mycobacterium-induced transmesothelial migration of monocytes into pleural space: Role of intercellular adhesion molecule-1 in tuberculous pleurisy. *J. Infect. Dis.* **1999**, *180*, 1616–1623. [CrossRef] [PubMed]
29. Choe, N.; Zhang, J.; Iwagaki, A.; Tanaka, S.; Hemenway, D.R.; Kagan, E. Asbestos exposure up regulates the adhesion of pleural leukocytes to pleural mesothelial cells via VCAM-1. *Am. J. Physiol.* **1999**, *277*, L292–L300.

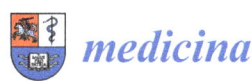

Article

Clinical Assessment of the Hyperbaric Oxygen Therapy Efficacy in Mild to Moderate Periodontal Affections: A Simple Randomised Trial

Alexandru Burcea [1], Laurenta Lelia Mihai [1,*], Anamaria Bechir [1,*], Mircea Suciu [2] and Edwin Sever Bechir [2]

[1] Faculty of Dental Medicine, Titu Maiorescu University of Bucharest, 031593 Bucharest, Romania; alexandru.burcea@helpdent.ro
[2] Faculty of Dental Medicine, George Emil Palade University of Medicine, Pharmacy, Science and Technology of Targu Mures, 540142 Targu Mures, Romania; oralmed2000@yahoo.com (M.S.); bechir.edwin@gmail.com (E.S.B.)
* Correspondence: lelia_mihai2000@yahoo.com (L.L.M.); anamaria.bechir@gmail.com (A.B.)

Abstract: *Background and Objectives:* Gum disease represents the condition due to the dental plaque and dental calculus deposition on the surfaces of the teeth, followed by ulterior destruction of the periodontal tissues through the host reaction to the pathogenic microorganisms. The aim of study was to present aspects regarding the efficacy of hyperbaric oxygen therapy (HBOT) as an adjuvant therapy for the treatment of periodontal disease, started from the already certified benefits of HBOT in the general medicine specialties. *Materials and Methods:* The participant patients in this study (71) required and benefited from specific periodontal disease treatments. All patients included in the trial benefited from the conventional therapy of full-mouth scaling and root planing (SRP) within 24 h. HBOT was performed on the patients of the first group (31), in 20 sessions, of one hour. The patients of the control group (40) did not benefit from HBO therapy. *Results:* At the end of study, the included patients in HBOT group presented significantly better values of oral health index (OHI-S), sulcus bleeding index (SBI), dental mobility (DM), and periodontal pocket depth (PD) than the patients of the control group. *Conclusions:* HBOT had beneficial effects on the oral and general health of all patients, because in addition to the positive results in periodontal therapy, some individual symptoms of the patients diminished or disappeared upon completion of this adjuvant therapy.

Keywords: periodontal disease; oral health index; dental mobility; periodontal pockets depth; hyperbaric oxygen therapy

1. Introduction

Dental biofilm is the main etiologic factor for caries, periodontal and peri-implant infections. Gum disease represents a disease with dental plaque and calculus formation on the surfaces of the teeth, followed by ulterior destruction of the periodontal tissues due to the host reaction to pathogenic microorganisms [1,2].

The spreading of periodontal disease is between 20 and 50% in the world, and represents one of important causes of indentations, which jeopardize the functions of oro-facial system, including mastication, aesthetics, self-reliability, and life quality [3]. This prevalence of periodontal disease is presumed to be rising in future years because of increased aging in population and of maintenance of natural teeth of dental arches in the elderly [4,5]. The development of periodontal disease in the context of the 2017 World Workshop on the Classification of Periodontal and Peri-Implant Diseases and Conditions presents four stages, defined based on severity (primarily periodontal breakdown with reference to root length and periodontitis-associated tooth loss), complexity of management (pocket depth, infrabony defects, furcation involvement, tooth hypermobility, masticatory dysfunction) and additionally described as extent (localized or generalized). The grade of periodontitis is estimated with direct or indirect evidence of progression rate in three categories:

Citation: Burcea, A.; Mihai, L.L.; Bechir, A.; Suciu, M.; Bechir, E.S. Clinical Assessment of the Hyperbaric Oxygen Therapy Efficacy in Mild to Moderate Periodontal Affections: A Simple Randomised Trial. *Medicina* **2022**, *58*, 234. https://doi.org/10.3390/medicina58020234

Academic Editor: Gaetano Isola

Received: 1 January 2022
Accepted: 1 February 2022
Published: 4 February 2022

Publisher's Note: MDPI stays neutral with regard to jurisdictional claims in published maps and institutional affiliations.

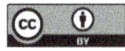

Copyright: © 2022 by the authors. Licensee MDPI, Basel, Switzerland. This article is an open access article distributed under the terms and conditions of the Creative Commons Attribution (CC BY) license (https://creativecommons.org/licenses/by/4.0/).

slow, moderate and rapid progression (Grade A–C). Risk factor analysis is used as grade modifier [6,7].

Cellular oxygenation is carried out by transporting the oxygen (that is fixed to haemoglobin), from inspired air to the tissues and cells, through the circulatory system. Disruption or interruption of oxygen transport induces hypoxia through changes in haemoglobin, capillary network, or blood flow [8–10]. Oxygen has a very small molecule, which allows its increased diffusibility in tissues, in comparison to any other substance [11]. Increasing the oxygen pressure in the environment over a certain point, increases the amount of dissolved oxygen in the plasma (quantitative increase) and the penetration rate of oxygen into the tissues (qualitative increase) [12].

The Undersea and Hyperbaric Medical Society (UHMS) defines hyperbaric oxygen therapy (HBOT) as a treatment in which the patient intermittently inspires 100% oxygen, in a pressurized treatment chamber at a higher pressure than at the sea level (1 atm absolute, ATA) [11,13,14]. In HBO therapy, the patient inspires pure or enriched oxygen, which causes a reduction in the amount of nitrogen in the blood [15]. The mechanisms of therapeutic action of HBOT are based on raising the partial pressure of inspired oxygen and increasing hydrostatic pressure, by compressing the gas in all spaces in the body, according to Boyle's law [16,17]. Increasing the oxygen's partial pressure raises its diffusibility in tissues. Even if there is a similar amount of oxygen in the plasma and in the transported oxygen by haemoglobin, by increasing the oxygen's partial pressure, its effectiveness is enhanced at a cellular level [18]. Increasing the pressure of the oxygen in the environment over a certain point induces the rising of the amount of oxygen dissolved in the plasma (increase in volume), and the penetration of the oxygen in the tissues (increase in quality) [19,20]. Therefore, HBO treatment leads to a considerable development in bone formation, so that the lamellar bone grows [21].

In the study effectuated by Giacon et al. [22], the authors consider that through HBO therapy pre-treatment, the protection proteins of oxidative stress are activated and tissues are prepared for surgery entailing transient ischemia. They presented a case report of an immediate dental implant, which depicted the utilisation of HBO therapy and of advanced platelet-rich fibrin (A-PRF) for pre-treating the implant site in a case of severe periodontitis with tooth attachment loss. Three sessions of HBO therapy effectuated for preconditioning by increasing the positive results, presumably through sterilization of surgical site and development of antioxidant protection. The authors underlined that future studies should specifically address this topic.

Altug et al. [23], studied the consequences of HBO therapy on implant osseointegration in experimental diabetes rabbits. The authors concluded that the disclosures in histomorphometry hint that HBO therapy has a certain impact on the osseointegration of dental implants, in the early healing time in diabetic rabbits. The authors underlined that dental implant stability is not influenced by HBO therapy.

The administration of oxygen in HBOT is realized in hyperbaric chambers, which can be multiplace (type A), and monoplace (type B, that provides treatment for a single patient) [24]. Both chambers are used to treat various diseases, from simple injuries to serious illness [25].

The comparative study started from the already certified benefits of HBOT in the general medicine specialties. The aim of this comparative study was to find out if the adjuvant HBO therapy presents beneficial effects in the treatment of adult patients affected by periodontal disease, after the conventional therapy of performing professional dental hygienization measures, and of full-mouth scaling and root planing (SRP) with EMS Piezon device and EMS Air-Flow Master. The expected result of the trial should potentially contribute to an advanced treatment strategy for periodontal disease, with an ideal clinical outcome.

2. Materials and Methods

The study was realized in conformity to the ethical principles of the Declaration of Helsinki and of the good clinical practice. The protocol was approved by the Ethics Committee of Dental Medicine Faculty, Titu Maiorescu University of Bucharest (No. 2 of 5 May 2017). All patients were informed about the research requirements, attended only by those that entered voluntarily in the research program. The study phases were explained to each recruited patient, including the need for monitoring. Included patients signed the written informed consent prior to the beginning of this study. The working hypothesis started from the premise that the benefits of HBOT are already certified in general medicine specialties, but can it be used as an adjuvant therapy in Romanian patients with periodontal disease?

The study was conducted in the Clinics of Dental Medicine Faculties, between of May 2017 and May 2021, but the COVID-19 pandemic epidemiological context determined a 12-month intermission. The authors followed calibration trainings to ensure: the precision and correctness of patients' anamneses, of clinical examination and diagnosis; the proper use of EMS Piezon and EMS Air-Flow Master Device; the use of the same standardized clinical measurements. The calibration trainings were realized in order to ensure the validity and reliability of clinical study and of obtained results. Adjuvant HBO therapy was performed in Hypermed Care SRL Clinic, by using the Revitalair®430 monoplace equipment, produced by Biobarica (Medley, FL, USA).

Clinical examinations and interviews were accomplished to evaluate eligibility. Patients were randomly screened, and then asked to participate in the study. Study initially enrolled 89 patients, but 12 subjects withdrawn voluntarily during the study and 6 subjects were excluded for lack of cooperation. The remaining patients in the study (71), had the age range of 38–59 years (means 48.5 years, ±10.5 years). Table 1 presents the sample patients and Figure 1 presents the flow diagram of the study.

Table 1. Sample patients.

	Group 1	Group 2
No of patients	31	40
Age (mean ± years)	48.5 ± 10.5	48.5 ± 10.5
Gender M/F	16/15	21/19
Confirmed periodontal disease	Mild to moderate	Mild to moderate

Oral examinations and X-rays were effectuated at the time of patients selection, to differentiate the periodontal affection from other diseases (e.g., apical periodontitis, tooth fracture, etc.). The oral examinations consisted of the assessment of periodontal status by determination of the oral hygiene conditions and of Simplified Oral Health Index (OHI-S), Sulcus Bleeding Index (SBI), examination of clinical attachment level (CAL), checking for dental mobility degree (MD), of the pocket depth (PD), and of furcation involvement. All periodontal examinations were effectuated by using mirrors, tweezers, probes, and a calibrated periodontal UNC-PCP15 Color-Coded Probe (Hu-Friedy Europe, The Netherlands) probe.

Inclusion criteria for this study consisted of non-smoking patients aged 38–59 years old, having at least 6 natural teeth on a half dental arch (excluding third molars), having periodontal symptomatology at the presentation in the dental office (like gum redness or/and bleeding, gum swelling, persistent metallic taste, halitosis, painful chewing, sensitive teeth, minimum 4 teeth with first or second degree of dental mobility, periodontal pockets), or with a confirmed diagnosis of mild to moderate periodontal disease.

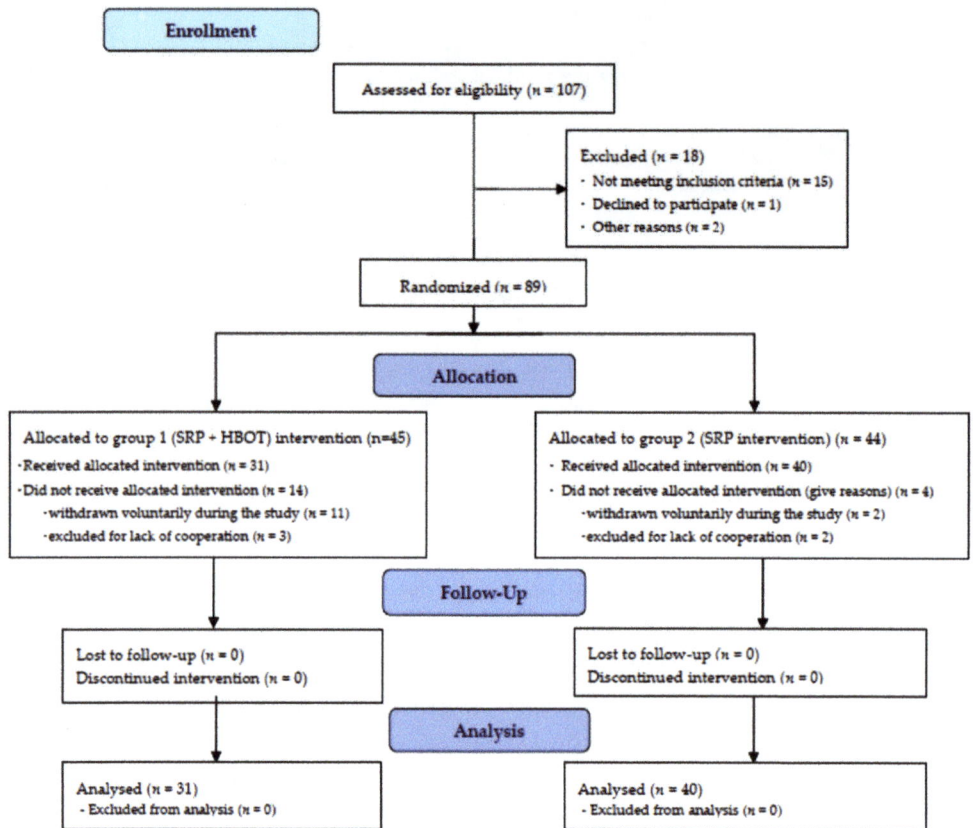

Figure 1. Flow Diagram of the study.

All selected patients for admission into the first group of patients with HBO therapy completed and signed a fact sheet with information regarding their general and specific health conditions (which contained affections which determined the exclusion criteria of study). Inclusion criteria of patients are depicted in Table 2.

Table 2. Inclusion criteria of patients in study.

Inclusion Criteria
Male and female patients between 38 and 59 years of age
Non-smokers
Having at least 6 natural teeth on a half dental arch, excluding third molars
Periodontal symptomatology/confirmed diagnosis of moderate periodontal disease
Patient's acceptance to participate in the study, with signed informed consent

Exclusion criteria for this study were represented by smoker patients, maximum scores of all studied periodontal indices, periodontal treatment and antibiotic therapy in the last six months, aggressive periodontitis, endodontic affections, orthodontic patients, patients with infections, systemic disorders, upper respiratory and pulmonary disorders (e.g., untreated pneumothorax, pneumonia, asthma, chronic obstructive pulmonary disease, etc.), cataract, Eustachian tube dysfunction, hereditary spherocytosis, fever, claustrophobia, convulsions, cardiac simulators or other implanted or external devices that control body functions, patients with unstable cardiovascular disease, pregnant woman, hospitalized patients, those with cancer, with uncontrolled diabetes mellitus, with parafunction of chewing habit, with severe malocclusion, those with missing data, patients with mental disability, uncooperative patients, and patients who refused to be included in the study.

According to the safety requirements of patients, those with general medical conditions presented in exclusion criteria of patients cannot be accepted for HBO therapy, thus patients with these affections were not be admitted in study group 1 (with HBOT). Exclusion criteria are presented in Table 3.

Table 3. Exclusion criteria of patients in study.

Exclusion Criteria	
Smoker patients	Hereditary spherocytosis
Maximum scores of all studied periodontal indices	Fever
Periodontal treatment and antibiotic therapy in the last six months	Claustrophobia
Aggressive periodontitis	Convulsions
Endodontic affections	Cardiac simulators
Orthodontic patients	Implanted or external devices that control body functions
Infections	Pregnancy
Systemic disorders	Hospitalized patients
Upper respiratory and pulmonary disorders	Patients with mental disability
Cataract	Uncooperative patients
Eustachian tube dysfunction	Patients who refused to be included in the study

Supra- and subgingival debridement, scaling, and root planing with EMS Piezon device and EMS Air-Flow Master device, followed by manual root planing were effectuated in every selected patient in 24 h. Guided Biofilm Therapy with EMS device is a treatment protocol built in conformity of each patient diagnosis and risk evaluation for achieving optimum outcomes. The treatment is realized in a minimally invasive way, with the highest comfort, safety and efficiency for the patients. Oral hygiene instructions were presented to every participant patient, and dental plaque disclosing gel (GC Tri Plaque ID Gel) was used before any assessment sessions. Patients included in the study used the same toothpaste (Colgate Total Gum Protection Toothpaste), same dental brush (Colgate Gum Health Extra Soft Toothbrush for Sensitive Gums with Deep Cleaning Floss-Tip Bristles), and same interdental pick (GUM-6326RA Soft-Picks Original Dental Picks, small). Participants brushed their teeth twice a day, morning and evening, at least two minutes each time (in conformity with the American Dental Association (ADA) suggestions), with Stillman method of tooth brushing. An amount of 1 cm tooth paste was used. The inter-dental pick was indicated to be utilized only in the evening, before teeth brushing. Two tubes of plaque revealing gel were handed to the patients participating in the study, for checking their dental hygiene 3 times weekly. The gel was applied after tooth brushing, and if the sanitization was not correct, the patients had to perform their tooth brushing again. At the end of the study, the used quantity of the plaque disclosing gel from the tubes was verified, in order to verify the compliance of participants to the study protocol.

The selected patients (71), were divided into two groups, the first group of patients (group I) who agreed upon and benefited of HBOT adjuvant therapy (31 patients, 15 women and 16 men), and the second group of patients (group II / control group), who did not undergo HBO therapy (40 patients, 19 women and 21 males). Both patient groups were selected according to the same inclusion/exclusion criteria and benefited from the same dental treatment protocol for periodontal disease, excepting HBO adjuvant therapy (which was realized only in 1st group of patients). The type of study design was simple randomized trial, by centralized randomization into groups, than participant patients were divided into the two groups by centralized randomization.

The applied clinical protocol to all patients consisted of: consultation and complementary radiographic examinations; diagnosis of general health and of oral/periodontal tissues; first clinical evaluation and registration of dental and periodontal status by determination of OHI-S index, of the sulcus bleeding index, the pathological tooth mobility and the depth of periodontal pockets; establishing of the treatment plan; filing the general and specific information sheet (by the patient for admission in the HBOT group), and signature on the informed consent; awareness of patients on the state of periodontal illness at presentation; training and insisting upon artificial oral hygiene procedures by using the Stillman technique of tooth brushing; taking of the same brand and type of toothbrushes, toothpastes, interdental brushes, and dental plaque disclosing gel; conducting of the corrective treatment (performing professional oral hygiene, and of specific therapy for dental and periodontal diseases with EMS devices); second clinical evaluation of the patients at 1 month after periodontal treatment; applying HBO therapy in the first group of patients; third clinical evaluation at 2 months after the completion of HBO therapy and recording of the results; comparison of results. Figure 2 depict the flow chart of the clinical study.

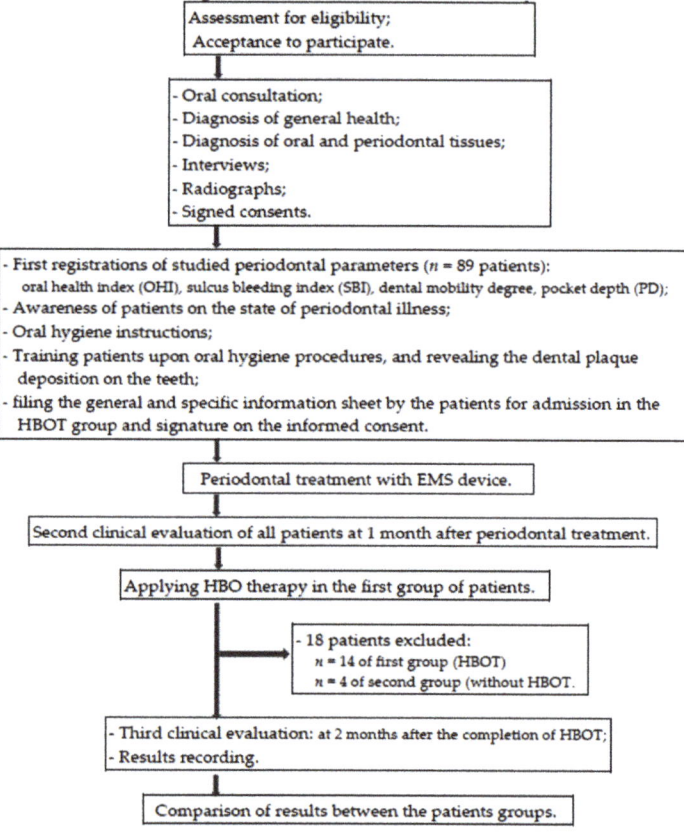

Figure 2. Flow chart of the clinical study.

After the effectuation of specific periodontal treatment in all patients, each patient belonging to the first group (with HBO adjuvant therapy) was set to perform 20 sessions of hyperbaric oxygen therapy for one hour, with the applied pressure of 1.4 ATM. The frequency of the therapy sessions was three sessions per week. HBO therapy was performed at the Biobarica Hypermed Care Clinic in Bucharest, in a monoplace hyperbaric chamber (Figure 3).

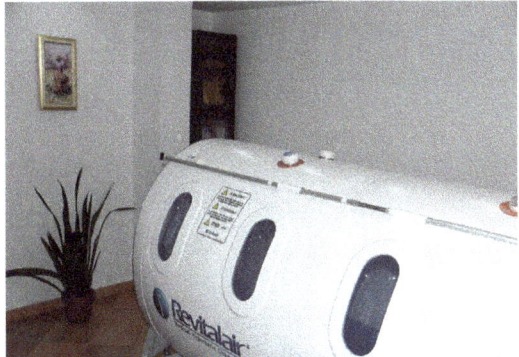 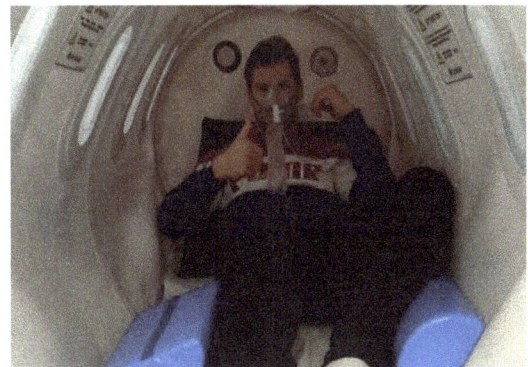

Figure 3. The monoplace hyperbaric chamber used in Biobarica Hypermed Care Clinic.

Stillman method of tooth brushing consists of thoroughly brushing around and under the gum line, and it helps to clean the debris deposited between the teeth, because the toothbrush bristles reach under the gums [25].

Oral hygiene status can be determined by using the oral health index (OHI), calculated by the oral debris score and the dental calculus score found on the buccal and lingual surfaces of each of the three segments of the dental arches. The calculation of the numerical values of simplified oral health index (OHI-S) is in conformity to the existing dental plaque and calculus deposits. The simplified oral hygiene index (OHI-S) allows the separate evaluation of the soft and hard deposits, present on the buccal/labial or oral dental crown surfaces of 6 teeth of both dental arches, one tooth for each sextant: maxillary dental arch, teeth 1.6, 1.1, 2.6 on buccal/labial surfaces, respectively mandibular dental arch teeth 3.6, 3.1, 4.6 on lingual surfaces (enumerated teeth are noted after FDI notation system). The selected surfaces used for scoring were the buccal for maxillary molar and the lingual for mandibular molars, respectively, the labial for the maxillary right central incisors and for the mandibular left central incisors. In the absence of first molar, the second or third molar were examined, and in the case of the incisors, the neighbouring incisor.

The quantification of dental deposits can be performed visually or by staining solution. The surfaces of dental crowns are examined with the probe, extending the examination to the level of contact points of the proximal coronary surfaces, including the subgingival area. Debris index-simplified (DI-S) calculation method: 0 = absence of dental plaque; 1 = microbial plaque present up to 1/3 of the tooth surface; 2 = microbial plaque present between 1/3 and 2/3 of the tooth surface; 3 = microbial plaque present over 2/3 of the tooth surface. Calculus index-simplified (CI-S) calculation method: 0 = absence of dental calculus; 1 = calculus present up to 1/3 of the tooth surface; 2 = calculus present between 1/3 and 2/3 of the tooth surface; 3 = calculus present over 2/3 of the tooth surface. The averages for the plaque and tartar indices will be calculated and then added together; their sum will represent the OHI-S index [26,27]. OHI-S score is summed and then divided to the number of examined dental crown surfaces, for the mean oral hygiene score [28,29]. An arithmetic mean of the individual scores for debris and calculus index was performed, and subsequently the highest determined score was taken into consideration. The values of OHI-S index, necessary for interpretation, are: excellent 0; good 0.1–1.2; satisfactory 1.3–3.0; and unsatisfactory 3.1–6 [30]. Index interpretation of OHI-S scores used in this study was: excellent = 0; good = 1; satisfactory = 2; and unsatisfactory = 3. The scores were calculated according to the results of the determinations performed on each patient. An arithmetic mean of the individual scores was performed on each tooth, and subsequently the highest determined final score was taken into consideration.

Sulcus Bleeding Index (SBI, Műhlemann and Son) on gentle probing of the sulcus represents one of the initial signs of periodontal disease. In SBI, four gingival units are scored systematically for each tooth: the labial and lingual marginal gingival (M units) and the mesial and distal gingival papilla (P units). After probing, the examiner should wait for 30 s for scoring. Scores for these units are summed and then distributed to 4. Adding the obtained scores of the studied teeth and dividing them by the number of studied teeth establishes the sulcus bleeding index (SBI). Criteria of SBI scoring are: 0—healthy aspect of papilla and of marginal gingiva, without bleeding on probing; 1—healthy gingival aspect, but bleeding on probing; 2—bleeding on probing, modified colour, without edema; 3—bleeding on probing, modified colour, slight edema; 4—bleeding on probing, modified colour, evident edema; 5—spontaneous bleeding, modified colour, pronounced edema. SBI scoring is effectuated on the eight upper and lower anterior teeth, and four gingival areas are included for each tooth: mesial-labial, mesial-lingual, oro-mesial, oro-distal [31]. Index interpretation of BSI scores in this study was: excellent = 0; very good = 1; good = 2; satisfactory = 3; and unsatisfactory = 4.

The clinical sign of dental/tooth mobility depicts the periodontal destruction degree determined by local affections of gums and surrounding structures of the teeth. Tooth mobility presents 4 degrees: grade 0 represents the physiological mobility; in grade 1, the teeth present more than 1 mm mobility in a buccal-oral direction: in grade 2, the teeth present more than 1 mm mobility in buccal-oral and mesial-distal direction; and in grade 3, the teeth present mobility in three directions, buccal-oral, mesial-distal and incisal/occlusal-apical direction. Tooth mobility can represent a possible aggravation factor of the establishment of periodontal disease [32].

Periodontal pockets represent a pathological feature characterized by the displacement of the gingival attachment, respectively, the deepening of the gingival sulcus apically, due to the expansion of dental plaque and dental calculus towards the dental root. It can be classified as supra-alveolar (when the bottom of the pocket is situated at the crown of the alveolar bone), and intra-alveolar (when the bottom of the periodontal pocket is situated apical to the alveolar bone). Periodontal pockets can imply one or more tooth surfaces, and they can present various depths on different surfaces of the tooth. Periodontal pocket depth (PD) is a primary sign of periodontitis. The size and severity can be divided into normal (1 to 3 mm), early/mild periodontitis (4 to 5 mm), moderate periodontitis (5 to 7 mm), and severe periodontitis (7 to 12 mm). Periodontal examinations are effectuated with a periodontal probe [33]. In this study, an arithmetic mean of the individual scores for pockets was performed on each tooth, and subsequently the highest determined score was taken into consideration. Rationale of classifying periodontal pockets is to realize a correct evaluation, and then a correct prognosis of periodontal disease after the stage and grade of the disease, including the contributory factors, and after that, to effectuate the adequate treatment management of disease [6].

All the statistical analysis were performed in SPSS 24 Software. The considered level of significance is 0.05, otherwise mentioned. Data was analysed through means of the Chi-Square test for group differences.

3. Results

Two months after the end of HBO therapy in the first group of patients, we summarized and compared the recorded data of all patients. The obtained results in both studied groups, according to the three clinical examinations, are presented in Table 4.

Table 4. Obtained results in the studied groups, according to the three clinical examinations.

	Selected Patients (71)		Group I HBOT 31 Patients	Group II Control 40 Patients
First clinical examination, at patients presentation	Oral health index (OHI-S)	Score 0	-	-
		Score 1	3 (=9.67%)	5 (=12.50%)
		Score 2	12 (=38.40%)	17 (=42.50%)
		Score 3	16 (=51.61%)	18 (=45.00%)
	Sulcus bleeding index (SBI)	Score 0	-	-
		Score 1	2 (=6.45%)	3 (=7.50%)
		Score 2	5 (=16.12%)	7 (=17.50%)
		Score 3	17 (=54.83%)	21 (=52.50%)
		Score 4	7 (=22.58%)	9 (=22.50%)
	Dental mobility degree (DM)	0-Physiological mobility	-	-
		1st degree mobility	15 (=48.38%)	19 (=47.50%)
		2nd degree mobility	16 (=51.61%)	21 (=52.50%)
	Pockets depth (PD)	Normal	-	-
		Early/mild periodontitis	12 (=38.40%)	15 (=37.50%)
		Moderate periodontitis	19 (=61.29%)	25 (=62.50%)
Second clinical examination of both groups patients, at 1 week after the finalization of periodontal treatments	Oral health index (OHI-S)	Score 0	4 (=12.90%)	6 (=15.00%)
		Score 1	8 (=25.80%)	11 (=27.50%)
		Score 2	10 (=32.25%)	12 (=30.00%)
		Score 3	9 (=29.03%)	11 (=27.50%)
	Sulcus bleeding index (SBI)	Score 0	3 (=9.67%)	5 (=12.50%)
		Score 1	5 (=16.12%)	7 (=17.50%)
		Score 2	7 (=22.58%)	9 (=22.50%)
		Score 3	14 (=45.16%)	16 (=40.00%)
		Score 4	2 (=6.45%)	3 (=7.50%)
	Dental mobility degree (DM)	Physiological mobility	4 (=12.90%)	7 (=17.50%)
		1st degree mobility	16 (=51.61%)	19 (=47.50%)
		2nd degree mobility	11 (=35.48%)	14 (=35.00%)
	Pockets depth (PD)	Normal	3 (=9.67%)	5 (=12.50%)
		Early/mild periodontitis	17 (=54.83%)	19 (=47.50%)
		Moderate periodontitis	11 (=35.48%)	16 (=40.00%)
Third clinical examination of both groups patients, at 2 months after the finalization of HBOT in first group of patients	Oral health index (OHI-S)	Score 0	12 (=38.40%)	9 (=22.50%)
		Score 1	11 (=35.48%)	12 (=30.00%)
		Score 2	5 (=16.12%)	11 (=27.50%)
		Score 3	3 (=9.67%)	8 (=20.00%)
	Sulcus bleeding index (SBI)	Score 0	8 (=25.80%)	5 (=12.50%)
		Score 1	9 (=29.03%)	8 (=20.00%)
		Score 2	8 (=25.80%)	11 (=27.50%)
		Score 3	6 (=19.35%)	14 (=35.00%)
		Score 4	-	2 (=5.00%)
	Dental mobility degree (DM)	Physiological mobility	8 (=25.80%)	9 (=22.50%)
		1st degree mobility	17 (=54.83%)	20 (=50.00%)
		2nd degree mobility	6 (=19.35%)	11 (=27.50%)
	Pockets depth (PD)	Normal	9 (=29.03%)	8 (=20.00%)
		Early/mild periodontitis	16 (=51.61%)	18 (=45.00%)
		Moderate periodontitis	5 (=16.12%)	14 (=35.00%)

By comparing the listed values in Table 4, we found the following:
- Oral health index (OHI-S): at the presentation, the patients of both groups had only values of 1, 2, and 3 in OHI-S score, without value 0; in the second clinical examination, we found that OHI-S scores were reduced in both study groups (HBOT and control), because of SRP treatment, but probably also as a result of patient awareness in the need for correct oral hygiene through brushing exercises (initially done at the clinic, until all patients have acquired the correct technique), respectively, by revealing the bacterial plaque (performed at each presentation of the patient in the practice); at the second and third determination, we found that the OHI-S decreased in the patients of both groups, to 0, 1, and 2; and in the third assessment, the OHI-S values were lower in the first group (which benefited from HBOT) compared to the control group. In Figure 4, the patient distribution based on OHI-S index, are presented at the first (a), second (b), and third (c) examination.
- Sulcus bleeding index (SBI): at their presentation, the patients of both groups had only values of 1, 2, 3, and 4 in SBI score, without value 0; in second clinical examination we found that SBI scores were significantly reduced in both study groups (HBOT and control), because of the same reasons (SRP treatment, correct teeth brushing); at the second and third determination, we found that the SBI scores decreased in the patients of both groups; and in third assessment, the SBI values were lower in the first group (HBOT) compared to the control group. In Figure 5, the patient distribution based on SBI index at first (a), second (b), and third (c) examination are depicted.
- Dental mobility (DM): We found that the DM has diminished in both groups; at the presentation all of patients had I-st and II-nd degree dental mobility; in the other two clinical examinations, we found that DM was reduced till physiological mobility, especially in patients who received HBO adjuvant therapy. Figure 6 depicts the patient distribution based on DM index at first (a), second (b), and third (c) examination.
- Pockets depth (PD): the measurements were effectuated with the periodontal probe and registered in the patients' record; we found that the PD values were reduced in both groups of patients in the second and third clinical examination, but the reduction of PD was more significant in patients belonging to the HBOT group. In Figure 7, the patient distribution based on PD index at first (a), second (b), and third (c) examination is presented.

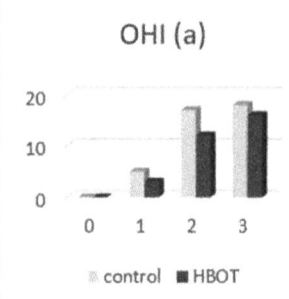 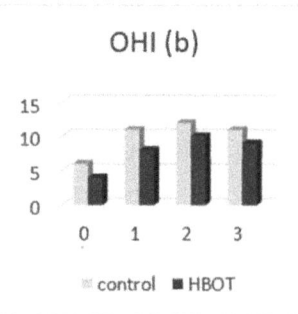 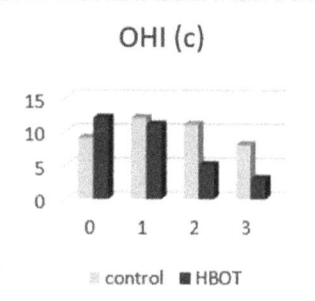

Figure 4. Patient distribution based on OHI index at (**a**) first examination, (**b**) second examination, and (**c**) third examination.

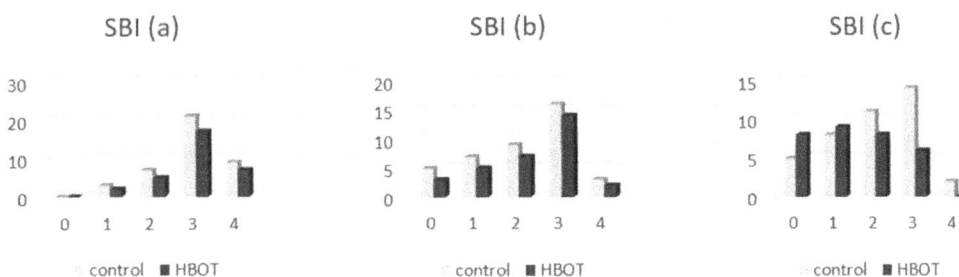

Figure 5. Patient distribution based on SB index at (**a**) first examination, (**b**) second examination, and (**c**) third examination.

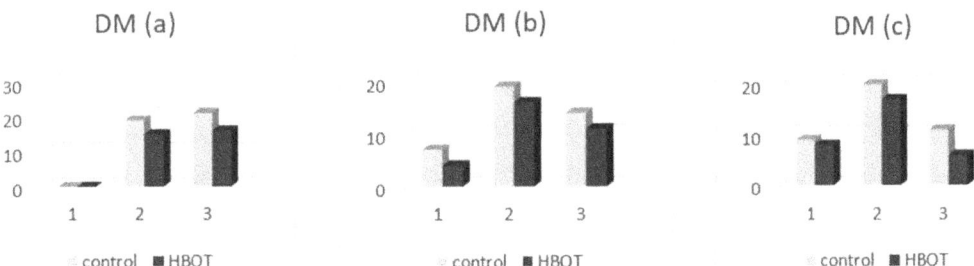

Figure 6. Patient distribution based on DM index at (**a**) first examination, (**b**) second examination, and (**c**) third examination.

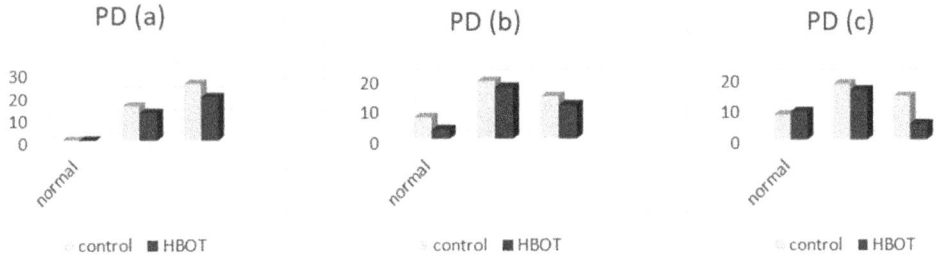

Figure 7. Patient distribution based on PD at (**a**) first examination, (**b**) second examination, and (**c**) third examination.

In conformity with the inclusion criteria, only patients with mild and moderate periodontal disease were admitted in study. Only two patients out of a total of 71 had a slight involvement of the furcation, therefore assessment of the involvement of furcation was not introduced in the study.

Table 5 present Chi-Square test p-values for test differences between control and test groups for all variables, at all three levels of investigation, with p-values. There are no significant differences, at any level, between the frequencies of the control and test groups, for any of the observed variables, no matter the treatment type.

Table 5. Chi-Square test *p*-values for test differences between groups, for all variables, at all "three levels of investigation".

Variable	*p*-Value	Variable	*p*-Value	Variable	*p*-Value	Variable	*p*-Value
OHI-S1	0.75	SBI1	0.99	DM1	0.65	PD1	0.91
OHI-S2	0.99	SBI2	0.91	DM2	0.82	PD2	0.81
OHI-S3	0.27	SBI3	0.21	DM3	0.66	PD3	0.28

In Table 6, Chi-Square test p-values are presented for test differences between groups for all variables, for test and control groups. The significance level is 0.1. Exceptions appear for the SBI index in the control group, which is significant at a 0.1 significance level, and all differences are significant at a 0.05 level. It can be noticed that there are significant differences in the effect of the three assessments, both in test or control groups.

Table 6. Chi-Square test *p*-values for test differences between both groups (SRP+HBOT and SRP) for all variables.

Variable	*p*-Value	
	Test	Control
OHI-S	0	0.016
SBI	0	0.078 *
DM	0.018	0.013
PD	0	0.026

* Significance level 0.1.

At the finalisation of study, it was noted that, although patients did not initially mention their mild vertigo, mild tinnitus, and fatigability, at the end of HBO therapy, 21 patients (= 67.74%) stated, without being asked, that they no longer had mild vertigo, mild tinnitus symptoms and that they no longer present signs of chronic fatigue.

4. Discussion

The current standards of periodontal disease for the assessment of periodontitis is based primarily upon attachment and bone loss, and classifies the disease into four stages based on severity (I, II, III or IV) and three grades based on disease susceptibility (A, B or C). Therefore, is possible to create a staging and grading system for periodontitis [34].

Complete radiographic examination represents a part of the initial periodontal assessment for establishing the degree of horizontal and vertical alveolar bone loss. According to the 2017 World Workshop on the Classification of Periodontal and Peri-Implant Diseases and Conditions, a new periodontitis classification categorizes the disease based on a multi-dimensional staging and grading system [6,7]. Staging is determined by the severity of the disease at initial presentation and the complexity of disease management [35]. Wandawa et al. [36] applied 16 HBOT meetings after SRP, and their results were not significant from a statistical point of view. Soranta et al. [37] studied the action of HBOT on MMP-8 level in the saliva of chronic periodontitis patients. They applied 8 HBOT sessions, and observed that the results were meaningfully better than in monotherapy with SRP. The study of Robo et al. [38] and Chen et al. [39] proved that HBOT meaningfully decreases the anaerobic flora in subgingival sulcus. In their research, Balestra et al. [40] consider that studies in reference with HBOT should be extended, because this therapy can produce a strong stimulus at the level of the molecular reactions, but the requirements are in reference with "how much", "how long", and "how often" should this adjuvant therapy be used.

HBOT has a triggering role in bone remodelling, and the research effectuated by Lu et al. [41] demonstrated that the major impact of oxygen pressure is at the incipient phase of differentiation of osteoblasts. Salmón-González et al. [42] consider that there is a correlation between increasing oxygen pressure and increasing osteoblastic and osteoclastic activity. Studies of Huang et al. [43] mention that HBOT stimulates the fibroblast activity, the angiogenesis, and proceeds on leukocyte function for promoting lesion healing. In the article published by El-Baz et al. [44], it is highlighted that HBOT is a treatment that has become quite popular in the community of autistic patients and that this type of therapy has many benefits. In the research conducted by Bennett et al. [45], it is emphasized that there was some evidence of HBOT efficacy in the treatment of acute migraine, although study participants belonged to an unselected population. Devaraj et al. [46] believe that although HBOT has broad indications in various medical cases, the effective use of this type of dental treatment requires evidence, so research should also be undertaken in the field of dentistry to develop adjunctive therapy options with hyperbaric oxygen.

During the Tenth European Consensus Conference on Hyperbaric Medicine, recommendations for accepted and non-accepted clinical indications and practice of HBOT have been established [47]. In certain situations, it is necessary to assess the cost–benefit ratio, especially when patients pay full treatment or in case of presumably long treatments.

HBOT can be used as a monotherapy, or as a multimodal therapeutic variant. After a study published in 2017, Chhabra et al. [48] concluded, that ensuring the local hyperbaric oxygen atmosphere, the administration of growth factors, skin-substitutes, electric stimulation and local drainage, may constitute the conditions for local wound healing, a fact which may be applicable in the treatment of periodontal diseases. Marcinkowska et al. [49] consider that through properly addressing and evaluating methodological issues referring to HBOT, this therapy may have potential for the treatment of neuropsychological deficits in a wide range of neurological states, with importance in the treatment of trigeminal nerve affections.

HBOT as a preventive therapy may diminish the peril of dental implant failures in the maxillofacial area, including the irradiated patients [50,51]. The research of Hollander et al. [52], show that HBOT could be beneficial in nonirradiated patients with intraoral compromised wound healing. The healing of wounds after application of HBOT is underlined by Re et al. [21], Hollander et al. [52], and Shih et al. [53], especially in periodontal disease and oral submucous fibrosis. HBOT as adjuvant therapy in dentistry, associated with the other specific dental treatments, has benefits and facilitates the healing process, notwithstanding the potential complications that may appear [21,54].

According to the safety requirements of patients, HBO therapy should not be accepted to those with general medical conditions presented in exclusion criteria of patients. Adverse effects and complications that may arise during HBO therapy can be absolute, relative or potential [55,56]. The most common complications during HBO therapy are represented by middle and inner ear barotrauma, pulmonary barotrauma, sinus/paranasal and dental barotrauma, claustrophobia, and ophthalmological manifestations (as progressive myopia, new cataracts) [56–58]. Potential contraindications of HBOT are represented by the presence of pacemakers or any implantable devices, hereditary spherocytosis, pregnancy, hypoglycaemia, chronic obstructive pulmonary disease, allergic rhinitis, asthma, upper respiratory infections, and acute pulmonary edema. In defiance to its numerous uses, potential adverse effects of HBOT, which represent a possible hazard for patients, should be taken into account. All these impose that this knowledge referring to the complications and adverse effects of HBO therapy should be presented in the informed consent [59,60].

Medical conditions along with the comprehension of necessity in preservation of dental and gingival health represent the potential predictable of general and oral health status [61]. Diseases of the periodontal tissues also affect the tooth mobility degree [2,62]. The mobility of the teeth represents a utilized symptom in the evaluation of the health status of periodontal tissues, respectively, in obtaining success or failure of the periodontal treatment [35,63]. The extension of periodontal disease cannot be correctly estimated without the evaluation of the mobility degree [64]. The used clinical method for determining the tooth mobility is based on individual's perception of tooth movement by application of a force on the tooth crown [65].

The acquaintances regarding the periodontal disease are significant for the prevention, and also for the preservation of the periodontal tissues health, in order to prevent severe subsequent disease. Incorrect oral hygiene induces the triggering of oral cavity tissue diseases, in particular of periodontal affections [5,66].

Future research directions will be correlated with the inclusion of a larger number of patients in clinical trial, longer duration of follow-up, thoroughgoing study of HBOT effects in severe periodontitis, respectively, by the enlargement of the researched items (such as patients which presents gingival recession, TMJ disorders).

The absence of assessments referring to severe periodontitis represents a limitation of this study. Another limitation of this clinical trial is represented by the relatively reduced number of patients in groups. The cost of HBO therapy is rather high, and represents another limitative reason. Additionally, because the price of HBO therapy in oral diseases is not discounted by the Romanian health care insurance system, the implementation of HBO therapy in real life presents difficulties.

5. Conclusions

Within the limits of the study, we concluded that the HBOT group of patients presented better values of OHI-S, SBI, DM and PD two months after the completion of HBO adjuvant therapy than patients in the second control group, but Chi-Square test p-values for test differences between groups, for all variables, at all the three levels of investigation, with p-values shown that there are no significant differences, at any level, between the frequencies of the control and test groups, for any of the observed variables, no matter the treatment type.

The majority of the patients of the first group declared that HBOT had beneficial effects on their general health status in symptoms prior to this adjuvant therapy, as tinnitus, vertigo, chronic fatigue, and migraines, but it is necessary to emphasise that all these are subjective statements.

Clinical trials with a greater the number of patients and longer follow-up time are required.

Author Contributions: Conceptualization, A.B. (Anamaria Bechir) and E.S.B.; methodology, L.L.M. and A.B. (Anamaria Bechir); software, M.S. and E.S.B.; validation, A.B. (Alexandru Burcea) and A.B. (Anamaria Bechir); investigation, A.B., A.B. (Alexandru Burcea), L.L.M. and E.S.B.; resources, M.S. and E.S.B.; original draft preparation, A.B. (Alexandru Burcea) and E.S.B.; review and editing, A.B. (Anamaria Bechir) and L.L.M.; supervision, A.B. (Alexandru Burcea) and A.B. (Anamaria Bechir). All authors have read and agreed to the published version of the manuscript.

Funding: This research received no external funding.

Institutional Review Board Statement: The study was conducted in accordance with the Declaration of Helsinki, and approved by the Ethics Committee of Dental Medicine Faculty, Titu Maiorescu University of Bucharest (No. 2/5 May 2017).

Informed Consent Statement: Informed consent was obtained from all subjects involved in the study.

Data Availability Statement: Not applicable.

Acknowledgments: The material, technical and administrative support for HBO therapy was covered by Biobarica Hypermed Care Clinic.

Conflicts of Interest: The authors declare no conflict of interest.

References

1. Newman, M.; Dragan, I.F.; Elangovan, S.; Karan, A.K. *Newman and Carranza's Essentials of Clinical Periodontology E-Book: An Integrated Study Companion*; Elsevier: Amsterdam, Netherlands, 2020; pp. 23–28, 31–37.
2. Könönen, E.; Gursoy, M.; Gursoy, U.K. Periodontitis: A Multifaceted Disease of Tooth-Supporting Tissues. *J. Clin. Med.* **2019**, *8*, 1135. [CrossRef]
3. Nazir, M.; Al-Ansari, A.; Al-Khalifa, K.; Alhareky, M.; Gaffar, B.; Almas, K. Global Prevalence of Periodontal Disease and Lack of Its Surveillance. *Sci. World J.* **2020**, *2020*, 2146160. [CrossRef]

4. Tonetti, M.S.; Bottenberg, P.; Conrads, G.; Eickholz, P.; Heasman, P.; Huysmans, M.C.; López, R.; Madianos, P.; Müller, F.; Needleman, L.; et al. Dental caries and periodontal diseases in the ageing population: Call to action to protect and enhance oral health and well-being as an essential component of healthy ageing—Consensus report of group 4 of the joint EFP/ORCA workshop on the boundaries between caries and periodontal diseases. *J. Clin. Periodontol.* **2017**, *44*, S135–S144.
5. Nazir, M.A. Prevalence of periodontal disease, its association with systemic diseases and prevention. *Int. J. Health Sci.* **2017**, *11*, 72–80.
6. Tonetti, M.S.; Greenwell, H.; Kornman, K.S. Staging and grading of periodontitis: Framework and proposal of a new classification and case definition. *J. Periodontol.* **2018**, *89*, S159–S172. [CrossRef]
7. Papapanou, P.N.; Sanz, M.; Buduneli, N.; Dietrich, T.; Feres, M.; Fine, D.H.; Flemmig, T.F.; Garcia, R.; Giannobile, W.V.; Filippo, G.; et al. Periodontitis: Consensus report of Workgroup 2 of the 2017 World Workshop on the Classification of Periodontal and Peri-Implant Diseases and Conditions. *J. Periodontol.* **2018**, *89*, S173–S182. [CrossRef]
8. Rhodes, C.E.; Varacallo, M. Physiology, Oxygen Transport. In *StatPearls [Internet]*; StatPearls Publishing: Tresure Island, FL, USA, 2021. Available online: https://www.ncbi.nlm.nih.gov/books/NBK538336/ (accessed on 20 December 2021).
9. Bosco, G.; Vezzani, G.; Mrakic Sposta, S.; Rizzato, A.; Enten, G.; Abou-samra, A.; Malacrida, S.; Quartesan, S.; Vezzoli, A.; Camporesi, E. Hyperbaric oxygen therapy ameliorates osteonecrosis in patients by modulating inflammation and oxidative stress. *J. Enzym. Inhib. Med. Chem.* **2018**, *33*, 1501–1505. [CrossRef]
10. Rech, F.V.; Negrini Fagundes, A.L.; Santos Simoes, R.; Rech, F.V.; Fagundes, A.L.N.; Simões, R.S.; Florencio-Silva, R.; da Silva Sasso, G.R.; Taha, M.O.; Fagundes, D.J. Action of hyperbaric oxygenation in the rat skin flap. *Acta Cirúrgica Bras.* **2015**, *30*, 235–241. [CrossRef]
11. Choudhury, R. Hypoxia and hyperbaric oxygen therapy: A review. *Int. J. Gen Med.* **2018**, *11*, 431–442. [CrossRef]
12. Lindenmann, J.; Smolle, C.; Kamolz, L.P.; Smolle-Juettner, F.M.; Graier, W.F. Survey of Molecular Mechanisms of Hyperbaric Oxygen in Tissue Repair. *Int. J. Mol. Sci.* **2021**, *22*, 11754. [CrossRef]
13. Indications for Hyperbaric Oxygen Therapy. Available online: https://www.uhms.org/resources/hbo-indications.html (accessed on 9 October 2021).
14. Jones, M.W.; Brett, K.; Han, N.; Wyatt, H.A. Hyperbaric Physics. In *StatPearls [Internet]*; StatPearls Publishing: Tresure Island, FL, USA, 2021. Available online: https://pubmed.ncbi.nlm.nih.gov/28846268/ (accessed on 9 November 2021).
15. Sen, S.; Sen, S. Therapeutic effects of hyperbaric oxygen: Integrated review. *Med. Gas. Res.* **2021**, *11*, 30–33. [CrossRef]
16. Chandan, G.; Cascella, M. Gas Laws and Clinical Application. [Updated 2 September 2021]. In *StatPearls [Internet]*; StatPearls Publishing: Tresure Island, FL, USA, 2021. Available online: https://www.ncbi.nlm.nih.gov/books/NBK546592/ (accessed on 17 December 2021).
17. Scheetz, A.M. New Developments in Hyperbaric Oxygen Therapy. *Stud. Publ.* **2021**. Available online: https://cupola.gettysburg.edu/student_scholarship/934 (accessed on 3 December 2021).
18. Hirota, K. Basic Biology of Hypoxic Responses Mediated by the Transcription Factor HIFs and Its Implication for Medicine. *Biomedicines* **2020**, *8*, 32. [CrossRef]
19. Keeley, T.P.; Mann, G.E. Defining Physiological Normoxia for Improved Translation of Cell Physiology to Animal Models and Humans. *Physiol Rev.* **2019**, *99*, 161–234. [CrossRef]
20. Gardin, C.; Bosco, G.; Ferroni, L.; Quartesan, S.; Rizzato, A.; Tatullo, M.; Zavan, B. Hyperbaric Oxygen Therapy Improves the Osteogenic and Vasculogenic Properties of Mesenchymal Stem Cells in the Presence of Inflammation In Vitro. *Int. J. Mol. Sci.* **2020**, *21*, 1452. [CrossRef]
21. Re, K.; Patel, S.; Gandhi, J.; Suh, Y.; Reid, I.; Joshi, G.; Smith, N.L.; Khan, S.A. Clinical utility of hyperbaric oxygen therapy in dentistry. *Med. Gas. Res.* **2019**, *9*, 93–100. [CrossRef]
22. Giacon, T.A.; Giancola, F.; Paganini, M.; Tiengo, C.; Camporesi, E.M.; Bosco, G. Hyperbaric Oxygen Therapy and A-PRF Pre-Treated Implants in Severe Periodontitis: A Case Report. *Int. J. Environ. Res. Public Health* **2021**, *18*, 413. [CrossRef]
23. Altug, H.A.; Tatli, U.; Coskun, A.T.; Erdogan, Ö.; Özkan, A.; Sencimen, M.; Kürkçü, M. Effects of hyperbaric oxygen treatment on implant osseointegration in experimental diabetes mellitus. *J. Appl. Oral Sci. Rev. FOB* **2018**, *26*, e20180083. [CrossRef]
24. Christiansen, S. An Overview of Hyperbaric Chamber Treatment. Available online: https://www.verywellhealth.com/hyperbaric-chamber-treatment-4582432 (accessed on 17 December 2021).
25. Bok, H.; Lee, C.H. Proper Tooth-Brushing Technique According to Patient's Age and Oral Status. *Int. J. Clin. Prev. Dent.* **2020**, *16*, 149–153. [CrossRef]
26. Katarzyńska-Konwa, M.; Obersztyn, I.; Trzcionka, A.; Mocny-Pachońska, K.; Mosler, B.; Tanasiewicz, M. Oral Status in Pregnant Women from Post-Industrial Areas of Upper Silesia in Reference to Occurrence of: Preterm Labors, Low Birth Weight and Type of Labor. *Healthcare* **2020**, *8*, 528. [CrossRef]
27. Bucur, S.A.; Raffanini Chiarati, C.; Avino, P.; Migliorino, I.; Cocoș, D.I.; Bud, E.S.; Bud, A.; Vlasa, A. Retrospective study regarding the status of the superficial marginal periodontium in adult patients wearing orthodontic retainers. *Rom. J. Oral Rehabil.* **2021**, *13*, 194–201.
28. Baishya, B.; Satpathy, A.; Nayak, R.; Mohanty, R. Oral hygiene status, oral hygiene practices and periodontal health of brick kiln workers of Odisha. *J. Indian Soc. Periodontol.* **2019**, *23*, 163–167. [CrossRef]

29. Bessa Rebelo, M.A.; Corrêa de Queiroz, A. Gingival Indices: State of Art, Gingival Diseases–Their Aetiology. In *Prevention and Treatment*; Panagakos, F., Ed.; IntechOpen: London, UK, 2011; pp. 42–43. Available online: http://www.intechopen.com/books/gingival-diseases-their-aetiology-prevention-andtreatment/gingival-indices-state-of-art (accessed on 5 October 2021).
30. Batista, N.C.; Paula, C.P.; Poiate, I.A.V.P.; Poiate, E., Jr.; Zuza, E.C.; Camargo, G.A.C.G. Evaluation of periodontal indices in young adults submitted to chlorhexidine 0.12% mouthwash: A randomized clinical trial. *Rev. Odontol UNESP* **2021**, *50*, e20210045. [CrossRef]
31. Nazaryan, R.; Kryvenko, L. Salivary oxidative analysis and periodontal status in children with atopy. *Interv. Med. Appl. Sci.* **2017**, *9*, 199–203. Available online: https://akjournals.com/view/journals/1646/9/4/article-p199.xml (accessed on 31 December 2021). [CrossRef]
32. Aminoshariae, A.; Mackey, S.A.; Palomo, L.; Kulild, J.C. Declassifying Mobility Classification. *J. Endod.* **2020**, *46*, 1539–1544. [CrossRef]
33. Bosshardt, D.D. The periodontal pocket: Pathogenesis, histopathology and consequences. *Periodontology* 2000, *76*, 43–50. [CrossRef]
34. Dietrich, T.; Ower, P.; Tank, M.; West, N.X.; Walter, C.; Needleman, I.; Hughes, F.J.; Wadia, R.; Milward, M.R.; Hodge, P.J.; et al. British Society of Periodontology. Periodontal diagnosis in the context of the 2017 classification system of periodontal diseases and conditions–implementation in clinical practice. *Br. Dent. J.* **2019**, *226*, 16–22. [CrossRef]
35. Kwon, T.H.; Lamster, I.B.; Levin, L. Current Concepts in the Management of Periodontitis. *Int. Dent. J.* **2021**, *71*, 462–476. Available online: https://www.sciencedirect.com/science/article/pii/S0020653920365606) (accessed on 11 October 2021). [CrossRef]
36. Wandawa, G.; Mustaqimah, D.N.; Sidik, S.; Saraswati, H.; Putri, F.A.; Ibrahim, E. Efficacy of hyperbaric oxygen therapy as an adjunctive therapy of chronic periodontitis. *J. Int. Dent. Med Res.* **2017**, *10*, 72–75.
37. Soranta, N.P.; Hendiani, I.; Rusminah, N.; Wandawa, G.; Suhadi. Effects of Hyperbaric Oxygen Therapy on MMP-8 Saliva Levels in Chronic Periodontis: A Preliminary Research. *Int. J. Sci. Basic Appl. Res. (IJSBAR)* **2021**, *60*, 45–55.
38. Robo, I.; Heta, S.; Karkanaqe, L.; Ostreni, V. HBOT Application at Cases of Gingival Inflammation. *J. Dent. Oral Sci.* **2019**, *1*, 1–16. [CrossRef]
39. Chen, T.L.; Xu, B.; Liu, J.C.; Li, S.G.; Li, D.Y.; Gong, G.; Wu, Z.F.; Lin, S.L.; Yi-Jun Zhou, Y.J. Effects of hyperbaric oxygen on aggressive periodontitis and subgingival anaerobes in Chinese patients. *J. Indian Soc. Periodontol.* **2012**, *16*, 492–497. [CrossRef] [PubMed]
40. Balestra, C.; Kot, J. Oxygen: A Stimulus, Not "Only" a Drug. *Medicina* **2021**, *57*, 1161. [CrossRef] [PubMed]
41. Lu, C.; Saless, N.; Wang, X.; Sinha, A.; Decker, S.; Kazakia, H.; Hou, H.; Williams, B.; Swuartz, T.K.; Hunt, T.; et al. The role of oxygen during fracture healing. *Bone* **2013**, *52*, 220–229. [CrossRef]
42. Salmón-González, Z.; Anchuelo, J.; Borregán, J.C.; del Real, A.; Sañudo, C.; García-Unzueta, M.T.; Riancho, J.A.; Valero, C. Hyperbaric Oxygen Therapy Does Not Have a Negative Impact on Bone Signaling Pathways in Humans. *Healthcare* **2021**, *9*, 1714. [CrossRef]
43. Huang, E.; Heyboer, M., 3rd; Savaser, D.J. Hyperbaric oxygen therapy for the management of chronic wounds: Patient selection and perspectives. *Chronic Wound Care Manag. Res.* **2019**, *6*, 27–37. [CrossRef]
44. El-baz, F.; Elhossiny, R.M.; Azeem, Y.A.; Abdelsayed, M.G.R. Study the effect of hyperbaric oxygen therapy in Egyptian autistic children: A clinical trial. *Egypt. J. Med. Hum. Genet.* **2014**, *15*, 155–162. [CrossRef]
45. Bennett, M.H.; French, C.; Schnabel, A.; Wasiak, J.; Kranke, P.; Weibel, S. Normobaric and hyperbaric oxygen therapy for the treatment and prevention of migraine and cluster headache. *Cochrane Database Syst. Rev.* **2015**, *12*, CD005219. [CrossRef]
46. Devaraj, D.; Srisakthi, D. Hyperbaric oxygen therapy–can it be the new era in dentistry? *J. Clin. Diagn. Res.* **2014**, *8*, 263–265. [CrossRef]
47. Mathieu, D.; Marroni, A.; Kot, J. Tenth European Consensus Conference on Hyperbaric Medicine: Recommendations for accepted and non-accepted clinical indications and practice of hyperbaric oxygen treatment *J. S. Pac. Underw. Med. Soc.* **2017**, *47*, 24–32.
48. Chhabra, S.; Chhabra, N.; Kaur, A.; Gupta, N. Wound Healing Concepts in Clinical Practice of OMFS. *J. Maxillofac. Oral Surg.* **2017**, *16*, 403–423. [CrossRef] [PubMed]
49. Marcinkowska, A.B.; Mankowska, N.D.; Kot, J. Impact of Hyperbaric Oxygen Therapy on Cognitive Functions: A Systematic Review. *Neuropsychol. Rev.* **2021**, 1–28. [CrossRef] [PubMed]
50. Shah, D.N.; Chauhan, C.J.; Solanki, J.S. Effectiveness of hyperbaric oxygen therapy in irradiated maxillofacial dental implant patients: A systematic review with meta-analysis. *J. Indian Prosthodont. Soc.* **2017**, *17*, 109–119. [CrossRef]
51. Benites Condezo, A.F.; Araujo, R.Z.; Koga, D.H.; Curi, M.M.; Cardoso, C.L. Hyperbaric Oxygen Therapy for the Placement of Dental Implants in Irradiated Patients: Systematic Review and Meta-Analysis. *Br. J. Oral Maxillofac. Surg.* **2021**, *59*, 59625–59632. [CrossRef]
52. Hollander, M.H.J.; Boonstra, O.; Timmenga, N.M.; Schortinghuis, J. Hyperbaric Oxygen Therapy for Wound Dehiscence After Intraoral Bone Grafting in the Nonirradiated Patient: A Case Series. *J. Oral Maxillofac Surg.* **2017**, *75*, 2334–2339. [CrossRef]
53. Shih, Y.H.; Wang, T.H.; Shieh, T.M.; Tseng, Y.H. Oral Submucous Fibrosis: A Review on Etiopathogenesis, Diagnosis, and Therapy. *Int. J. Mol. Sci.* **2019**, *20*, 2940. [CrossRef]
54. Meligy, S.S.; Shehadat, S.A.A.I.; Samsudin, A.R. Hyperbaric oxygen therapy: A review of possible new era in dentistry. *J. Dent. Health Oral Disord Ther.* **2018**, *9*, 174–179. [CrossRef]
55. Side Effects. Available online: https://www.uhms.org/2-side-effects.html (accessed on 28 December 2021).

56. Heyboer, M., 3rd; Sharma, D.; Santiago, W.; McCulloch, N. Hyperbaric Oxygen Therapy: Side Effects Defined and Quantified. *Adv. Wound Care* **2017**, *6*, 210–224. [CrossRef]
57. Olex-Zarychta, D. Hyperbaric Oxygenation as Adjunctive Therapy in the Treatment of Sudden Sensorineural Hearing Loss. *Int. J. Mol. Sci.* **2020**, *21*, 8588. [CrossRef]
58. Gawdi, R.; Cooper, J.S. Hyperbaric Contraindications. [Updated 9 May 2021]. In *StatPearls [Internet]*; StatPearls Publishing: Tresure Island, FL, USA, 2021. Available online: https://www.ncbi.nlm.nih.gov/books/NBK557661/ (accessed on 28 December 2021).
59. Ortega, M.A.; Fraile-Martinez, O.; García-Montero, C.; Callejón-Peláez, E.; Sáez, M.A.; Álvarez-Mon, M.A.; García-Honduvilla, N.; Monserrat, J.; Álvarez-Mon, M.; Bujan, J.; et al. A General Overview on the Hyperbaric Oxygen Therapy: Applications, Mechanisms and Translational Opportunities. *Medicina* **2021**, *57*, 864. [CrossRef]
60. Bennett, M.H.; Mitchell, S.J. Hyperbaric and Diving Medicine. In *Harrison's Principles of Internal Medicine, 20e*; McGraw Hill: New York, NY, USA, 2018. Available online: https://accessmedicine.mhmedical.com/content.aspx?bookid=2129&sectionid=192510342 (accessed on 28 December 2021).
61. Peres, M.A.; Macpherson, L.M.D.; Weyant, R.J.; Daly, B.; Venturelli, R.; Mathur, M.R.; Listl, S.; Celeste, R.K.; Guarnizo-Herreño, C.; Kearns, C.; et al. Oral diseases: A global public health challenge. *Lancet* **2019**, *394*, 249–260, Erratum in *Lancet* **2019**, *394*, 1010. [CrossRef]
62. Lang, N.P.; Bartold, P.M. Periodontal health. *J. Clin. Periodontol.* **2018**, *45*, S9–S16. [CrossRef] [PubMed]
63. Giannakoura, A.; Pepelassi, E.; Kotsovilis, S.; Nikolopoulos, G.; Vrotsos, I. Tooth mobility parameters in chronic periodontitis patients prior to periodontal therapy: A cross-sectional study. *Dent. Oral Craniofac. Res.* **2019**, *5*, 1–8. Available online: https://www.oatext.com/tooth-mobility-parameters-in-chronic-periodontitis-patients-prior-to-periodontal-therapy-a-cross-sectional-study.php#Article (accessed on 27 October 2021). [CrossRef]
64. Ko, T.J.; Byrd, K.M.; Kim, S.A. The Chairside Periodontal Diagnostic Toolkit: Past, Present, and Future. *Diagnostics* **2021**, *11*, 932. [CrossRef]
65. Varadhan, K.B.; Parween, S.; Bhavsar, A.K.; Prabhuji, M.L.V. Tooth mobility measurements- realities and limitations. *J. Evol. Med. Dent. Sci.* **2019**, *8*, 1342–1350. [CrossRef]
66. Astuti, I.A.; Yunus, M.; Warih Gayatri, R. Effect of Patient's Knowledge and OHI-S on Periodontal Disease Among Age Group 19–64 Years in the Dental Clinic at the Community Health Centre, Bareng, Malang. ISMoPHS 2020. *KnE Life Sci.* **2020**, *2021*, 115–128. [CrossRef]

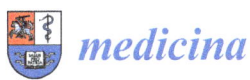

Article

Hyperbaric Oxygen Therapy with Iloprost Improves Digit Salvage in Severe Frostbite Compared to Iloprost Alone

Marie-Anne Magnan [1,*], Angèle Gayet-Ageron [2], Pierre Louge [1], Frederic Champly [3], Thierry Joffre [4], Christian Lovis [5] and Rodrigue Pignel [1]

1. Hyperbaric Medicine Unit, Department of Acute Medicine, University Hospitals of Geneva, 1205 Geneva, Switzerland; pierre.louge@hcuge.ch (P.L.); rodrigue.pignel@hcuge.ch (R.P.)
2. CRC & Division of Clinical-Epidemiology, Department of Health and Community Medicine, University of Geneva & University Hospitals of Geneva, 1205 Geneva, Switzerland; angele.gayet-ageron@hcuge.ch
3. Emergency Department of Mont-Blanc Hospitals, The Mont-Blanc Hospitals, 74700 Chamonix-Sallanches, France; f.champly@ch-sallanches-chamonix.fr
4. Hyperbaric Center, Hospices Civils de Lyon, University Hospitals of Lyon-1, 69003 Lyon, France; thierry.joffre@chu-lyon.fr
5. Division of Medical Information Sciences, Geneva University Hospitals and University of Geneva, 1205 Geneva, Switzerland; christian.lovis@hcuge.ch
* Correspondence: marie-anne.magnan-rondot@hcuge.ch

Abstract: *Background and Objectives*: Frostbite is a freezing injury that can lead to amputation. Current treatments include tissue rewarming followed by thrombolytic or vasodilators. Hyperbaric oxygen (HBO) therapy might decrease the rate of amputation by increasing cellular oxygen availability to the damaged tissues. The SOS-Frostbite study was implemented in a cross-border program among the hyperbaric centers of Geneva, Lyon, and the Mont-Blanc hospitals. The objective was to assess the efficacy of HBO + iloprost among patients with severe frostbite. *Materials and Methods:* We conducted a multicenter prospective single-arm study from 2013 to 2019. All patients received early HBO in addition to standard care with iloprost. Outcomes were compared to a historical cohort in which all patients received iloprost alone between 2000 and 2012. Inclusion criteria were stage 3 or 4 frostbite and initiation of medical care <72 h from frostbite injury. Outcomes were the number of preserved segments and the rate of amputated segments. *Results:* Thirty patients from the historical cohort were eligible and satisfied the inclusion criteria, and 28 patients were prospectively included. The number of preserved segments per patient was significantly higher in the prospective cohort (mean 13 ± SD, 10) compared to the historical group (6 ± 5, $p = 0.006$); the odds ratio was significantly higher by 45-fold (95%CI: 6-335, $p < 0.001$) in the prospective cohort compared to the historical cohort after adjustment for age and delay between signs of freezing and treatment start. *Conclusions:* This study demonstrates that the combination of HBO and iloprost was associated with higher benefit in patients with severe frostbite. The number of preserved segments was two-fold higher in the prospective cohort compared to the historical group (mean of 13 preserved segments vs. 6), and the reduction of amputation was greater in patients treated by HBO + iloprost compared with the iloprost only.

Keywords: frostbite; classification; hyperbaric oxygen therapy; cold disease; prognosis; amputation; medical outcome

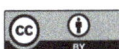

1. Introduction

Frostbite is an injury caused by freezing of the skin and underlying tissues. Severe frostbite is a relatively uncommon event that can lead to early arthritis, tissue loss, or amputation. Frostbite comprises on average 2% of mountain emergencies in the western Alps [1]. Frostbite takes place in three phases: pre-freeze/freezing, thawing/rewarming, and mummification.

Pre/freeze is an acute ischemia with peripheral vasoconstriction. During freezing, cell death is triggered by intracellular dehydration and direct damage to cell membrane by ice microcrystals. Thawing is best accomplished by the immersion of frozen limbs in warm water. After blood flow is restored, cyanotic lesions can occur. During rewarming, there is a vascular stasis with a prothrombotic environment (hypoxia and acidosis), interstitial edema, and ischemia–reperfusion injuries. It leads to the destruction of microcirculation and cell death [2,3]. Frostbite outcome is related to the initial cyanotic lesion. The Cauchy classification defines four grades that predict the amputation risk after rapid thawing in warm water when there is no targeted frostbite care [3]. It is based on the extent of the initial cyanotic lesion. Frostbite is classified as grade 1 if cyanosis disappears, grade 2 if only distal phalanges are cyanotic (amputation risk below 1%), grade 3 if cyanosis involves the intermediate or proximal phalanges (amputation risk: 30–83% greater in the hands than feet), and grade 4 if cyanosis involves the metacarpals or metatarsals (amputation risk: 99%) [3] (Figure 1).

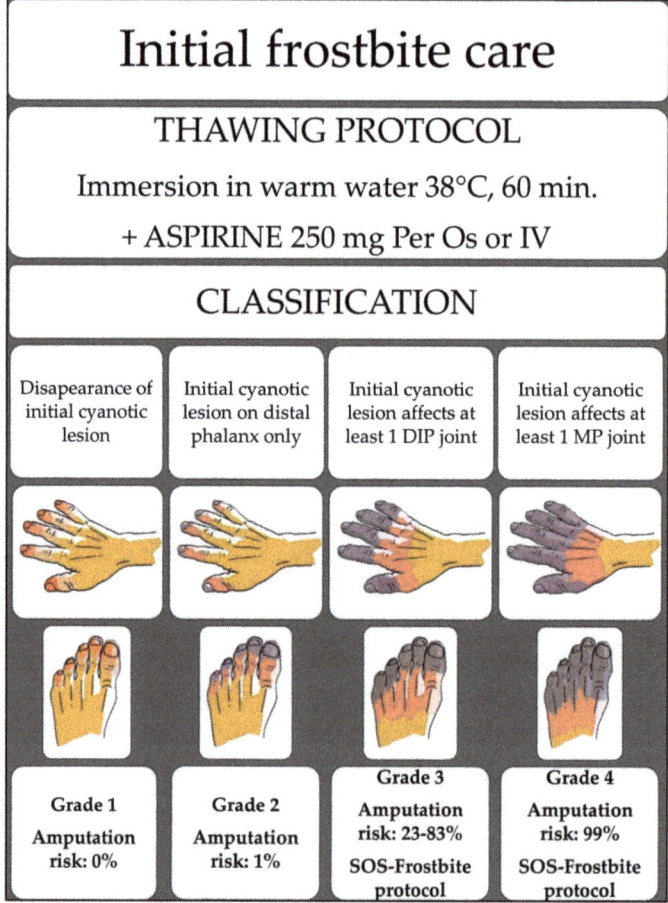

Figure 1. The frostbite classification by E. Cauchy (*drawings@copyright ifremmont*).

The goal of treatment is to limit tissue damage from hypoxia and acidosis, mitigate the subsequent prothrombotic cascade, reduce edema and the inflammatory response, and minimize the impact of the ischemic–reperfusion syndrome. Prior studies have demonstrated the efficacy of thrombolytics such as recombinant tissue plasminogen activator (rt-PA) [4] and vasodilator such as iloprost [5–7] in improving outcome [8]; medical care must be initiated within 24 h for rt-PA [9,10] and 48 h for iloprost [11]. Currently, the Wilderness Medical Society guidelines do not recommend HBO treatment for frostbite [8]. However, HBO may improve frostbite outcome by increasing the cellular oxygen availability to the damaged tissues. This may help to mitigate the negative impact of the inflammatory cascade and the ischaemia–reperfusion syndrome [12]. Few case reports suggest that HBO might improve frostbite injury outcome [13–23]. There are no randomized controlled trials (RCT) with HBO conducted so far. It is arduous to carry out a double-blinded RCT for HBO because frostbite is uncommon, and blinding subjects to HBO or not HBO could be difficult.

We implemented a cross-border European program (INTERREG-IV FRANCE-SUISSE) to foster and coordinate the care management of patients who suffer frostbite in the French and Swiss Alps.

2. Materials and Methods

2.1. Study Oversight

The SOS-Frostbite research program was a multicenter prospective, non-randomized study from 2013 to 2019. The study was conducted by the hyperbaric centers of Geneva and Lyon, and the Mont-Blanc hospitals in Chamonix and Sallanches. The statistical analysis was performed independently by the unit of methodological support from the CTU of Geneva University Hospital. The study aim was to assess whether the early addition of HBO to standard care with iloprost (prospective group) was associated with better frostbite outcomes compared to standard care alone (retrospective group).

2.2. Setting and Participants

Patients were eligible for the SOS-Frostbite protocol after screening determined no contraindication to aspirin, iloprost, or HBO. The inclusion criteria for both groups were grade 3 or 4 frostbite according to the Cauchy classification [3] and start of medical care within 72 h from frostbite injury, which was defined previously in the historical cohort as the onset of frostbite. Physicians involved in the study systematically searched for the onset of loss of sensitivity in the fingers or toes through the medical history to determine this time period.

To identify the historical cohort, we retrospectively collected data of all frostbite medical files treated at the Mont-Blanc hospital from 2000 to 2012. Before 2000, as the Cauchy classification had not yet been established, no patients could be included. All eligible patients who met the inclusion criteria from the retrospective analysis were included in the historical cohort. They were all grade 3 or 4 frostbitten patients who received a standardized protocol including iloprost, which was initiated no longer than 72 h from frostbite injury.

The standardized frostbite treatment: frostbitten extremities were rewarmed by immersion in warm water (38 °C) for 60 min, and patients were given aspirin 250 mg orally. During the hour following the rewarming, the frostbite classification was determined. Grade 3 or 4 frostbite patients received the first iloprost infusion immediately (by infusion pump, 8–10 mcg/h for 6 h, 48–60 mcg/day). Patients were hospitalized for 7 days to continue daily iloprost (by infusion pump, 8 to 10 mcg/h for 6 h, 48–60 mcg/day), aspirin (250 mg/day; orally), antibiotics (amoxicillin/clavulanate: 1 g/125 mg 3 times daily, orally for 7 days), and daily wound care with topical hyaluronic acid.

To identify the SOS-Frostbite group, data were prospectively collected from patients satisfying inclusion criteria who received the same standardized frostbite treatment protocol plus early HBO from 2013 to 2019.

The SOS Frostbite protocol: The SOS-Frostbite protocol was initiated upon hospital arrival. Patients were treated with the same standardized protocol as the historical cohort with the addition of HBO. The first HBO (150 min at 2.5ATA) session was done as soon as possible after the first iloprost infusion (from 1 to 6 h after the end of the iloprost infusion, as some patients were transferred from other hospitals to the Geneva or Lyon hyperbaric chamber for HBO). Then, patients were hospitalized for 7 days and received the same treatment protocol as in the historical cohort plus HBO sessions (150 min, 2.5 ATA, 1 daily) (Appendix A, Figure A1). After hospital discharge, the patient completed daily HBO sessions for 7 additional days (14 HBO session in total). Hyperbaric chambers involved in the study used multiplace chambers and patients breathed oxygen via a mask or a hood.

2.3. The Follow-Up

A Technecium 99 (Tc99) bone scan was performed at day 3 and day 7 (control group and prospective cohort). Results were considered pathological when the bone scan demonstrated absent or markedly decreased uptake of the Tc99 tracer in the bone tissue (severe bone ischemia). An additional Tc 99 bone scan was conducted at the end of the HBO sessions if radiological improvement (recovery of bone activity) was identified on the day 7 Tc99 bone scan compared to the day 3 Tc99 bone scan. All patients had a clinical examination at 6 months, 1 year. Patients enrolled in the first 4 years of the study also had a follow-up at 2 years and 3 years to evaluate early and delayed sequelae such as arthritis.

2.4. Outcomes

The study's primary outcome was the number of preserved segments at 12 months, which was defined as the difference between the number of segments with frostbite after rewarming and lost segments. Each phalanx and each metacarpal or metatarsal is defined as a segment; 4 segments comprise a ray (3 segments for the thumb or the hallux), and 3 out 4 segments make a digit (2 out 3 segments make the digit for the thumb or the hallux). To align with the eligibility criteria regarding frostbite severity (grade 3 or 4), we only considered rays with at least 2 segments damaged. The secondary outcomes were the number of amputated segments at 12 months and the ratio of the number of amputated segments at 12 months divided by the number of segments with initial frostbite injury.

2.5. Data Collection

All data from the prospective and the historical cohorts were collected on site using a standardized case report form. All observations were coded to preserve patient anonymity and data confidentiality.

2.6. Statistical Analysis

There was no preliminary estimation of study sample size; we used all available data on 31 December 2019 and obtained a fixed sample size of 58 patients. In the control group, we described 6 (mean ± SD, 5.3) preserved segments at 12 months post-treatment. We had 80% power to detect a two-fold increase in the number of preserved segments (+6) in the standard care plus HBO group, considering a larger variability of the difference of number of preserved segments (±10).

Continuous variables were reported as mean ± SD, median, and interquartile range. Categorical variables are reported as frequencies and percentages. We compared two cohorts of patients: those included between 2000 and 2012 (historical cohort) and those included after 2013 (prospective cohort). We compared continuous variables between the two cohorts of patients with the use of nonparametric Mann–Whitney test, as we anticipated that continuous variables are non-normally distributed and do not respect the assumptions for using Student's t-test; we compared categorical variables between the two cohorts with the use of chi-square or Fisher's exact tests, depending on assumptions, and p-values of less than 0.05 were considered to indicate statistical significance. Since the main outcome (number of preserved segments) was an ordinal variable (0, 1, 2, 3, and 4 preserved segments) and because one patient could have several data points for the main outcome (repeated measurements), we performed mixed ordinal logistic regressions with the patient identifier as a random factor. We compared the main outcome between the two cohorts of patients (HBO plus standard care vs. standard care alone). We adjusted the analysis for patient age, delay between signs of freezing and medical treatment received (<6 h, 6–12 h, 12–24 h, 24–48 h, and 48–72 h). For secondary outcome, we also performed mixed ordinal logistic regressions models as the number of amputations was also ordinal (3–4, 2, 1, 0 amputation), and we also adjusted the analysis for patient age and the delay between signs of freezing and medical treatment received. All analyses were performed with the use of STATA 16 IC (StatCorp, College Station, TX, USA).

3. Results
3.1. Description
3.1.1. Patients

The prospective cohort: Thirty-nine patients with grade 3 or 4 frostbite were treated from 2013 to 2019 with the SOS-Frostbite protocol; 11 patients were excluded because medical care delay was over 72 h from frostbite injury or the treatment protocol was interrupted or changed. For statistical analysis, 28 patients were prospectively included in the SOS-Frostbite group. None of the patients from the prospective cohort suffered from HBO side effects.

The retrospective cohort (control group): After reviewing all frostbite medical files in the Mont-Blanc hospitals (168 medical files), 30 patients met the inclusion criteria (standardized frostbite treatment with iloprost, grade 3 or 4 frostbite and medical care initiated within 72 h from frostbite injury) (Figure 2).

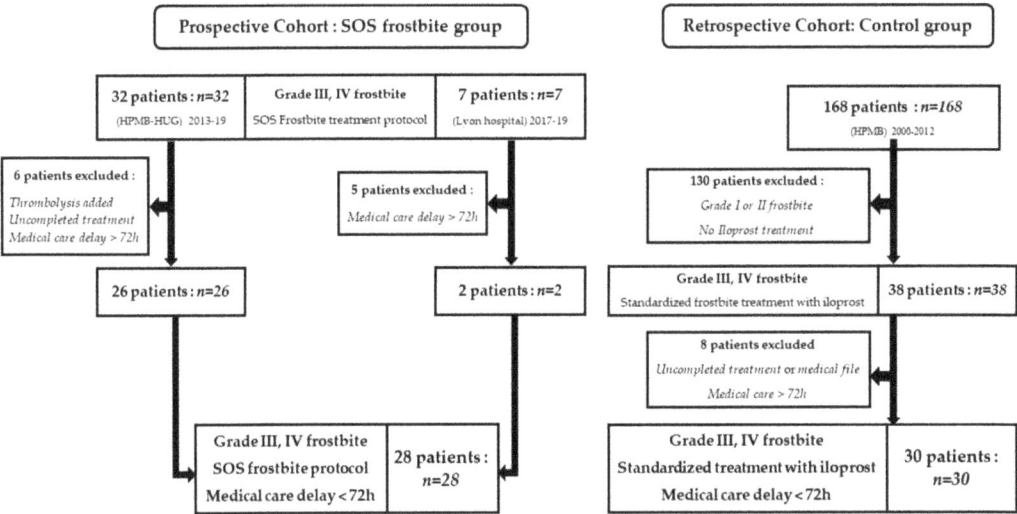

Figure 2. Study flow chart.

The SOS-Frostbite group and the historical control group both consisted of a similar number of patients with identical inclusion criteria.

The comparison of patient characteristics is presented in Table 1. Percentages of patients with delays of 12 to 24 h or 24 to 48 h were more frequent in the prospective cohort compared to the historical cohort. Patients were significantly older in the prospective than in the historical cohort. A higher proportion of patients with three or four segments with frostbite were observed in the prospective cohort compared to the control group ($p < 0.001$).

Table 1. Description of patients included in the study (n = study), the number of preserved digits, and the number of amputated segments.

Variables	Overall	Control Group (n = 30)	SOS Frostbite Group (n = 28)	p
Age at enrollment, mean ± SD (median: interquartile range), years	33 ± 11 (31: 26–40)	30 ± 9 (27: 25–35)	37 ± 12 (32: 28–43)	0.024 *
Sex, n (%)				
Male	54 (93)	29 (97)	25 (89)	0.344 **
Female	4 (7)	1 (3)	3 (11)	
Delay between frostbite and treatment, n (%)				
<6 h	6 (10)	5 (17)	1 (4)	
6–12 h	13 (22)	12 (40)	1 (4)	<0.001 **
12–24 h	19 (33)	10 (33)	9 (32)	
24–48 h	18 (31)	3 (10)	15 (54)	
48–72 h	2 (4)	0 (0)	2 (7)	
Frostbite location, n (%)				
Right hand	21 (18)	10 (15)	11 (22)	
Left hand	25 (22)	12 (18)	13 (27)	0.424 ***
Right foot	36 (32)	22 (34)	14 (29)	
Left foot	32 (28)	21 (33)	11 (22)	
Number of segments with frostbite, n (%)				
2	128 (54)	72 (67)	56 (43)	
3	89 (37)	32 (30)	57 (43)	<0.001 **
4	21 (9)	3 (3)	18 (14)	

* Mann–Whitney nonparametric test; ** Fisher's exact test; *** Chi-square test.

3.1.2. Outcomes

A significantly higher mean number of preserved segments per patient was observed in the prospective SOS-Frostbite group (13 SD ± 10) compared to the historical control group (6 SD ± 5) ($p = 0.006$). In the prospective cohort, 57% of patients had three to four preserved segments (respectively 43% for three segments and 14% for four segments) compared to 13% in the control group (respectively 13% for three segments and 0% for four segments). ($p < 0.001$, Table 2). At baseline, a higher but not statistically significant number of frostbitten segments was observed in the prospective than in the control group. However, a significantly higher number of frostbitten amputated segments was observed in the control than in the prospective group ($p = 0.014$, Table 2).

The odds ratio of the number of preserved segments was significantly higher by 20-fold (95%CI: 4-101, $p < 0.001$) in the prospective group who received standard care plus HBO compared to the control group (Table 3, model 1). This association remained after adjustment for patient age and delay between signs of freezing and medical treatment start (Table 3, model 2).

The association between the treatment received (cohort group) and a lower number of amputated segments was assessed. The odds of fewer amputated segments were significantly higher in the prospective group with standard care plus HBO compared to the control group with standard care alone (odds ratio 0.015; 95% CI: 0.0009; 0.25, $p = 0.003$). This association was reinforced after adjustment for patient age and delay between signs of freezing and onset of medical treatment, but due to very small numbers, the imprecision of the estimates was very large (odds ratio 0.0004; 95% CI: 0.00003; 0.06, $p = 0.002$).

Table 2. Comparison of outcomes between retrospective and prospective cohort studies.

Variables	Overall	Control Group (n = 30)	SOS Frostbite Group (n = 28)	p
Number of preserved segments per patient, mean ± SD (median: interquartile range)	9 ± 9 (6: 3–14)	6 ± 5 (4: 2–9)	13 ± 10 (8: 4–22.5)	0.006 *
Number of segments preserved, n (%)				
0	17 (7)	17 (16)	0 (0)	
1	12 (5)	10 (9)	2 (1)	<0.001 **
2	121 (51)	66 (62)	55 (42)	
3	70 (29)	14 (13)	56 (43)	
4	18 (8)	0 (0)	18 (14)	
Total number of rays among frostbite at baseline (n = 387), n (%)	21 (5)	3 (1)	18 (10)	0.124 ***
Total number of rays amputated among rays with frostbite at baseline (n = 21), n (%)	2 (10)	2 (40)	0 (0)	0.014 ****
Amputations per patient ±SD (median: interquartile range)	1 ± 4 (0: 0–0)	2 ± 6 (0: 0–1)	0.1 ± 0.3 (0: 0–0)	0.044 *
Ratio of amputation/injured digits				
nil	353 (92)	179 (85)	174 (98)	
One-third	4 (1)	3 (1)	1 (1)	
One-half	8 (2)	6 (3)	2 (1)	<0.001 ****
Two-thirds	5 (1)	5 (24)	0 (0)	
1	17 (4)	17 (8)	0 (0)	

* Mann–Whitney nonparametric test. ** Mixed ordinal logistic regression model with number of preserved digits coded as 0, 1, 2, 3, and 4 (five categories) as the dependent variable and group as the independent variable. *** Mixed logistic regression model with beam with frostbite (yes/no) as the dependent variable and group as the independent variable among observations with at least one segment with frostbite. **** Fisher's exact test.

Table 3. Association between treatment group and study outcome, univariate and multivariate analyses.

Number of Preserved Digits (Primary Outcome)	Odds Ratio	95%CI	p-Value
Model 1 (univariate analysis)			
Treatment received			
Standard	1	-	<0.001
Standard + HBOT	20	4–101	
Model 2 (multivariable analyses)			
Treatment received			<0.001
Standard	1	-	
Standard + HBOT	45	6–335	
Delay between signs of freezing and medical treatment			0.406
<6 h	1	-	-
6–12 h	2	0.08–40	0.702
12–24 h	1	0.06–21	0.951
24–48 h	0.3	0.01–6	0.389
48–72 h	3	0.03–259	0.659
Age of patient at enrollment	1	0.93–1	0.941

If we consider the ratio of segment amputation to all injured segments, a higher proportion of patients with one-third, half, two-thirds, or the total of segments amputated in the control group were observed compared to the standard care plus HBO group after 1-year follow-up (Table 2).

4. Discussion

This observational study is the first published prospective study reporting data on severe frostbite treated by early HBO.

In this study, HBO is a positive adjunct to treatment with iloprost. When started within 48 h from injury, iloprost can increase the segment salvage rate up to 78% in severe frostbite [24]. Iloprost has the highest recommendation level in frostbite treatment [8] and should be considered on grade 3 or 4 frostbites when rt-PA is contraindicated or is used in the field. Frostbite treatment with iloprost is strongly recommended, as it decreases the risk of amputation; HBO further improves segment salvage even if initiated after 48 h from frostbite injury.

This study did not compare the combined effect of thrombolytics and HBO. Thrombolytics are another recommended treatment that can lower the amputation rate from 41% to 10% when done within 24 h from frostbite injury [4]; a risk–benefit analysis should always be performed regarding bleeding risk and all contraindication to the treatment.

HBO is a non-invasive treatment; side effects are self-limiting and can mostly be avoided with appropriate screening [25]. In appropriate indications, the benefits of HBO frequently outweigh the risks. The US Food and Drug administration approved HBO for the treatment of acute ischemia, whereas iloprost has not yet been approved for such treatment. It can be performed on some people with contraindication to rt-PA due to the bleeding risk or in children. When available, HBO may be considered as an alternative treatment when there are contraindications to iloprost or thrombolytics. In our study, we showed that HBO plus standard care including iloprost significantly reduced the amputation risk even over 48h from frostbite injury.

The physiological mechanism of HBO action is well known [12–23], but there are no previous randomized controlled trials conducted to evaluate the added value of HBO on frostbite injury outcomes. Regarding frostbite physiopathology, there are good reasons as to why HBO could improve frostbite injury outcomes. HBO has a direct action on tissue ischemia, increasing dissolved oxygen and improving oxygen transportation in the blood. The HBO decreases blood viscosity and minimizes the inflammatory cascade. There is a hyperoxic vasoconstriction in the micro vascularization of healthy tissues, inducing a redistribution of blood to hypoxic territories. Those effects of HBO on vasoconstriction decrease edema and the incidence of compartment syndrome. There is a reduction of the deleterious influences of ischemia–reperfusion [12,26,27] besides diminishing damages due to the thaw–rewarming phase; HBO has an anti-infective activity due to its bactericidal effect on anaerobic germs and bacteriostatic action on aerobic germs so it can prevent infection during the mummification phase [12,28]. Finally, when repeated every day, HBO sessions induce vascular endothelium growth factor activation, fibroblast and collagen production, and thus the progression toward the resolution of tissue damage. HBO promotes the formation of the healing sulcus between necrotic and healthy tissues [12,28]. These clinical effects were described in recent retrospective studies [13].

Regarding the longer delay for medical care in the prospective cohort, the second aim of this INTERREG project was to set up a network for severe frostbite management. A SOS-Frostbite call center has been created. Some patients have been repatriated from far away to benefit from this research protocol, which could explain the longer delay for medical care from frostbite injury in the SOS-Frostbite group. Despite the longer delay for medical care in the SOS-Frostbite group, segment salvage was still significantly improved.

5. Conclusions

The SOS-Frostbite program is the first controlled prospective study that evaluates the effect of early HBO additive to iloprost on severe frostbite. Results show more favorable outcome in terms of the functionality and quality of life in patients treated by HBO: HBO added to the standard care with iloprost might improve frostbite injury outcomes by doubling the chance to preserve the number of injured segments from amputation.

Moreover, the benefits of HBO frequently outweigh the risks as contraindications and side effects are limited, in comparison to standard treatments such as rt-PA and iloprost. Transferring the patient suffering from severe frostbite to a hyperbaric center could be considered even if it implies delayed HBO, as it still improves frostbite outcomes after 48 h. Our findings should be tested in a randomized controlled trial before concluding that HBO should be added to standard care of severe frostbite in patients receiving iloprost.

6. Patents

The decision to design a prospective single arm study instead of two-arm randomized study was made because severe frostbite is an infrequent event [1,2]. We collected data on a small sample of 28 patients prospectively and compared the prospective cohort with data from a retrospective cohort from a previous double blinded RCT [5]. In both series, patients were mostly healthy, had little comorbidity, and had good access to medical care. Frostbite also occurs secondary to occupational exposure and in the homeless and migrant populations. The prognosis and outcome of frostbite for members of socially disadvantaged groups is likely much more severe. The fact our patients were healthy was an advantage, as frostbite was the only injury studied, inducing less bias from other pathologies. The Lyon hyperbaric site was more focused on the treatment of occupational accidents and injuries sustained by homeless patients. These patients were often hospitalized on medical services to treat comorbid conditions with an unfortunate delay in frostbite treatment. These patients were excluded if frostbite treatment was not initiated with 72 h.

Our study was not a randomized controlled trial. We tried to minimize selection and information biases using strict eligibility criteria. The allocation of the treatment group was not at random in our study, but we prespecified a list of criteria to select patients with very similar characteristics in this observational study in order to allow an unbiased comparison of treatment effects between the two treatment groups.

The two groups have a comparable number of patients, but those from the prospective group were older, had more severe frostbite, and the medical care delay was longer in comparison with the control group.

Another hypothesis is that HBO might prevent other side effects such as early arthritis by augmenting the healing process. It is still too early to present data, and it will not be possible to compare data with the historical cohort as there was no long-term follow up over 12 months.

Author Contributions: Conceptualization M.-A.M., R.P. and F.C.; methodology M.-A.M., R.P., P.L. and F.C.; software: C.L.; validation, M.-A.M., A.G.-A., P.L., F.C., T.J., C.L. and R.P.; formal analysis, A.G.-A.; investigation M.-A.M., P.L., F.C. and T.J.; data curation R.P. and M.-A.M.; writing—original draft preparation M.-A.M. and A.G.-A.; writing—review and editing, M.-A.M., A.G.-A., P.L. and R.P.; visualization M.-A.M., R.P. and P.L.; supervision M.-A.M. and R.P.; project administration: M.-A.M.; funding acquisition M.-A.M., R.P. and F.C. All authors have read and agreed to the published version of the manuscript.

Funding: The SOS-Frostbite program had financial support by the Interreg IV France-Switzerland and the Swiss Confederation. The Interreg committee and the Swiss Confederation had no influence on the design and the conduct of the trial and were not involved in data collection or analysis in writing of or submitting the manuscript. There was no commercial support for this study.

Institutional Review Board Statement: This trial was conducted according to the guidelines of the Declaration of Helsinki and was approved by the institutional review board at the University of Geneva and the French Committee on the Protection of the Persons in Biomedical Research (CCPPRB) approved the study protocol (protocol code 14-053 on 14 October 2015).

Informed Consent Statement: Informed consent was obtained from all subjects involved in the study and written informed consent form has been obtained from the patient(s) to publish this paper. Each patient received oral and written information about the treatment and signed a written consent form.

Data Availability Statement: All data from the prospective and the historical cohorts were collected on site using a standardized case report form in the international frostbite registry. All observations were coded to preserve patient anonymity and data confidentiality.

Acknowledgments: We honor the memory of Emmanuel Cauchy, who unfortunately died in an avalanche in 2018. He was a medical doctor specialized in mountain medicine and a mountain guide. He initiated the SOS-Frostbite program in 2013. We thank the INTERREG France-Suisse IV program and the Swiss Confederation for its financial support.

Conflicts of Interest: The authors declare no conflict of interest. The Interreg committee and the Swiss Confederation had no role in the design of the study; in the collection, analyses, or interpretation of data; in the writing of the manuscript, or in the decision to publish the results.

Appendix A

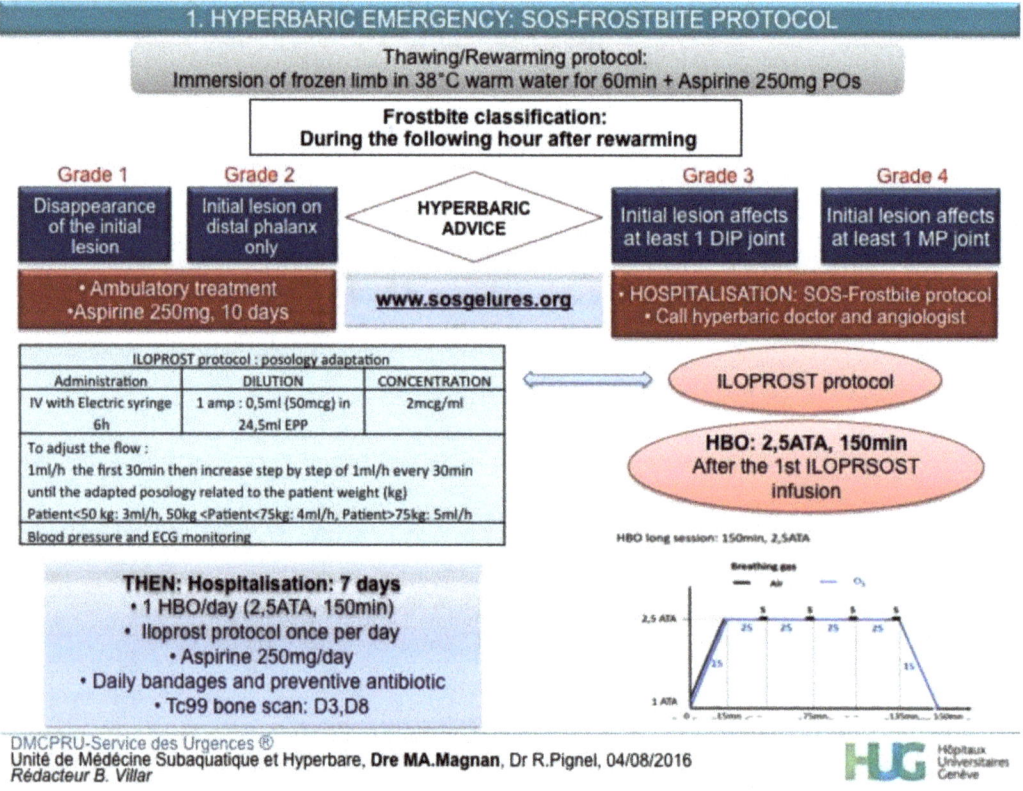

Figure A1. The SOS-Frostbite protocol during hospitalization at university hospitals of Geneva.

References

1. Brustia, R.; Enrione, G.; Catuzzo, B.; Cavoretto, L.; Campagnoni, M.P.; Visetti, E.; Cauchy, E.; Ziegler, S.; Giardini, G.; on behalf of RESAMONT 2 Project Group. Results of a Prospective Observational Study on Mountaineering Emergencies in Western Alps: Mind Your Head. *High Alt. Med. Biol.* **2016**, *17*, 116–121. [CrossRef]
2. Hallam, M.-J.; Cubison, T.; Dheansa, B.; Imray, C. Managing frostbite. *BMJ* **2010**, *341*, c5864. [CrossRef] [PubMed]
3. Cauchy, E.; Chetaille, E.; Marchand, V.; Marsigny, B. Retrospective study of 70 cases of severe frostbite lesions: A proposed new classification scheme. *Wilderness Environ. Med.* **2001**, *12*, 248–255. [CrossRef]
4. Bruen, K.J. Reduction of the Incidence of Amputation in Frostbite Injury with Thrombolytic Therapy. *Arch. Surg.* **2007**, *142*, 546–553. [CrossRef]

5. Cauchy, E.; Cheguillaume, B.; Chetaille, E. A Controlled Trial of a Prostacyclin and rt-PA in the Treatment of Severe Frostbite. *N. Engl. J. Med.* **2011**, *364*, 189–190. [CrossRef]
6. Irarrázaval, S.; Besa, P.; Cauchy, E.; Pandey, P.; Vergara, J. Case Report of Frostbite with Delay in Evacuation: Field Use of Iloprost Might Have Improved the Outcome. *High Alt. Med. Biol.* **2018**, *19*, 382–387. [CrossRef]
7. Cauchy, E.; Davis, C.B.; Pasquier, M.; Meyer, E.F.; Hackett, P.H. A New Proposal for Management of Severe Frostbite in the Austere Environment. *Wilderness Environ. Med.* **2016**, *27*, 92–99. [CrossRef] [PubMed]
8. McIntosh, S.E.; Freer, L.; Grissom, C.K.; Auerbach, P.S.; Rodway, G.W.; Cochran, A.; Giesbrecht, G.G.; McDevitt, M.; Imray, C.H.; Johnson, E.L.; et al. Wilderness Medical Society Practice Guidelines for the prevention and treatment of Frostbite: 2019 up-date. *Wilderness Environ. Med.* **2019**, *30*, S19–S32. [CrossRef]
9. Millet, J.D.; Brown, R.K.J.; Levi, B.; Kraft, C.T.; Jacobson, J.A.; Gross, M.D.; Wong, K.K. Frostbite: Spectrum of Imaging Findings and Guidelines for Management. *Radiographics* **2016**, *36*, 2154–2169. [CrossRef] [PubMed]
10. Gonzaga, T.; Jenabzadeh, K.; Anderson, C.P.; Mohr, W.J.; Endorf, F.W.; Ahrenholz, D.H. Use of Intra-arterial Thrombolytic Therapy for Acute Treatment of Frostbite in 62 Patients with Review of Thrombolytic Therapy in Frostbite. *J. Burn. Care Res.* **2016**, *37*, e323–e334. [CrossRef] [PubMed]
11. Poole, A.; Gauthier, J. Treatment of severe frostbite with iloprost in northern Canada. *Can. Med Assoc. J.* **2016**, *188*, 1255–1258. [CrossRef]
12. Camporoso, E.; Bosco, G. Mechanisms of action of hyperbaric oxygen therapy. *Undersea Hyperb. Med.* **2014**, *41*, 247–252. [PubMed]
13. Ghumman, A.; Denis-Katz, H.S.; Ashton, R.; Wherrett, C.; Malic, C. Treatment of Frostbite With Hyperbaric Oxygen Therapy: A Single Center's Experience of 22 Cases. *Wounds* **2019**, *31*, 322–325. [PubMed]
14. Gage, A.A.; Ishikawa, H.; Winter, P.M. Experimental frostbite. The effect of hyperbaric oxygenation on tissue survival. *Cryo Biol.* **1970**, *7*, 1–8. [CrossRef]
15. Okuboye, A.J.; Ferguson, C.C. The use of hyperbaric oxygen in the treatment of experimental frostbite. *Can. J. Surg.* **1968**, *11*, 78–84. [PubMed]
16. Higdon, B.; Youngman, L.; Regehr, M.; Chiou, A. Deep Frostbite Treated With Hyperbaric Oxygen and Thrombolytic Thera-pies. *Wounds* **2015**, *27*, 215–223. [PubMed]
17. Singhal, S.; Dwivedi, D.A.; Alasinga, S.; Malhotra, V.K.; Kotwal, A. Successful treatment of frostbite with hyperbaric oxygen treatment. *Indian J. Occup. Environ. Med.* **2015**, *19*, 121–122. [CrossRef]
18. Lansdorp, A.C.; Roukema, G.R.; Boonstra, O.; Dokter, J.; Van Der Vlies, C.H. Delayed treatment of frostbite with hyperbaric oxygen: A report of two cases. *Undersea Hyperb. Med.* **2017**, *44*, 365–369. [CrossRef]
19. Kemper, T.C.P.M.; De Jong, V.M.; Anema, A.H.; Brink, A.V.D.; Van Hulst, A.R. Frostbite of both first digits of the foot treated with delayed hyperbaric oxygen:a case report and review of literature. *Undersea Hyperb. Med.* **2014**, *41*, 65–70.
20. Finderle, Z.; Cankar, K. Delayed treatment of frostbite injury with hyperbaric oxygen therapy: A case report. *Aviat. Space Environ. Med.* **2002**, *73*, 392–394.
21. Robins, M. Early treatment of frostbite with hyperbaric oxygen and pentoxifylline: A case report. *Undresea Hyperb. Med.* **2019**, *46*, 521–526.
22. Robins, M.; Cooper, J.S. *Hyperbaric Management of Frostbite*; StatPearls (Internet); StatPearls: Treasure Island, FL, USA, 2019.
23. Cauchy, E.; Leal, S.; Magnan, M.-A.; Nespoulet, H. Portable Hyperbaric Chamber and Management of Hypothermia and Frostbite: An Evident Utilization. *High Alt. Med. Biol.* **2014**, *15*, 95–96. [CrossRef] [PubMed]
24. Lindford, A.; Valtonen, J.; Hult, M.; Kavola, H.; Lappalainen, K.; Lassila, R.; Aho, P.; Vuola, J. The evolution of the Helsinki frostbite management protocol. *Burn* **2017**, *43*, 1455–1463. [CrossRef] [PubMed]
25. Heyboer, M.; Sharma, D.; Santiago, W.; McCulloch, N. Hyperbaric Oxygen Therpay/Side Effects Defined and Quantified. *Adv. Wound Care* **2017**, *6*, 210–224. [CrossRef]
26. Haapaniemi, T.; Nylander, G.; Sirsjö, A.; Larsson, J. Hyperbaric Oxygen Reduces Ischemia-Induced Skeletal Muscle Injury. *Plast. Reconstr. Surg.* **1996**, *97*, 602–607. [CrossRef]
27. Hentia, C.; Rizzato, A.; Camporesi, E.; Yang, Z.; Muntean, D.M.; Săndesc, D.; Bosco, G. An overview of protective strategies against ischemia/reperfusion injury: The role of hyperbaric oxygen preconditioning. *Brain Behav.* **2018**, *8*, e00959. [CrossRef]
28. Mark, W.J.; Jeffrey, S.C. *Hyperbaric Therapy for Wound Healing*; Statpearls Publishing: Treasure Island, FL, USA, 2021.

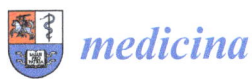

Systematic Review

A Systematic Review to Assess the Impact of Hyperbaric Oxygen Therapy on Glycaemia in People with Diabetes Mellitus

Sudhanshu Baitule [1,*,†], Aaran H. Patel [1,2,*,†], Narasimha Murthy [1,2], Sailesh Sankar [1,2], Ioannis Kyrou [1,2,3,4], Asad Ali [1,2], Harpal S. Randeva [1,2] and Tim Robbins [1,2,3,5,*]

1. Warwickshire Institute for the Study of Diabetes, Endocrinology & Metabolism, University Hospitals Coventry & Warwickshire NHS Trust, Clifford Bridge Road, Coventry CV2 2DX, UK; narasimha.murthy@uhcw.nhs.uk (N.M.); Sailesh.Sankaranarayanan@uhcw.nhs.uk (S.S.); kyrouj@gmail.com (I.K.); Asad.Ali@uhcw.nhs.uk (A.A.); harpal.randeva@uhcw.nhs.uk (H.S.R.)
2. Warwick Medical School, Faculty of Science, Engineering and Medicine, University of Warwick, Coventry CV4 7AL, UK
3. Faculty of Health & Life Sciences, Coventry University, Coventry CV1 5FB, UK
4. Aston Medical School, College of Health and Life Sciences, Aston University, Birmingham B4 7ET, UK
5. Institute of Digital Healthcare, WMG, University of Warwick, Coventry CV4 7AL, UK
* Correspondence: Sudhanshu.Baitule@uhcw.nhs.uk (S.B.); Aaran.Patel@uhcw.nhs.uk (A.H.P.); Timothy.Robbins@uhcw.nhs.uk (T.R.)
† Joint first authors.

Abstract: *Background and Objectives*: Hyperbaric oxygen is a recognised treatment for a range of medical conditions, including treatment of diabetic foot disease. A number of studies have reported an impact of hyperbaric oxygen treatment on glycaemic control in patients undergoing treatment for diabetic foot disease. There has been no systematic review considering the impact of hyperbaric oxygen on glycaemia in people with diabetes. *Materials and Methods*: A prospectively PROSPERO-registered (PROSPERO registration: CRD42021255528) systematic review of eligible studies published in English in the PUBMED, MEDLINE, and EMBASE databases, based on the following search terms: hyperbaric oxygen therapy, HBO2, hyperbaric oxygenation, glycaemic control, diabetes, diabetes Mellitus, diabetic, HbA1c. Data extraction to pre-determined piloted data collection form, with individual assessment of bias. *Results*: In total, 10 eligible publications were identified after screening. Of these, six articles reported a statistically significant reduction in blood glucose from hyperbaric oxygen treatment, while two articles reported a statistically significant increase in peripheral insulin sensitivity. Two articles also identified a statistically significant reduction in HbA1c following hyperbaric oxygen treatment. *Conclusions*: There is emerging evidence suggesting a reduction in glycaemia following hyperbaric oxygen treatment in patients with diabetes mellitus, but the existing studies are in relatively small cohorts and potentially underpowered. Additional large prospective clinical trials are required to understand the precise impact of hyperbaric oxygen treatment on glycaemia for people with diabetes mellitus.

Keywords: diabetes; hyperbaric oxygen therapy; glycaemia

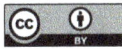

1. Introduction

The use of hyperbaric oxygen in treating decompression sickness in deep-sea divers and people with carbon monoxide poisoning is well-established [1]. Hyperbaric oxygen therapy (HBOT) is also an approved medical treatment for various conditions including necrotizing soft tissue infection, diabetic wounds, osteomyelitis, compartment syndrome, crush and reperfusion injuries, and acute sensorineural hearing loss [1]. HBOT has been postulated to have a positive impact on diabetic foot ulcers, suggesting its incorporation as an adjunct treatment with further scope for research in this area [2,3].

HBOT involves oxygen delivery at a concentration of 100% with a pressure of 2 to 3 atmosphere absolute (ATA) in a hyperbaric chamber. The mechanism of HBOT is to increase tissue oxygen levels resulting in accelerated wound healing, decreased oedema, and killing of anaerobic bacteria [4,5].

In diabetes, meticulous glycaemic control has been shown to reduce the risk of microvascular, macrovascular, and neurological complications [6,7]. There is emerging evidence demonstrating blood glucose level changes in people with diabetes undergoing hyperbaric oxygen treatment [8–12]. However, these studies have involved diverse methodologies, whilst, to date, there has been no systematic review of the impact of HBOT on glycaemia in people with diabetes.

Here, we present the first systematic review considering the effect of HBOT on the glycaemia in people with diabetes. We also explore the proposed mechanisms involved in the potential impact of HBOT on glycaemia in diabetes.

2. Materials and Methods

The systematic review was performed according to the PRISMA protocol as shown in Figure 1 [13]. The review was prospectively registered on the NIHR PROSPERO Database (PROSPERO registration ID: CRD42021255528).

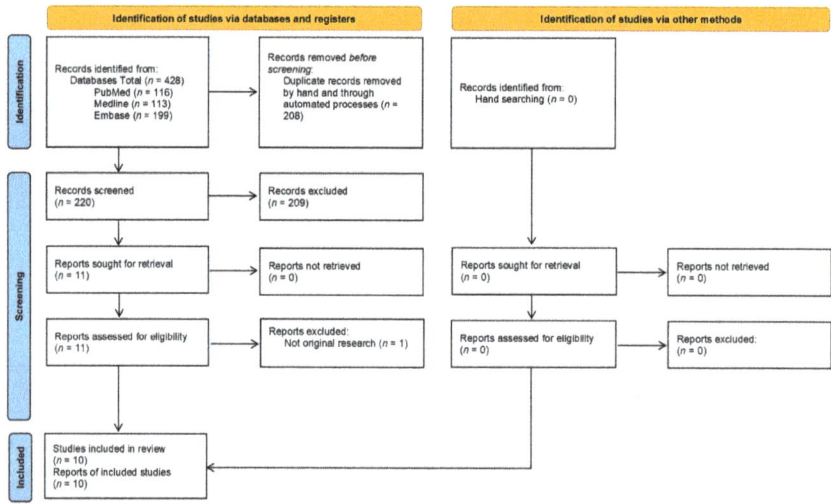

Figure 1. Diagram demonstrating the search strategy used according to the PRISMA protocol [13].

2.1. Study Selection

The literature search was conducted in the PUBMED, MEDLINE, and EMBASE databases. The search terms used to identify the relevant medical literature were Hyperbaric oxygen therapy/HBO2/hyperbaric oxygenation; Glycaemic control; Diabetes/diabetic/diabetes mellitus; HbA1c. The search strategies used are detailed in the Appendix A(Tables A1–A3). Only studies involving humans whichwere published in English language journals were considered eligible, with no restriction to the publication date. Furthermore, filters were applied to set participant's age as 18 years and above, as this research looked at only the adult population with any type of diabetes (excluding diabetes insipidus) who had undergone HBOT. Any study that focused only on animals, children, or hyperbaric combination therapies was excluded. Any studies focusing on wound care and insulin sensitivity were also excluded. Studies focused on insulin sensitivity but mentioning glycaemia as an outcome in their abstracts were included.

2.2. Data Extraction

Data were extracted to a pre-defined, data-extraction proforma which was based on the following variables: year of publication, type of study, location of research and publication, sample size including the baseline characteristics of the population, any biases, single centre or multicentre study, length of follow up comprising of a number of session of interventions, statistical methods used for analysis showing the statistically significant outcome. Miscellaneous variables relevant to this systematic review were also extracted. Data extraction was performed independently by two authors (S.B. and A.P.), with any discrepancies resolved by a third author (T.R.).

2.3. Quality Assessment

All studies included in the review were assessed for study quality. Due to the small number of studies and diverse methodologies a single formal tool was not used. Instead, a narrative review was conducted for bias considering sample size, study methodology, any evidence of randomisation, and blinding. All studies were assessed independently for bias by two authors (S.B. and A.P.). Papers were not excluded based on producing a negative outcome or being of low-quality.

2.4. Data Synthesis

The diversity among the identified eligible studies, in terms of their study design, sample size and population, did not allow a meta-analysis to be conducted. A qualitative analysis and narrative summary of the studies reporting any change or any factors that pre-dispose to changes in HbA1c were performed. Where possible, these changes have then been grouped under broader categories in a tabulated form.

3. Results

The performed systematic search yielded 428 records. Of these, 208 were duplicates and, thus, were removed prior to screening of titles and abstracts. Of the 220 records screened, 11 articles were selected for a detailed review. One of these was excluded after detailed review as it was a letter to editor and not an original research article [10]. In total, 10 studies were eligible for inclusion in this systematic review, which were all available as full text articles. The designs and locations of these studies are summarised in Tables 1 and 2. The characteristics and findings of the individual eligible studies are summarised in Table 3.

Table 1. Summary of study designs included in this systematic review.

Study Design	Number of Studies	Percentage of Studies (%)
Prospective cohort	7	70
Randomised placebo-controlled trial	1	10
Retrospective analysis	2	20

Table 2. Summary of locations (countries) of the studies included in this systematic review.

Study Location	Number of Studies
United States	3
Australia	3
China	1
Indonesia	1
Israel	1
Portugal	1

Table 3. Summary of the characteristics and findings of the ten eligible original research studies included in this review. DM = Diabetes Mellitus HTN = Hypertension, HBOT = Hyperbaric oxygen therapy, HbA1c = Glycated haemoglobin, IQR = Interquartile range, OGTT = oral glucose tolerance test, T1DM = type 1 diabetes mellitus, T2DM = type 2 diabetes mellitus.

	Data Collection	Study Design	Study Location	Sample Size	Sub-Population	Length of HBOT	Controls	Statistically Significant Outcomes	Other Notable Outcomes
Heyboer et al.2019 [8]	Single Centre	Retrospective analysis	United States	77 patients	Patients with diabetes mellitus undergoing HBOT for various indications	Median 19 sessions (IQR = 31)	None	Statistically significant greater percentage of treatments of patients with T2DM resulted in a decrease in blood glucose levels (77.5%) vs. T1DM ($p < 0.001$)	Blood glucose decreased in 75.4% of treatments in this group with a median decrease of 25 mg/dL (IQR = 54 mg/dL)
Irawan et al. 2018 [14]	Single Centre	Prospective cohort study	Indonesia	15 patients	Patients with diabetes mellitus and diabetic foot ulcers	10 sessions	No HBOT	Significant decrease in HbA1c after 10 session from 10.98 ± 2.37 % to 9.70 ± 2.46 % ($p = 0.006$)	None
Xu et al. 2017 [15]	Single Centre	Randomised, prospective, placebo controlled	China	23 patients	Patients with T2DM suffering from intracerebral haemorrhage	30 sessions	Normobaric oxygen therapy	A significant increase in insulin sensitivity during the HBOT sessions after 30 sessions ($p < 0.05$). Significant decreases in insulin, fasting glucose (11.3 ± 1.5 vs. 9.6 ± 1.1 mmol/L), and HbA1c (9.2 ± 1.6 vs. 7.8 ± 1.3%) in the HBOT group after 30 sessions ($p < 0.05$)	No change in insulin sensitivity, fasting plasma glucose of HbA1c in normobaric conditions.
Vera-Cruz et al. 2015 [16]	Single Centre	Prospective cohort study	Portugal	16 patients	Patients with T2DM and indications for HBOT	20 sessions	Patients without T2DM	Glycaemia measured following OGTT significantly decreased from 280.25 ± 22.29 mg/dL to 185.78 ± 11.70 mg/dL after 20 sessions of HBOT in patients with T2DM	HBOT decreased fasting plasma glucose levels to 119.1 ± 4.80 mg/dL in patients with T2DM, however without reaching statistical significance ($p = 0.089$)
Stevens et al. 2015 [17]	Single Centre	Retrospective analysis	United States	190 patients	Patients with diabetes mellitus receiving HBOT for various indications	1 session	None	None relevant	In-chamber glucose was higher than pre-HBOT glucose in 1708 of the 3136 HBOT sessions (54%)
Peleg et al. 2013 [11]	Single Centre	Prospective cohort crossover study	Israel	13 patients	Patients with insulin-and non-insulin-dependent diabetes mellitus with HBOT indicated for non-healing wound	1 session	Room air conditions at sea level pressure 13 patients with traumatic brain injury or stroke treated for neurological deficit 13 healthy volunteers	The non-insulin dependent diabetes mellitus patients had a significant decrease in their blood glucose levels during both sessions: from 9.2 ± 3.0 mmol/L to 7.3 ± 3.0 mmol/L during HBOT and from 9.9 ± 2.9 to 7.8 ± 3.4 mmol/L ($p = 0.004$) during the control normobaric session	The insulin-dependent patients had no change in blood glucose either during HBOT (13.0 ± 4.0 mmol/L before to 13.2 ± 5.7 mmol/L after, $p = 0.88$) or during the control session (13.15 ± 2.7 before to 13.2 ± 4.7 mmol/L after, $p = 0.96$)

Table 3. Cont.

	Data Collection	Study Design	Study Location	Sample Size	Sub-Population	Length of HBOT	Controls	Statistically Significant Outcomes	Other Notable Outcomes
Wilkinson et al. 2012 [18]	Single Centre	Prospective cohort study	Australia	5 patients	Obese patients with T2DM and indications for HBOT	30 sessions	Non-obese individuals without T2DM	Peripheral insulin sensitivity was significantly increased by HBOT at 3 and 30 visits in patients with T2DM. ($p = 0.008$). HbA1c was significantly reduced only in subjects without diabetes ($p < 0.05$)	No significant change in HbA1c after 30 visits in patients with T2DM. No change in fasting plasma glucose and insulin after 30 visits
Al-Waili et al. 2006 [19]	Single Centre	Prospective cohort study	United States	23 patients	Patients with diabetes mellitus and indications for HBOT	15–30 sessions	None	HBOT caused a significant drop in mean blood glucose approximately to the same extent in patients with diabetes mellitus alone or in patients with both diabetes mellitus and hypertension	Significant drop in blood glucose in 12 patients without HTN, and diabetes mellitus.
Trytko & Bennet 2003 [9]	Single Centre	Prospective cohort study	Australia	27 patients	Patients over 18 years old with diabetes mellitus and indications for HBOT	Up to 10 consecutive sessions	None	Mean reduction in blood glucose for each individual following HBOT of 2.04 ($p < 0.0001$)	T2DM were 102 of the recorded sessions and 80 of these had a reduction in blood glucose. Mean blood glucose reduction following HBOT did not significantly alter with treatment number during the course. In 17/23 patients who completed 10 sessions, there was a small and non-significant reduction in the mean HbA1c by 0.22% ($p = 0.06$)
Ekanayake & Doolette 2001 [12]	Single Centre	Prospective cohort crossover study	Australia	5 patients	Patients with diabetes mellitus of >6 years duration and indications for HBOT	1 session	Normobaric air conditions 5 patients without diabetes mellitus	Decline in glucose levels in both HBOT and normobaric conditions in patients with diabetes mellitus. Decline only reaches significance between time points after 45 min in HBOT	No change in serum insulin levels under any condition

Of the included studies, seven were prospective studies in cohorts of patients with diabetes, two presented retrospective analyses of prospectively collected data, and one study was a randomised, prospective, placebo-controlled trial in patients with type 2 diabetes mellitus. Most of these studies included participants with diabetes mellitus who were receiving HBOT for various indications, including non-healing wounds, diabetic foot ulcers, radio-induced cystitis and neurological deficits such as sudden deafness.

The majority of the included studies demonstrated a reduction in blood glucose levels following a single session of HBOT in patients with type 2 diabetes mellitus. This effect was consistent across different session lengths and treatment conditions used in the different studies. A prospective cross-over study by Ekanayake & Doolette demonstrated that blood glucose levels in five patients with diabetes mellitus reduced following exposure to both hyperbaric and normobaric conditions, but this decrease only reached significance following exposure to HBOT for at least 45 min [12]. However, this study did not find a significant reduction in blood glucose levels in control subjects without diabetes mellitus in either condition. A significant reduction in blood glucose following a HBOT session in patients with diabetes mellitus was also shown in a prospective study conducted by Trytko & Bennett, which assessed mean blood glucose change across up to 10 consecutive HBOT sessions per participant [9]. This study analysed 226 HBOT sessions across 27 patients, and reported that there was a decrease in blood glucose levels in 80 of the 102 sessions which were in patients with type 2 diabetes mellitus. A prospective cohort study in 23 patients with diabetes mellitus by Al-Waili et al. also demonstrated significant reduction in blood glucose levels as a mean across 15–30 HBOT sessions per participant [19]. Peleg et al. also showed statistically significant decrease in blood glucose levels after a HBOT session in patients with type 2 diabetes mellitus [11], while no significant reduction in blood glucose levels was noted in healthy volunteers without diabetes following HBOT, agreeing with the earlier findings by Ekanayake & Doolette. Moreover, the study by Peleg et al. did not find any significant reduction in blood glucose levels in patients with type 1 diabetes mellitus following exposure to both hyperbaric and normobaric conditions. A retrospective review by Heyboer et al. also found a greater impact of HBOT in patients with type 2 diabetes mellitus as opposed to those with type 1 diabetes mellitus [8]. This retrospective review of prospectively collected data showed that blood glucose levels in patients with diabetes mellitus decreased in 75.4% of 1825 HBOT cycles surveyed. However, on further analysis, a statistically significant greater percentage of treatments of patients with type 2 diabetes mellitus resulted in a decrease in blood glucose levels (77.5%) compared to treatments of patients with type 1 diabetes mellitus (51.5%).

Contrary, the study by Stevens et al. does not support this general finding of a reduction of blood glucose in patients with type 2 diabetes mellitus following HBOT [17]. This retrospective review of prospectively collected data from 190 patients with diabetes mellitus found that in-chamber glucose was higher than pre-HBOT glucose in 54% of sessions. However, there is no evidence in this study of statistical analysis of change in blood glucose levels following HBOT.

The potential mechanism for a reduction in blood glucose levels caused by HBOT appears to be mediated by increased insulin sensitivity, as opposed to enhanced insulin secretion. The study by Ekanayake & Doolette measured insulin levels in patients with diabetes mellitus during both a single session under hyperbaric and normobaric conditions, and found no change in insulin levels following treatment in either condition [12]. This finding was also seen in the study by Wilkinson, Chapman & Heilbronn; demonstrating that there was no change in fasting insulin levels measured in five patients with type 2 diabetes mellitus even after 30 sessions of HBOT performed over five weeks [18]. This study also demonstrated a statistically significant increase in peripheral insulin sensitivity after both 3 and 30 sessions of HBOT measured using a hyperinsulinaemic clamp in those patients with type 2 diabetes mellitus. A further study by Xu et al. subjected 23 patients with type 2 diabetes mellitus to 30 sessions of either hyperbaric or normobaric conditions and assessed peripheral insulin sensitivity using hyperinsulinaemic-euglycaemic clamps [15]. This study also demonstrated a significant increase in peripheral insulin sensitivity in patients with type 2 diabetes mellitus after 30 HBOT sessions, which was not seen in those exposed to normobaric conditions. However, this study also showed a significant decrease in insulin levels after 30 sessions in both HBOT and normobaric condition groups. This evidence further supports HBOT-induced increased insulin sensitivity as the proposed mechanism for reducing blood glucose levels in patients with type 2 diabetes mellitus.

The reduction in blood glucose levels in patients with type 2 diabetes mellitus attributed to HBOT appears to be longitudinal. The study by Xu et al. demonstrated a significant reduction in fasting plasma glucose after 30 sessions of HBOT [15]. A study by Vera-Cruz et al., which measured fasting plasma glucose and performed an oral glucose tolerance test (OGTT) at baseline and after 20 sessions of HBOT over four weeks, found that whilst fasting plasma glucose did not significantly decrease, there was a significant decrease in glycaemia following an OGTT after 20 sessions of HBOT in patients with type 2 diabetes mellitus [16]. Similarly, Wilkinson, Chapman & Heilbronn also showed no significant reduction in fasting plasma glucose after 30 sessions of HBOT [18].

HbA1c was used as an outcome measure in three studies following up participants after multiple sessions of HBOT. The study by Trytko & Bennett found that in 17 patients with type 2 diabetes mellitus who completed 10 sessions of HBOT, there was a small, non-significant reduction in HbA1c [9]. The study by Wilkinson, Chapman & Heilbronn also found no significant change in HbA1c after 30 sessions of HBOT [18]. However, the study by Xu et al. demonstrated a significant reduction in HbA1c after 30 sessions of HBOT, which was not seen in those exposed to normobaric conditions [16]. The study by Irawan et al. corroborates this finding of a reduction in HbA1c, with a significant reduction after 10 HBOT sessions [14].

Some studies suggest that the reduction in blood glucose levels in patients with type 2 diabetes mellitus following HBOT may be independent of the hyperbaric conditions. Peleg et al. found that there was a significant decrease in blood glucose for patients with type 2 diabetes after a session under normobaric control conditions [11]. Ekanayake & Doolette also identified a decrease in blood glucose levels following a session under normobaric conditions. However, this decrease did not reach significance [12]. Both of these studies had relatively small participant numbers and only considered the change in blood glucose after a single session. On the contrary, Xu et al. did not find any change in fasting plasma glucose or HbA1c after 30 sessions under control normobaric conditions [15]. This study by Xu et al. had a larger number of participants and considered the longitudinal impact on glycaemia after multiple sessions. The outcomes measured by Xu et al. could therefore be considered more reliable when considering the clinical utility of HBOT in type 2 diabetes mellitus as a treatment adjunct. However, these discrepancies highlight the need for further controlled trials with larger participant numbers to ascertain the true impact of HBOT on glycaemia in patients with type 2 diabetes mellitus compared to normobaric conditions.

Moreover, four of the studies do have a consideration for the incidence of hypoglycaemic events during or immediately after HBOT. The retrospective review by Heyboer et al. found that none of the patients with diabetes mellitus experienced a hypoglycaemic episode following a HBOT session [8]. However, the retrospective review by Stevens et al. found an incidence of 1.5% for hypoglycaemia during or immediately after HBOT in the 3136 sessions reviewed, but noted that severe or symptomatic hypoglycaemic events were rare [17]. The prospective study by Trytko & Bennett had symptomatic hypoglycaemia occur in 11 out of 237 HBOT treatments in patients with diabetes mellitus; only two of these occurring in patients not requiring insulin treatment [9]. Al-Waili et al. also reported occurrences of symptomatic hypoglycaemic episodes in two of the 41 study participants undergoing HBOT; one of these being an insulin-treated diabetes mellitus patient [19]. Patients with type 1 diabetes mellitus are at an increased risk of hypoglycaemic episodes with HBOT, as found in the study by Stevens et al. and suggested by the results of the Trytko & Bennett study [9,17]. A suggestion is made for a threshold blood glucose level below which the risk of hypoglycaemia during HBOT is increased, with Al-Waili et al. noting this threshold level to be 120 mg/dL, whilst the data from Stevens et al. suggesting that this threshold blood glucose level is 150 mg/dL [17,19].

There are a number of sources of bias to consider when interpreting these studies. The most significant would be the presence of sampling bias. Moreover, most of the studies included for analysis in this review had relatively small sample sizes. Even those with large numbers of HBOT sessions often sourced these from a small number of participants. The small sample sizes used may reduce the reliability of the obtained results and the external validity of the reported findings. These small sample sizes may have also impacted the power of the studies to identify significant changes in glycaemic variables, such as HbA1c, which HBOT may impact in the longer-term.

A number of the studies included patients with both type 1 and type 2 diabetes mellitus that were analysed together in a single diabetes mellitus group. Evidence presented suggests that the effects of HBOT on blood glucose differ between type 1 and type 2 diabetes mellitus when the subgroups are analysed. Therefore, including both patients with type 1 and type 2 diabetes together may impact the demonstrated effects of HBOT.

The patients included in the majority of these studies received HBOT for treatment of diverse conditions. Common indications for HBOT included non-healing ulcers and diabetic foot ulcers. These indications for HBOT can be associated with poorly controlled diabetes mellitus or long-standing disease, with most studies also having an older age range of participants. These factors could also have an effect on the impact of HBOT on glycaemia.

Another source of bias to consider is that the identified studies have included different HBOT protocols. This included different hyperbaric conditions, different lengths of treatments, and different numbers of treatment sessions per patient. Heyboer et al. have adjusted for this by using each treatment as a unit of analysis as opposed to each participant [8]. Al-Waili et al. and Trytko & Bennet have taken this into account by measuring the mean for each patient as the unit of analysis [9,19]. Trytko & Bennet also found that mean blood glucose reduction following treatment did not significantly alter with treatment number during the course. However, the methodology used by Peleg et al. suggests that the number of treatment sessions is an important factor. Peleg et al. suggest that factors such as anxiety when first introduced to the chamber environment may act as a confounding factor, and so recruited only patients who had already received at least 10 sessions of HBOT to limit this [11]. Ekanayake & Doolette incorporated a similar principle into their methodology for the same reason, only sampling blood glucose and insulin on the third to fifth day of HBOT [12]. Indeed, the findings from the study by Xu et al. also suggest that the number of treatment sessions is influential, with significant changes in insulin sensitivity, HbA1c and fasting plasma glucose only after 30 session of HBOT [15]. Whilst an increase in insulin sensitivity and decreases in fasting plasma glucose and HbA1c were also observed after 10 sessions of HBOT, these changes were not significant.

Finally, two of the prospective studies were cross-over in design [11,12]. Ekanayake & Doolette had all participants exposed to control normobaric conditions on the day of their HBOT session. Peleg et al. had all participants receive their HBOT session before their normobaric session between 1–14 days later. Randomising the sequence of exposures for participants may have helped to ensure that the sequence of exposures is not influencing the results seen.

4. Discussion

The impact of HBOT on glycaemia in people with diabetes mellitus is an area of contention as demonstrated by several published studies [8–12]. This review represents the first systematic review conducted on the published research literature to explore the potential impact of HBOT on glycaemic control in people with diabetes. A total of 10 studies were eligible to be included in this systematic review which comprised of seven prospective cross-over and cohort studies; two retrospective reviews of prospectively collected quality data; and one randomised, prospective, placebo-controlled trial.

The majority of the studies demonstrated a reduction in blood glucose levels following HBOT in patients with diabetes, mainly for people with type 2 diabetes mellitus [8,9,15]. The nine original studies reviewed showcased various results involving different methodologies. Variables observed included the use of HBOT and normobaric conditions in people with diabetes mellitus (mainly those with type 2 diabetics mellitus) with assessment of changes in insulin levels, insulin sensitivity, OGTT, and HbA1c (Table 4). Whilst most of the studies support the hypothesis that HBOT reduces blood glucose levels in patients with type 2 diabetes mellitus, there was one study that demonstrated high in-chamber glucose levels contrasting the other study findings [17]. Blood glucose levels, both basal and following an OGTT, were also reduced in people with type 2 diabetes mellitus after several sessions of HBOT [18,19]. Whilst some studies did show a significant reduction in HbA1c following HBOT, the impact seen was not consistent [9,14,15,18]. This highlights the need for large prospective trials to ascertain the precise longer-term effects of HBOT on glycaemia in people with type 2 diabetes mellitus.

Table 4. Summary of the eligible studies reviewed with their outcomes for this systematic review.

Year	Study Reference	Impact on Fasting Blood Glucose	Change in Insulin Levels	Peripheral Insulin Sensitivity	Impact on OGTT 2-h Glucose Level	HbA1c Change
2019	Heyboer et al. [8]	Decrease *	NA	NA	NA	NA
2018	Irawan et al. [14]	NA	NA	NA	NA	Decrease *
2017	Xu et al. [15]	Decrease *	Decrease *	Increased *	NA	Decrease *
2015	Vera-Cruz et al. [16]	Decrease	NA	NA	Decrease *	NA
2015	Stevens et al. [17]	Increase †	NA	NA	NA	NA
2013	Peleg et al. [11]	Decrease *	NA	NA	NA	NA
2012	Wilkinson et al. [18]	No change	No change	Increased *	NA	No change
2006	Al-Waili et al. [19]	Decrease *	NA	NA	NA	NA
2003	Trytko & Bennet. [9]	Decrease *	NA	NA	NA	Decrease
2001	Ekanayake & Doolette. [12]	Decrease *	No change	NA	NA	NA

* Indicates statistical significance. † There is no evidence in this study of statistical analysis of change in blood glucose levels following HBOT. OGTT = Oral Glucose Tolerance Test, HbA1c = Glycated haemoglobin. Green background colour indicates a positive impact, red background colour indicates a negative impact and an orange background colour indicates no impact.

The mechanism responsible for the reduction in blood glucose levels caused by HBOT appears to be, at least in part, attributed to increased insulin sensitivity as opposed to enhanced insulin secretion, with two studies demonstrating a significant increase in peripheral insulin sensitivity [15,18]. This finding was particularly noted for people with type 2 diabetes mellitus.

This review has several strengths. These include prospective Prospero registration, independent two author identification, and extraction, a rigorous PRISMA-based approach to reporting, an individualised approach to quality assessment of each paper, no restriction to publication date.

However, there are also certain limitations to consider regarding this systematic review. Indeed, this research only considers the literature published in the English language, thus excluding relevant studies that may have been published in other languages. Accordingly, only 10 studies published in the English language were eligible for inclusion, whilst the small sample sizes included in these studies may reduce the reliability and generalisability of the relevant findings. Finally, due to the small sample sizes and diverse methodology involved in the eligible studies, a meta-analysis was not possible, and rather, an individualised approach to conducting this systematic review was considered.

5. Conclusions

This systematic review suggests that HBOT can impact glycaemia for people with diabetes. Indeed, this systematic review brings together articles demonstrating the impact of HBOT in lowering blood glucose and improving insulin sensitivity in people with type 2 diabetes mellitus. Despite these findings, there remains uncertainty as to the clinical significance of these HBOT-induced effects on glycaemic control. There is, therefore, a need for further research to consider the longer-term clinical impact of HBOT on glycaemia for people with type 2 diabetes mellitus, which could be considered as a potential adjunctive therapy to potentially improve glycaemic control in selected cases.

Author Contributions: Conceptualization, H.S.R. and T.R.; methodology, S.B., A.H.P. and T.R.; formal analysis, S.B. and A.H.P.; data curation, S.B., A.H.P. and T.R.; writing—original draft preparation, S.B. and A.H.P.; writing—review and editing, N.M., S.S., I.K., A.A., H.S.R. and T.R.; supervision, H.S.R. and T.R.; S.B. and A.H.P. are joint first authors. All authors have read and agreed to the published version of the manuscript.

Funding: This research received no external funding.

Institutional Review Board Statement: Not applicable.

Informed Consent Statement: Not applicable.

Acknowledgments: Clinical Evidence Based Information Service at University Hospitals Coventry and Warwickshire NHS Trust for assisting in developing the search terms.

Conflicts of Interest: The authors declare no conflict of interest.

Appendix A

Table A1. Demonstrating the search strategy used on the PubMed database.

Search Number	Query	Results
17	#15 AND #16	116
16	#3 AND #6	931
15	#7 OR #8 OR #9 OR #10 OR #11 OR #12 OR #13 OR #14	624,093
14	"hypoglycemia"[MeSH Terms]	28,951
13	hypoglycaemia[Title/Abstract] OR hypoglycemia[Title/Abstract] OR hypoglycaemic[Title/Abstract] OR hypoglycemic[Title/Abstract]	59,161
12	"hyperglycemia"[MeSH Terms]	37,247
11	hyperglycaemia[Title/Abstract] OR hyperglycemia[Title/Abstract] OR hyperglycaemic[Title/Abstract] OR hyperglycemic[Title/Abstract]	65,507
10	"glycemic control"[MeSH Terms]	270
9	glycemic[Title/Abstract] OR glycaemic[Title/Abstract]	50,821
8	"blood glucose"[MeSH Terms]	168,266
7	"blood sugar"[Title/Abstract] OR glucose[Title/Abstract]	502,819
6	#4 OR #5	16,145
5	"Hyperbaric Oxygenation"[Mesh]	12,056
4	"hyperbaric oxygen*"[Title/Abstract] OR HBO2[Title/Abstract] OR HBO[Title/Abstract]	12,164
3	#1 OR #2	729,572
2	"Diabetes Mellitus"[Mesh]	440,904
1	diabetes[Title/Abstract] OR diabetic*[Title/Abstract]	669,965

Table A2. Demonstrating the search strategy used on the Medline database.

#	Query	Results
S17	S15 AND S16	113
S16	S3 AND S6	919
S15	S7 OR S8 OR S9 OR S10 OR S11 OR S12 OR S13 OR S14	597,728
S14	(MH "Hypoglycemia+")	28,914
S13	TI (hypoglycaemia OR hypoglycemia OR hypoglycaemic OR hypoglycemic) OR AB (hypoglycaemia OR hypoglycemia OR hypoglycaemic OR hypoglycemic)	58,437
S12	(MH "Hyperglycemia+")	37,174
S11	TI (hyperglycaemia OR hyperglycemia OR hyperglycaemic OR hyperglycemic) OR AB (hyperglycaemia OR hyperglycemia OR hyperglycaemic OR hyperglycemic)	63,950
S10	(MH "Glycemic Control")	257
S9	TI (glycemic OR glycaemic) OR AB (glycemic OR glycaemic)	50,265
S8	(MH "Blood Glucose")	167,965
S7	TI ("blood sugar" OR glucose) OR AB ("blood sugar" OR glucose)	473,206
S6	S4 OR S5	15,885
S5	(MH "Hyperbaric Oxygenation")	12,048
S4	TI ("hyperbaric oxygen*" OR HBO2 OR HBO) OR AB ("hyperbaric oxygen*" OR HBO2 OR HBO)	11,723
S3	S1 OR S2	727,311
S2	(MH "Diabetes Mellitus+")	439,985
S1	TI (diabetes OR diabetic*) OR AB (diabetes OR diabetic*)	663,799

Table A3. Demonstrating the search strategy used on the Embase database.

#	Query	Results
17	15 and 16	199
16	3 and 6	1303
15	7 or 8 or 9 or 10 or 11 or 12 or 13 or 14	864,384
14	exp hypoglycemia/	82,561
13	(hypoglycaemia or hypoglycemia or hypoglycaemic or hypoglycemic).ti. or (hypoglycaemia or hypoglycemia or hypoglycaemic or hypoglycemic).ab.	86,203
12	exp hyperglycemia/	101,038
11	(hyperglycaemia or hyperglycemia or hyperglycaemic or hyperglycemic).ti. or (hyperglycaemia or hyperglycemia or hyperglycaemic or hyperglycemic).ab.	94,423
10	exp glycemic control/	53,870
9	(glycemic or glycaemic).ti. or (glycemic or glycaemic).ab.	81,559
8	exp glucose blood level/	260,424
7	((blood adj1 sugar) or glucose).ti. or ((blood adj1 sugar) or glucose).ab.	658,030
6	4 or 5	14,749
5	exp hyperbaric oxygen/ or exp hyperbaric oxygen therapy/	3230
4	((hyperbaric adj1 oxygen*) or HBO2 or HBO).ti. or ((hyperbaric adj1 oxygen*) or HBO2 or HBO).ab.	13,775
3	1 or 2	1,195,748
2	exp diabetes mellitus/	1,014,391
1	(diabetes or diabetic*).ti. or (diabetes or diabetic*).ab.	995,738

References

1. Mathieu, D.; Marroni, A.; Kot, J. Tenth European Consensus Conference on Hyperbaric Medicine: Recommendations for accepted and non-accepted clinical indications and practice of hyperbaric oxygen treatment. *Diving Hyperb. Med. J.* **2017**, *47*, 24–32. [CrossRef] [PubMed]
2. Kaya, A.; Aydin, F.; Altay, T.; Karapinar, L.; Ozturk, H.; Karakuzu, C. Can major amputation rates be decreased in diabetic foot ulcers with hyperbaric oxygen therapy? *Int. Orthop.* **2008**, *33*, 441–446. [CrossRef] [PubMed]
3. Duzgun, A.P.; Satır, H.Z.; Ozozan, O.; Saylam, B.; Kulah, B.; Coskun, F. Effect of Hyperbaric Oxygen Therapy on Healing of Diabetic Foot Ulcers. *J. Foot Ankle Surg.* **2008**, *47*, 515–519. [CrossRef] [PubMed]
4. Flood, M. Hyperbaric oxygen therapy for diabetic foot ulcers. *J. Lanc. Gen. Hosp.* **2007**, *2*, 140–145.
5. Bhutani, S.; Vishwanath, G. Hyperbaric oxygen and wound healing. *Indian J. Plast. Surg.* **2012**, *45*, 316–324. [CrossRef] [PubMed]
6. Skyler, J.S. Effects of Glycemic Control on Diabetes Complications and on the Prevention of Diabetes. *Clin. Diabetes* **2004**, *22*, 162–166. [CrossRef]
7. Ketema, E.B.; Kibret, K.T. Correlation of fasting and postprandial plasma glucose with HbA1c in assessing glycemic control; systematic review and meta-analysis. *Arch. Public Health* **2015**, *73*, 1–9. [CrossRef] [PubMed]
8. Heyboer III, M.; Wojcik, S.M.; Swaby, J.; Boes, T. Blood glucose levels in diabetic patients undergoing hyperbaric oxygen therapy. *Undersea Hyperb. Med.* **2019**, *46*, 437–445.
9. Trytko, B.; Bennett, M.H. Blood sugar changes in diabetic patients undergoing hyperbaric oxygen therapy. *South Pac. Underw. Med. Soc. J.* **2003**, *33*, 62–69.
10. Vote, D.; Ekanayake, L.; Doolette, D. Blood sugar levels and hyperbaric oxygen. *South Pac. Underw. Med. Soc. J.* **2001**, *31*, 81–82.
11. Peleg, R.K.; Fishlev, G.; Bechor, Y.; Bergan, J.; Friedman, M.; Koren, S.; Tirosh, A.; Efrati, S. Effects of hyperbaric oxygen on blood glucose levels in patients with diabetes mellitus, stroke or traumatic brain injury and healthy volunteers: A prospective, crossover, controlled trial. *Diving Hyperb. Med. J.* **2013**, *43*, 218–221.
12. Ekanayake, L.; Doolette, D. Effects of hyperbaric oxygen treatment on blood sugar levels and insulin levels in diabetics. *South Pac. Underw. Med. Soc. J.* **2001**, *31*, 16–20.
13. Page, M.J.; McKenzie, J.E.; Bossuyt, P.M.; Boutron, I.; Hoffmann, T.C.; Mulrow, C.D.; Shamseer, L.; Tetzlaff, J.M.; Akl, E.A.; Brennan, S.E.; et al. The PRISMA 2020 statement: An updated guideline for reporting systematic reviews. *BMJ* **2021**, *372*, n71. [CrossRef]
14. Irawan, H.; Semadi, I.N.; Widiana, I.G.R. A Pilot Study of Short-Duration Hyperbaric Oxygen Therapy to Improve HbA1c, Leukocyte, and Serum Creatinine in Patients with Diabetic Foot Ulcer Wagner 3–4. *Sci. World J.* **2018**, *2018*, 1–6. [CrossRef]
15. Xu, Q.; Wei, Y.-T.; Fan, S.-B.; Wang, L.; Zhou, X.-P. Repetitive hyperbaric oxygen treatment increases insulin sensitivity in diabetes patients with acute intracerebral hemorrhage. *Neuropsychiatr. Dis. Treat.* **2017**, *13*, 421–426. [CrossRef]
16. Vera-Cruz, P.; Guerreiro, F.; Ribeiro, M.J.; Guarino, M.P.; Conde, S.V. Hyperbaric Oxygen Therapy Improves Glucose Homeostasis in Type 2 Diabetes Patients: A Likely Involvement of the Carotid Bodies. *Adv. Exp. Med. Biol.* **2015**, *860*, 221–225. [CrossRef] [PubMed]
17. Stevens, S.L.; Narr, A.J.; Claus, P.L.; Millman, M.P.; Steinkraus, L.W.; Shields, R.C.; Buchta, W.G.; Haddon, R.; Wang, Z.; Murad, M.H. The incidence of hypoglycemia during HBO2 therapy: A retrospective review. *Undersea Hyperb. Med.* **2015**, *42*, 191–196. [PubMed]
18. Wilkinson, D.; Chapman, I.M.; Heilbronn, L.K. Hyperbaric oxygen therapy improves peripheral insulin sensitivity in humans. *Diabet. Med.* **2012**, *29*, 986–989. [CrossRef] [PubMed]
19. Al-Waili, N.S.; Butler, G.J.; Beale, J.; Abdullah, M.S.; Finkelstein, M.; Merrow, M.; Rivera, R.; Petrillo, R.; Carrey, Z.; Lee, B.; et al. Influences of Hyperbaric Oxygen on Blood Pressure, Heart Rate and Blood Glucose Levels in Patients with Diabetes Mellitus and Hypertension. *Arch. Med. Res.* **2006**, *37*, 991–997. [CrossRef] [PubMed]

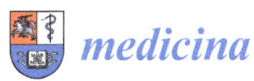

Review

Critical Flicker Fusion Frequency: A Narrative Review

Natalia D. Mankowska [1,*], Anna B. Marcinkowska [1,2,3], Monika Waskow [3], Rita I. Sharma [4,5], Jacek Kot [6] and Pawel J. Winklewski [2,3,4]

1. Applied Cognitive Neuroscience Lab, Department of Human Physiology, Medical University of Gdansk, 80-210 Gdansk, Poland; anna.marcinkowska@gumed.edu.pl
2. 2nd Department of Radiology, Medical University of Gdansk, 80-210 Gdansk, Poland; pawel.winklewski@gumed.edu.pl
3. Institute of Health Sciences, Pomeranian University in Slupsk, 76-200 Slupsk, Poland; monika.waskow@apsl.edu.pl
4. Department of Human Physiology, Medical University of Gdansk, 80-210 Gdansk, Poland; rita.sharma@gumed.edu.pl
5. Department of Anaesthesiology and Intensive Care, Medical University of Gdansk, 80-210 Gdansk, Poland
6. National Centre for Hyperbaric Medicine, Institute of Maritime and Tropical Medicine in Gdynia, Medical University of Gdansk, 80-210 Gdansk, Poland; jkot@gumed.edu.pl
* Correspondence: natalia_mankowska@gumed.edu.pl; Tel./Fax: +48-58-3491515

Abstract: This review presents the current knowledge of the usage of critical flicker fusion frequency (CFF) in human and animal model studies. CFF has a wide application in different fields, especially as an indicator of cortical arousal and visual processing. In medicine, CFF may be helpful for diagnostic purposes, for example in epilepsy or minimal hepatic encephalopathy. Given the environmental studies and a limited number of other methods, it is applicable in diving and hyperbaric medicine. Current research also shows the relationship between CFF and other electrophysiological methods, such as electroencephalography. The human eye can detect flicker at 50–90 Hz but reports are showing the possibility to distinguish between steady and modulated light up to 500 Hz. Future research with the use of CFF is needed to better understand its utility and application.

Keywords: critical flicker fusion frequency; threshold of flicker fusion; neuropsychology; diving and hyperbaric medicine; minimal hepatic encephalopathy

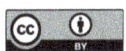

1. Introduction

Critical flicker fusion frequency (CFF or CFFF) is defined as the frequency at which flickering light can be perceived as continuous and it is used to assess the processing of temporal vision. The upper level of one's abilities in visual processing is described as the critical flicker fusion threshold (or threshold for flicker fusion, TFF), which represents the maximum speed of flickering light that can be perceived by the visual system [1,2]. Because of its efficiency in detecting rapid changes, it is used as an index of cerebral nervous system (CNS) function that is described as alertness and cortical arousal in humans [3,4].

The ability to detect flicker fusion is dependent on: (1) frequency of the modulation, (2) the amplitude of the modulation, (3) the average illumination intensity, (4) the position on the retina at which the stimulus occurs, (5) the wavelength or colour of the LED, (6) the intensity of ambient light [3,5,6] or (7) the viewing distance and (8) size of the stimulus [7]. Moreover, there are also internal factors of individuals that can affect CFF measures: age, sex, personality traits, fatigue, circadian variation in brain activity [4] and cognitive functions like visual integration, visuomotor skills and decision-making processes [3]. The performance of CFF in humans and predators alike is dependent on these factors. Umeton et al. also describe preys' features like a pattern or even the way they move as relevant in perceiving the flicker fusion effect [2].

It is believed that the human eye cannot detect flicker above 50 to 90 Hz and it depends on intensity and contrast, but some reports indicate people can distinguish between modulated and steady light at up to 500 Hz [8].

In recent years, there have been many studies with animal models. The pioneers of these studies were Shure and Halstead who investigated the influence of brain lesions in monkeys on TFF [9]. The reason for this decision was Halstead's finding that the removal of the specific brain localisation relates to CFF performance. Nowadays, not only monkeys are of interest to scientists. Lisney and colleagues used electroretinograms and indicated that flicker from fluorescent lamps may be a stress factor for hens [10,11]. The limitation of these studies is the number of included chickens (4 to 15), thus future research is needed.

A high CFF threshold is crucial for flying animals (like pigeons—143 Hz or peregrine falcons—129 Hz) that need an efficient visual system, e.g., to detect rapidly approaching objects to avoid colliding with them, but there are some studies with shrimps that need similar skills. The shrimp TFF is about 160 Hz, although there are individuals with a threshold of 200 Hz [12]. These are just a few examples of the use of CFF in animal studies; in the literature, reports may be found on its usage in dogs, mice, rats or snakes and more. Researchers typically use two types of method to determine the CFF of an animal—electroretinograms and behavioural methods, like two-alternative forced-choice procedure [13,14], e.g., pecking at the lit panel by a bird [15].

Flicker has its countertype in a different sensory modality, i.e., hearing. A few researchers have done a comparison of visual and auditory stimuli. Shipley found that in healthy and young individuals, critical flicker frequency is worse than a critical flutter frequency (which is "the frequency at which a clicking sound appears steady") [16]. Shams et al. point out that the perception of visual stimulus intensity may be modulated by the occurrence of sound [5]. Moreover, the frequency of flickering light is prone to change under the influence of the frequency of fluttering sound; multiple audio signals with a single flash result in perceiving this as multiple flashes.

The CFF test may be used in different forms, but the instruction is usually the same; a subject has to focus their vision on a light-emitting diode when the light frequency is increased at a constant rate (e.g., 1 Hz) and has to press a button when it seems to be continuous light in their opinion. It is also possible to reverse the order of the task to one in which the light frequency decreases and the subject has to report when they see flicker.

In some studies, the CFF test is used as a computer program where participants have to report altered vision by pressing a button [17]; in others, it is a device that can be described as similar to virtual reality glasses, for example, the HEPAtonorm Analyzer [18] or with the addition of other methods like electroretinograms or functional magnetic image resonance, among others [10]. The choice of (1) the device to measure TFF and (2) additional methods should depend on the research hypotheses and the research group.

2. Arousal as an Indicator of Cognitive Performance

The relationship between arousal and cognitive performance has been known since 1908, when two psychologists, Robert M. Yerkes and John D. Dodson, did a series of experiments with mice and described the Yerkes-Dodson Law, which states that cognitive performance increases with both physiological and mental arousal, but when it becomes too high, the performance decreases. This law could be illustrated in a bell-shaped curve [19]. The critical flicker fusion frequency test can be used as a tool to monitor these changes in brain function and to assess cortical arousal in various environmental conditions [3,20,21]. Additionally, arousal can be modulated by physical activity. Based on this knowledge, several experiments investigated the impact of physical exercise on the CFF performance and found that arousal increases directly after exercise and returns to the output level during recovery [21].

Tomporowski et al. compared results from the Paced Auditory Serial Addition Test (PASAT) before and after exercise. In Experiment 1, nine men completed two sessions of a 40-min bout of cycling, and in Experiment 2, 10 women completed four 120-min sessions of cycling [22]. Researchers have proven that arousal is exercise-induced and may induce better PASAT performance, which means that acute aerobic exercise may affect working memory and attention.

Lambourne and colleagues assessed the influence of aerobic exercises (on cycle ergometer) on two mental processes: sensory discrimination and executive functions in 19 young adults [21]. They used the CFF test as a visual sensory-discrimination task. The measures of the CFF performance were made five times during 40 min of cycling at a moderate level and three times during the 30-min post-exercise period. The results showed an improvement in cognitive performance after physical exercise. However, the CFF results rapidly decreased after the termination of exercise. This means that the increasing level of CFF may result from enhancing receptiveness to sensory stimulation involved in stimulus detection. The arousal probably does not influence executive processing, but the effect of acute exercise on higher-level processes is unclear.

3. Use of the Critical Flicker Fusion Test in Neuropsychology

The use of CFF for CNS function assessment is postulated by Casey et al. [23]. In experimental procedures with electroretinogram and functional magnetic resonance imaging researchers found that subjects report fusion much longer after the retina and visual cortex responded to flicker [24,25] which means that the human perception of flicker is associated with the activity of higher cortical regions [26,27].

The Halstead-Reitan Battery of Neuropsychological Tests was initially used as a method to assess cognitive functioning in individuals with brain lesions above 15 years old. It was created in 1947 [28] and included two critical flicker fusion measures that were dropped later because of insufficient discrimination between groups of patients with or without brain lesions [29].

CFF as a method to assess cognitive functions is objective, simple, quick, low-cost and it is not affected by factors such as a level of education or language [30–33]. A significant advantage of CFF performance is its resistance to the learning effect [34–36].

Studies with CFF can be performed in 3-month-old infants [37]. They estimate infant TFF by a two-alternative forced-choice preferential looking technique. The researcher (observer) estimates the location of the flickering target (left or right side of the visual field) based on cues given by the infant (e.g., gaze direction or length of looking time to each side). If 75% or more trials were well estimated, then it was inferred that the infant was able to detect flicker at that frequency. The location of light was semi-randomised, and the first trials began at 20 Hz. The findings indicate a significant improvement in development is occurring between 3 to 4.5 months of age, which then may slow or even plateau. The forced-choice preferential looking procedure is not the only method used in research involving infants; researchers also use visual evoked potentials and electroretinograms [38].

The differences in CFF performance (as an index of processing speed) in children might be a predictor of future cognitive functioning. Visual processing speed, however, is not the only predictor of cognitive abilities in the future [1]. Saint and colleagues examined 54 children with CFF and the Woodcock-Johnson III Tests of Cognitive Abilities and observed that psychomotor coordination became better with age (younger children had longer reaction time latency) [1].

The CFF test in children or adolescents has also been used in studies with groups with brain injuries [18], diabetes [39] and reading disabilities [40].

4. The Diagnostic Values of CFF

Several studies have investigated the effect of dietary supplementation, especially with compounds that are naturally found throughout the CNS (e.g., lutein, fatty acids or plant pigments, xanthophylls, found in the brain and retina in particular), with the threshold of CFF [41–43]. Bovier et al. have indicated improvements in reaction times and increasing CFF thresholds in adults after lutein and zeaxanthin supplementation [41,42].

Other research projects support this hypothesis [44,45] and even use CFF to find drug effects on psychomotor performance, attention and concentration [46].

Lauridsen et al. compared a continuous reaction times test (CRT) with CFF for the diagnosis of minimal hepatic encephalopathy [47]. The CRT test was a measure of the subject's ability to perform motor reactions adequately and repeatedly. The CFF test reflected biological activity in retinal cells and provided information about visual processing, arousal and attention. The patient's CFF threshold was the average of the nine measurements at 60 Hz, and if it was lower than 39 Hz, then it was considered cerebral dysfunction. In the trial with CRT, participants were asked to press the button as soon as they heard the signal at 500 Hz and 90 dB. A reaction time above 2 s was registered as a lack of response. Both CRT and CFF tests gave false positives and inconsistent results. These two measures describe different aspects of minimal hepatic encephalopathy so the choice between the CRT or CFF test should be made carefully.

The CFF threshold may be a useful measure to follow cognitive processing abilities in patients with implanted vagus nerve stimulators (VNSs) for epilepsy treatment and Alzheimer's disease [17,48]. After a 12-month treatment with a VNS, all epilepsy patients showed significant improvement in CFF compared to baseline ($p < 0.05$).

Some research has suggested that a reduced CFF threshold could be used to detect individuals with Alzheimer's disease [27,48–51]. In these patients, impairment of short-term memory is observed, which could be enhanced by the 10 Hz flicker. This result confirms previous ones that found memory dysfunction correlated with the loss of the 10 Hz alpha rhythm [52,53]. The EEG frequency and amplitude fall with age, especially in those with mild memory problems [54]. These problems may be partially solved by cholinesterase inhibitors that enhance alpha rhythms as flicker probably does [51,55]. There is a possibility that activity induced by flicker enhances mouse hippocampus activity and the human cortico-cortical and cortico-thalamic loops [56–58].

The use of the CFF was considered in subjects with obstructive sleep apnoea syndrome who may have cognitive impairment. This syndrome may affect attention, memory and executive functions that are associated with brain changes, especially in frontal regions [59]. Depending on the existence and size of brain lesions, CFF performance may vary, but the results of previous studies were inconclusive, and there is a need for future research with a larger sample size [60,61].

5. Diving and Hyperbaric Medicine

Neuropsychological assessment may be difficult in the underwater environment. The number of available tests for these conditions is limited so CFF seems to be a good solution due to its advantages. In recent years, many studies have focused on examining the impact of both recreational and professional diving on cognitive functions and take into consideration both acute and chronic effects.

CFF is widely used in experiments involving divers [34,62] and provides a reliable assessment that can be compared to psychometric testing (e.g., trail-making tasks or math processing) under normobaric—10 min of breathing air or oxygen in a quiet room at a constant temperature of 22 °C [35]—and hyperbaric-dry chamber—breathing air or enriched air nitrox for 20 min at 4 ATA—conditions [63]. A decrease in cerebral performance was reported in association with a decreasing level of CFF and vice versa [3,63]. Balestra and colleagues highlighted that breathing pure oxygen in normobaric conditions has an impact on CFF performance and proved that CFF results are dependent on cortical arousal because of increased brain blood flow in occipital regions and modification of pupil size induced by scopolamine, a muscarinic antagonist [64].

While breathing hyperbaric oxygen, it seems that neuronal excitability measured by CFF depends on the oxygen dose. During a study on professional military divers from the Special Forces, the CFF was increased while breathing a PPO_2 of 2.8 ATA, which represents augmented neuronal excitability, while CFF was decreased at a PPO_2 of 1.4 ATA, which represents attention and alertness deterioration [65]. Interestingly results at the lower PPO$_2$ (1.4 ATA) in this group seem contradictory to those observed in recreational divers [35]. Differences in performance might be explained by investigated populations (elite, experienced, combat vs. occasional, recreational divers). Hyperbaric oxygen induces neuromuscular hyperexcitability in normal volunteers, while attenuates such an effect in elite military divers frequently exposed to oxygen and pressure [66].

Recreational diving (generally to 40 m of seawater, msw; in the mentioned literature the depth is 33 msw) may result in changes in the CFF performance even at 30 min post-dive [35,36,67].

Another risk in diving is nitrogen narcosis, which in the course of the hyperbaric exposure can be compared to alcohol intoxication and may cause a neurologic syndrome characterised by an impairment of cerebral performance or increased arousal [3]. The influence of the depth narcosis can be compared to the effect of a glass of Martini for every 15 m of depth [68]. Actually, the inert gas (nitrogen) penetration in the lipids of the brain's nerve cells and interference with nerve cells' signal transmission (according to the Meyer-Overton rule) might be further strengthened by the pressure effect [69]. Consequently, it is likely that the depth interval between subsequent "glasses of Martini" would be possibly presented with a smaller value and 10 m is probably more realistically correlated to the increase in the narcotic risk in diving. Impaired cerebral performance includes dysfunction of time perception, reaction speed and ability to think, calculate and react [70].

High-pressure nervous syndrome (HPNS) may appear especially in professional divers who dive deeper than 150 msw due to rapidly increasing pressure in the CNS during compression [20,71]. Nowadays, advanced diving equipment with closed-circuit breathing apparatuses allows recreational divers to also reach depths previously unreachable. Therefore, HPNS becomes a real hazard also for sport and recreational underwater activities [72].

The negative effects of HPNS (e.g., impairment of motor, sensory, behavioural and cognitive function) are known, but there is still a need to conduct future research to understand better its influence on humans. A significant decrease of CFF was observed in divers exposed to high pressures while breathing heliox at 62 ATA, which is equivalent to a depth of 610 m [73].

Quite recently, Ardestani and colleagues asked two groups of divers (reported or non-reported HPNS symptoms) to complete a few tests from the Physiopad package to measure their working memory, vigilance and decision making at 180 to 207 msw [20]. The Physiopad package includes HPNS questionnaires, a hand dynamometry test, a CFF test, an adaptive visual analog scale (AVAS), a simple math process (MathProc test), a perceptual vigilance task (PVT) and a time estimation task (time-wall). The CFF was performed daily and showed no differences between these two groups of divers, which means that the association between psychometric tests and subjective measurements may not exist. These results may arise from one of the limitations of this study; namely, none of the participants was medically diagnosed with HPNS.

Interestingly, the CFF correlates with hypoxemia, as shown during experimental exposures in hypobaric chambers for aviation purposes [74].

6. CFF and Its Connection with Brainwaves

CFF performance is related to other measures of brain activity. Some electrophysiological experiments have shown that the human visual cortex is sensitive to the frequency of flickering light, which induces neural activity changes in electroencephalogram (EEG) at the same level. Adrian and Matthews discovered " ... that regular potential waves at frequencies other than 10 a second can be induced by flicker" [75] (p. 377). Authors recorded the EEG activity from the occipital lobe of subjects exposed to flickering light with frequencies up to 25 Hz, and that was the first time when steady-state visually evoked potentials were recorded [76,77].

In healthy older people, alpha-like EEG (8–12 Hz) can be induced by flicker and may even strengthen memory [78]. This relationship is highly specific for frequency. Williams et al. asked participants to identify the real word in 10 pairs of trigrams (three-letter words). After the practice task, the learning phase ensued (48 pairs of trigrams) [51]. Two minutes later the participants had to choose the "old" word in a pair of "old"-"new" trigrams (this time all of the words were real). Flickering light occurred in the learning phase (1000 ms in the beginning when the screen was blank); then the flicker was continued for 500 ms before and after the trigrams appeared. The frequency and intensity of flickers were randomised and unique for each participant. Six pairs of trigrams occurred after flickering at each frequency (two at each frequency-intensity combination). Results showed that flicker frequencies close to 10.0 Hz have a positive effect on recognition, unlike 8.7 and 11.7 Hz, which were ineffective.

Similar conclusions were made by Herrmann, who observed that 10 Hz visual stimulation has the strongest impact on the visual cortex and induces the strongest neural entrainment (brainwave frequency synchronisation) [79].

Sauseng et al. also showed the connection of alpha-frequency (around 10 Hz) stimulation with memory [80]. They concluded that repetitive transcranial magnetic stimulation might increase the capacity of short-term memory by enhancing the ability to ignore distractors. They emphasised that memory capacity also relied on a larger number of skills such as successful retention of the most important information as well as attention and executive functions.

7. Conclusions

To conclude, critical flicker fusion frequency has been a widely used method to assess cortical arousal and visual system parameters for many years. It may be successfully used in research involving both human and animal subjects. The CFF test may measure cognitive functioning just as well as other psychometric methods, although it must be considered carefully. As a simple and quick method, resistant to the learning effect, it may be used in many groups, from new-borns to the elderly, from healthy people to people with various diseases, such as epilepsy, dementia, minimal hepatic encephalopathy, etc. Despite these advantages, there is a need to conduct future research to compare the CFF test with other measures, especially neuropsychological ones, to verify its reliability and to better understand its advantages and limitations.

Author Contributions: Conceptualization, A.B.M. and P.J.W.; methodology, N.D.M.; validation, A.B.M., R.I.S. and M.W.; formal analysis, N.D.M. and A.B.M.; investigation, N.D.M.; resources, M.W., J.K. and P.J.W.; writing—original draft preparation, N.D.M.; writing—review and editing, all authors; supervision, A.B.M., J.K. and P.J.W.; project administration, N.D.M.; funding acquisition, M.W., J.K. and P.J.W. All authors have read and agreed to the published version of the manuscript.

Funding: This research was funded by Pomeranian University in Slupsk, 76-200 Slupsk, Poland and the Medical University of Gdansk, 80-210 Gdansk, Poland.

Institutional Review Board Statement: Not applicable.

Informed Consent Statement: Not applicable.

Data Availability Statement: No new data were created or analyzed in this study. Data sharing is not applicable to this article.

Conflicts of Interest: The authors declare no conflict of interest.

References

1. Saint, S.E.; Hammond, B.R., Jr.; Khan, N.A.; Hillman, C.H.; Renzi-Hammond, L.M. Temporal vision is related to cognitive function in preadolescent children. *Appl. Neuropsychol. Child* **2019**, *10*, 1–8. [CrossRef]
2. Umeton, D.; Read, J.C.A.; Rowe, C. Unravelling the illusion of flicker fusion. *Biol. Lett.* **2017**, *13*, 20160831. [CrossRef]
3. Balestra, C.; Machado, M.-L.; Theunissen, S.; Balestra, A.; Cialoni, D.; Clot, C.; Besnard, S.; Kammacher, L.; Delzenne, J.; Germonpré, P.; et al. Critical flicker fusion frequency: A marker of cerebral arousal during modified gravitational conditions related to parabolic flights. *Front. Physiol.* **2018**, *9*. [CrossRef]
4. Hindmarch, I. Critical Flicker Fusion Frequency (CFF): The Effects of Psychotropic Compounds. *Pharmacopsychiatry* **1982**, *15*, 44–48. [CrossRef]

5. Shams, L.; Kamitani, Y.; Shimojo, S. Visual illusion induced by sound. *Cogn. Brain Res.* **2002**, *14*, 147–152. [CrossRef]
6. Walter, W.G.; Dovey, V.J.; Shipton, H. Analysis of the electrical response of the human cortex to photic stimulation. *Nature* **1946**, *158*, 540–541. [CrossRef]
7. Brenton, R.S.; Thompson, H.S.; Maxner, C. Critical flicker frequency: A new look at an old test. In *New Methods of Sensory Visual Testing*; Springer: New York, NY, USA, 1989; pp. 29–52.
8. Davis, J.; Hsieh, Y.-H.; Lee, H.-C. Humans perceive flicker artifacts at 500 Hz. *Sci. Rep.* **2015**, *5*, srep07861. [CrossRef] [PubMed]
9. Shure, G.H.; Halstead, W.C. Cerebral localization of intellectual processes. *Psychol. Monogr. Gen. Appl.* **1958**, *72*, 1–40. [CrossRef]
10. Lisney, T.J.; Ekesten, B.; Tauson, R.; Håstad, O.; Ödeen, A. Using electroretinograms to assess flicker fusion frequency in domestic hens Gallus gallus domesticus. *Vis. Res.* **2012**, *62*, 125–133. [CrossRef]
11. Lisney, T.J.; Rubene, D.; Rózsa, J.; Løvlie, H.; Håstad, O.; Ödeen, A. Behavioural assessment of flicker fusion frequency in chicken Gallus gallus domesticus. *Vis. Res.* **2011**, *51*, 1324–1332. [CrossRef] [PubMed]
12. Kingston, A.C.N.; Chappell, D.R.; Speiser, D.I. A snapping shrimp has the fastest vision of any aquatic animal. *Biol. Lett.* **2020**, *16*, 20200298. [CrossRef]
13. D'Eath, R.B. Can video images imitate real stimuli in animal behaviour experiments? *Biol. Rev.* **1998**, *73*, 267–292. [CrossRef]
14. Railton, R.C.R.; Foster, T.M.; Temple, W. A comparison of two methods for assessing critical flicker fusion frequency in hens. *Behav. Process.* **2009**, *80*, 196–200. [CrossRef]
15. Rubene, D.; Håstad, O.; Tauson, R.; Wall, H.; Ödeen, A. The presence of UV wavelengths improves the temporal resolution of the avian visual system. *J. Exp. Biol.* **2010**, *213*, 3357–3363. [CrossRef] [PubMed]
16. Shipley, T. Auditory flutter-driving of visual flicker. *Science* **1964**, *145*, 1328–1330. [CrossRef] [PubMed]
17. Achinivu, K.; Staufenberg, E.; Cull, C.; Cavanna, A.E.; Ring, H. Cognitive function during vagus nerve stimulation for treatment-refractory epilepsy: A pilot study using the critical flicker fusion test. *J. Neurother.* **2012**, *16*, 32–36. [CrossRef]
18. Yadav, S.K.; Srivastava, A.; Srivastava, A.; Thomas, M.A.; Agarwal, J.; Pandey, C.M.; Lal, R.; Yachha, S.K.; Saraswat, V.A.; Gupta, R.K. Encephalopathy assessment in children with extra-hepatic portal vein obstruction with MR, psychometry and critical flicker frequency. *J. Hepatol.* **2010**, *52*, 348–354. [CrossRef] [PubMed]
19. Yerkes, R.M.; Dodson, J.D. The relation of strength of stimulus to rapidity of habit-formation. In *Punishment: Issues and Experiments*; Appleton-Century-Crofts Division of Meredith Corporation: New York, NY, USA, 1908; pp. 27–41.
20. Ardestani, S.B.; Balestra, C.; Bouzinova, E.V.; Loennechen, Ø.; Pedersen, M. Evaluation of divers' neuropsychometric effectiveness and high-pressure neurological syndrome via computerized test battery package and questionnaires in operational setting. *Front. Physiol.* **2019**, *10*, 1386. [CrossRef]
21. Lambourne, K.; Audiffren, M.; Tomporowski, P.D. Effects of Acute Exercise on Sensory and Executive Processing Tasks. *Med. Sci. Sports Exerc.* **2010**, *42*, 1396–1402. [CrossRef]
22. Tomporowski, P.D.; Cureton, K.; Armstrong, L.E.; Kane, G.M.; Sparling, P.B.; Millard-Stafford, M. Short-term effects of aerobic exercise on executive processes and emotional reactivity. *Int. J. Sport Exerc. Psychol.* **2005**, *3*, 131–146. [CrossRef]
23. Casey, B.; Tottenham, N.; Liston, C.; Durston, S. Imaging the developing brain: What have we learned about cognitive development? *Trends Cogn. Sci.* **2005**, *9*, 104–110. [CrossRef] [PubMed]
24. Carmel, D.; Lavie, N.; Rees, G. Conscious awareness of flicker in humans involves frontal and parietal cortex. *Curr. Biol.* **2006**, *16*, 907–911. [CrossRef] [PubMed]
25. Jiang, Y.; Zhou, K.; He, S. Human visual cortex responds to invisible chromatic flicker. *Nat. Neurosci.* **2007**, *10*, 657–662. [CrossRef] [PubMed]
26. Skottun, B.C. On using very high temporal frequencies to isolate magnocellular contributions to psychophysical tasks. *Neuropsychologia* **2013**, *51*, 1556–1560. [CrossRef]
27. Wooten, B.R.; Renzi, L.M.; Moore, R.; Hammond, B.R. A practical method of measuring the human temporal contrast sensitivity function. *Biomed. Opt. Express* **2010**, *1*, 47–58. [CrossRef]
28. Mazur-Mosiewicz, A.; Dean, R.S. Halstead-Reitan neuropsychological test battery. In *Encyclopedia of Child Behavior and Development*; Springer: Boston, MA, USA, 2011; pp. 727–731.
29. Reed, J.C.; Reed, H.B.C. Contributions to neuropsychology of reitan and associates: Neuropsychology laboratory, Indiana University Medical Center, 1960s. *Arch. Clin. Neuropsychol.* **2015**, *30*, 751–753. [CrossRef]
30. Córdoba, J. New assessment of hepatic encephalopathy. *J. Hepatol.* **2011**, *54*, 1030–1040. [CrossRef]
31. Gencdal, G.; Gunsar, F.; Meral, C.E.; Salman, E.; Gürsel, B.; Oruc, N.; Karasu, Z.; Ersoz, G.; Akarca, U.S. Diurnal changes of critical flicker frequency in patients with liver cirrhosis and their relationship with sleep disturbances. *Dig. Liver Dis.* **2014**, *46*, 1111–1115. [CrossRef]
32. Torlot, F.J.; McPhail, M.J.W.; Taylor-Robinson, S.D. Meta-analysis: The diagnostic accuracy of critical flicker frequency in minimal hepatic encephalopathy. *Aliment. Pharmacol. Ther.* **2013**, *37*, 527–536. [CrossRef]
33. Wunsch, E.; Post, M.; Gutkowski, K.; Marlicz, W.; Szymanik, B.; Hartleb, M.; Milkiewicz, P. Critical flicker frequency fails to disclose brain dysfunction in patients with primary biliary cirrhosis. *Dig. Liver Dis.* **2010**, *42*, 818–821. [CrossRef]
34. Germonpré, P.; Balestra, C.; Hemelryck, W.; Buzzacott, P.; Lafère, P. Objective vs. subjective evaluation of cognitive performance during 0.4-MPa dives breathing air or nitrox. *Aerosp. Med. Hum. Perform.* **2017**, *88*, 469–475. [CrossRef] [PubMed]
35. Hemelryck, W.; Rozloznik, M.; Germonpré, P.; Balestra, C.; Lafère, P. Functional comparison between critical flicker fusion frequency and simple cognitive tests in subjects breathing air or oxygen in normobaria. *Diving Hyperb. Med. J.* **2013**, *43*, 138–142.

36. Lafère, P.; Balestra, C.; Hemelryck, W.; Guerrero, F.; Germonpré, P. Do environmental conditions contribute to narcosis onset and symptom severity? *Int. J. Sports Med.* **2016**, *37*, 1124–1128. [CrossRef] [PubMed]
37. Saint, S.E.; Hammond, B.R.; O'Brien, K.J.; Frick, J.E. Developmental trends in infant temporal processing speed. *Vis. Res.* **2017**, *138*, 71–77. [CrossRef]
38. Rasengane, T.A.; Allen, D.; Manny, R.E. Development of temporal contrast sensitivity in human infants. *Vis. Res.* **1997**, *37*, 1747–1754. [CrossRef]
39. Ryan, C.; Vega, A.; Longstreet, C.; Drash, A. Neuropsychological changes in adolescents with insulin-dependent diabetes. *J. Consult. Clin. Psychol.* **1984**, *52*, 335–342. [CrossRef]
40. Edwards, V.T.; Giaschi, D.E.; Dougherty, R.F.; Edgell, D.; Bjornson, B.H.; Lyons, C.; Douglas, R.M. Psychophysical indexes of temporal processing abnormalities in children with developmental Dyslexia. *Dev. Neuropsychol.* **2004**, *25*, 321–354. [CrossRef]
41. Bovier, E.R.; Hammond, B.R. A randomized placebo-controlled study on the effects of lutein and zeaxanthin on visual processing speed in young healthy subjects. *Arch. Biochem. Biophys.* **2015**, *572*, 54–57. [CrossRef]
42. Bovier, E.R.; Renzi, L.M.; Hammond, B.R. A Double-Blind, Placebo-Controlled Study on the Effects of Lutein and Zeaxanthin on Neural Processing Speed and Efficiency. *PLoS ONE* **2014**, *9*, e108178. [CrossRef]
43. Mewborn, C.; Renzi, L.M.; Hammond, B.R.; Miller, L.S. Critical flicker fusion predicts executive function in younger and older adults. *Arch. Clin. Neuropsychol.* **2015**, *30*, 605–610. [CrossRef]
44. Hammond, B.R.; Wooten, B.R. CFF thresholds: Relation to macular pigment optical density. *Ophthalmic Physiol. Opt.* **2005**, *25*, 315–319. [CrossRef]
45. Renzi, L.M.; Bovier, E.R.; Hammond, B.R. A role for the macular carotenoids in visual motor response. *Nutr. Neurosci.* **2013**, *16*, 262–268. [CrossRef]
46. Dixon, R.; Hughes, A.; Nairn, K.; Sellers, M.; Kemp, J.; Yates, R. Effects of the antimigraine compound zolmitriptan ('Zomig') on psychomotor performance alone and in combination with diazepam in healthy volunteers. *Cephalalgia* **1998**, *18*, 468–475. [CrossRef]
47. Lauridsen, M.M.; Jepsen, P.; Vilstrup, H. Critical flicker frequency and continuous reaction times for the diagnosis of minimal hepatic encephalopathy. A comparative study of 154 patients with liver disease. *Metab. Brain Dis.* **2011**, *26*, 135–139. [CrossRef]
48. Merrill, C.A.; Jonsson, M.A.G.; Minthon, L.; Ejnell, H.; Silander, H.C.-S.; Blennow, K.; Karlsson, M.; Nordlund, A.; Rolstad, S.; Warkentin, S.; et al. Vagus nerve stimulation in patients with Alzheimer's disease. *J. Clin. Psychiatry* **2006**, *67*, 1171–1178. [CrossRef]
49. Curran, S.; Wattis, J. Critical flicker fusion threshold: A potentially useful measure for the early detection of Alzheimer's disease. *Hum. Psychopharmacol.* **2000**, *15*, 103–112. [CrossRef]
50. Renzi, L.M.; Hammond, B.R. The relation between the macular carotenoids, lutein and zeaxanthin, and temporal vision. *Ophthalmic Physiol. Opt.* **2010**, *30*, 351–357. [CrossRef] [PubMed]
51. Williams, J.; Ramaswamy, D.; Oulhaj, A. 10 Hz flicker improves recognition memory in older people. *BMC Neurosci.* **2006**, *7*, 1–7. [CrossRef] [PubMed]
52. Locatelli, T.; Cursi, M.; Liberati, D.; Franceschi, M.; Comi, G. EEG coherence in Alzheimer's disease. *Electroencephalogr. Clin. Neurophysiol.* **1998**, *106*, 229–237. [CrossRef]
53. Miyauchi, T.; Hagimoto, H.; Ishii, M.; Endo, S.; Tanaka, K.; Kajiwara, S.; Endo, K.; Kosaka, K. Quantitative EEG in patients with presenile and senile dementia of the Alzheimer type. *Acta Neurol. Scand.* **1994**, *89*, 56–64. [CrossRef]
54. Niedermeyer, E. Alpha rhythms as physiological and abnormal phenomena. *Int. J. Psychophysiol.* **1997**, *26*, 31–49. [CrossRef]
55. Balkan, S.; Yaraş, N.; Mihçi, E.; Dora, B.; Ağar, A.; Yargıçoğlu, P. Effect of donepezil on eeg spectral analysis in Alzheimer's disease. *Acta Neurol. Belg.* **2003**, *103*, 164–169. [PubMed]
56. Watabe, A.M.; O'Dell, T.J. Age-related changes in theta frequency stimulation-induced long-term potentiation. *Neurobiol. Aging* **2003**, *24*, 267–272. [CrossRef]
57. Perlstein, W.M.; Cole, M.A.; Larson, M.; Kelly, K.; Seignourel, P.; Keil, A. Steady-state visual evoked potentials reveal frontally-mediated working memory activity in humans. *Neurosci. Lett.* **2003**, *342*, 191–195. [CrossRef]
58. Silberstein, R.B.; Nunez, P.L.; Pipingas, A.; Harris, P.; Danieli, F. Steady state visually evoked potential (SSVEP) topography in a graded working memory task. *Int. J. Psychophysiol.* **2001**, *42*, 219–232. [CrossRef]
59. Caporale, M.; Palmeri, R.; Corallo, F.; Muscarà, N.; Romeo, L.; Bramanti, A.; Marino, S.; Buono, V.L. Cognitive impairment in obstructive sleep apnea syndrome: A descriptive review. *Sleep Breath.* **2020**, *25*, 29–40. [CrossRef]
60. Guzel, A.; Gunbey, E.; Koksal, N. The performance of critical flicker frequency on determining of neurocognitive function loss in severe obstructive sleep apnea syndrome. *J. Sleep Res.* **2017**, *26*, 651–656. [CrossRef]
61. Schneider, C.; Fulda, S.; Schulz, H. Daytime variation in performance and tiredness/sleepiness ratings in patients with insomnia, narcolepsy, sleep apnea and normal controls. *J. Sleep Res.* **2004**, *13*, 373–383. [CrossRef]
62. Lafère, P.; Balestra, C.; Hemelryck, W.; Donda, N.; Sakr, A.; Taher, A.; Marroni, S.; Germonpré, P. Evaluation of critical flicker fusion frequency and perceived fatigue in divers after air and enriched air nitrox diving. *Diving Hyperb. Med. J.* **2010**, *40*, 114–118.
63. Lafère, P.; Hemelryck, W.; Germonpré, P.; Matity, L.; Guerrero, F.; Balestra, C. Early detection of diving-related cognitive impairment of different nitrogen-oxygen gas mixtures using critical flicker fusion frequency. *Diving Hyperb. Med. J.* **2019**, *49*, 119–126. [CrossRef]

64. Grasby, P.M.; Frith, C.D.; Paulesu, E.; Friston, K.; Frackowiak, R.; Dolan, R. The effect of the muscarinic antagonist scopolamine on regional cerebral blood flow during the performance of a memory task. *Exp. Brain Res.* **1995**, *104*, 337–348. [CrossRef]
65. Kot, J.; Winklewski, P.; Sicko, Z.; Tkachenko, Y. Effect of oxygen on neuronal excitability measured by critical flicker fusion frequency is dose dependent. *J. Clin. Exp. Neuropsychol.* **2015**, *37*, 276–284. [CrossRef]
66. Jammes, Y.; Arbogast, S.; Faucher, M.; Montmayeur, A.; Tagliarini, F.; Meliet, J.L.; Robinet, C. Hyperbaric hyperoxia induces a neuromuscular hyperexcitability: Assessment of a reduced response in elite oxygen divers. *Clin. Physiol. Funct. Imaging* **2003**, *23*, 149–154. [CrossRef] [PubMed]
67. Balestra, C.; Lafère, P.; Germonpré, P. Persistence of critical flicker fusion frequency impairment after a 33 mfw SCUBA dive: Evidence of prolonged nitrogen narcosis. *Eur. J. Appl. Physiol.* **2012**, *112*, 4063–4068. [CrossRef] [PubMed]
68. Conference for National Cooperation in Aquatics. *The New Science of Skin and Scuba Diving: A Revision of the Widely Used Science of Skin and Scuba Diving*; Chairman, B.E.E., Lanphier, E.H., Young, J.E., Goff, L.G., Eds.; Association Press: New York, NY, USA, 1962.
69. Tonner, P.H.; Scholz, J.; Koch, C.; am Esch, J.S. The anesthetic effect of dexmedetomidine does not adhere to the Meyer-Overton rule but is reversed by hydrostatic pressure. *Anesth. Analg.* **1997**, *84*, 618–622. [PubMed]
70. Levett, D.Z.H.; Millar, I.L. Bubble trouble: A review of diving physiology and disease. *Postgrad. Med. J.* **2008**, *84*, 571–578. [CrossRef]
71. Ozgok-Kangal, M.K.; Murphy-Lavoie, H.M. High Pressure Diving Nervous Syndrome. In *StatPearls*; StatPearls Publishing: Treasure Island, FL, USA, 2021.
72. Kot, J. Extremely deep recreational dives: The risk for carbon dioxide (CO_2) retention and high pressure neurological syndrome (HPNS). *Int. Marit. Health* **2012**, *63*, 49–55.
73. Seki, K.; Hugon, M. Critical flicker frequency (CFF) and subjective fatigue during an oxyhelium saturation dive at 62 ATA. *Undersea Biomed. Res.* **1976**, *3*, 235–247.
74. Truszczyński, O.; Wojtkowiak, M.; Biernacki, M.; Kowalczuk, K. The effect of hypoxia on the critical flicker fusion threshold in pilots. *Int. J. Occup. Med. Environ. Health* **2009**, *22*, 13–18. [CrossRef]
75. Adrian, E.D.; Matthews, B.H.C. The Berger rhythm: Potential changes from the occipital lobes in man. *Brain* **1934**, *57*, 355–385. [CrossRef]
76. Herrmann, C.; Strüber, D.; Helfrich, R.F.; Engel, A.K. EEG oscillations: From correlation to causality. *Int. J. Psychophysiol.* **2016**, *103*, 12–21. [CrossRef] [PubMed]
77. Silberstein, R.B. Steady-state visually evoked potentials, brain resonance, and cognitive processes. In *Neocortical Dynamics and EEG Rhythms*; Oxford University Press: Oxford, England, 1995; pp. 272–303.
78. Williams, J. Frequency-specific effects of flicker on recognition memory. *Neuroscience* **2001**, *104*, 283–286. [CrossRef]
79. Herrmann, C.S. Human EEG responses to 1–100 Hz flicker: Resonance phenomena in visual cortex and their potential correlation to cognitive phenomena. *Exp. Brain Res.* **2001**, *137*, 346–353. [CrossRef]
80. Sauseng, P.; Klimesch, W.; Heise, K.-F.; Gruber, W.R.; Holz, E.; Karim, A.; Glennon, M.; Gerloff, C.; Birbaumer, N.; Hummel, F.C. Brain oscillatory substrates of visual short-term memory capacity. *Curr. Biol.* **2009**, *19*, 1846–1852. [CrossRef] [PubMed]

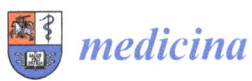

Comment

Comment on Mankowska et al. Critical Flicker Fusion Frequency: A Narrative Review. *Medicina* 2021, 57, 1096

Xavier C. E. Vrijdag [1,*], Hanna van Waart [1], Jamie W. Sleigh [1,2] and Simon J. Mitchell [1,3]

1 Department of Anaesthesiology, School of Medicine, University of Auckland, Private Bag 92019, Auckland 1142, New Zealand; hanna.van.waart@auckland.ac.nz (H.v.W.); jamie.sleigh@waikatodhb.health.nz (J.W.S.); sj.mitchell@auckland.ac.nz (S.J.M.)
2 Department of Anaesthesia, Waikato Hospital, Hamilton 3240, New Zealand
3 Department of Anaesthesia, Auckland City Hospital, Auckland 1023, New Zealand
* Correspondence: x.vrijdag@auckland.ac.nz

We have read with great interest the review by Mankowska et al. and congratulate the authors on providing an overview of the use of critical flicker fusion frequency (CFFF) in medicine and particularly in diving medicine [1]. In their diving and hyperbaric medicine section they discuss CFFF as a measure of cognitive performance, and how this could be influenced by hyperbaric oxygen, nitrogen narcosis, and high-pressure neurologic syndrome. We would like to comment specifically on the diving medicine section of the article and point out some missing literature that provides important context for the use of CFFF in measuring nitrogen narcosis.

First, the paragraph describing nitrogen narcosis mentions the penetration of nitrogen into the lipids of neurons acting to interfere with signal transmission. This is an outdated view on the cellular mechanism of narcosis. Research on anaesthetic gases suggest an effect on ligand-gated ion-channels in the postsynaptic membrane of excitable neurones [2]. Specifically, the $GABA_A$-receptor is known for binding sedative anaesthetics with consequent opening of the ionophore for chloride-ions, causing hyperpolarization of the cell membrane and thereby signal inhibition [2]. Nitrogen is also known to bind to this $GABA_A$-receptor [3]. This indicates that nitrogen narcosis is not a phenomenon of a gas-lipid reaction in the bilayer but is more likely to be a gas-protein reaction within the receptors in the synapses [4].

Second, an incomplete description is given of the effects of air breathing at different diving depths on CFFF. The authors describe several studies that found a reduction in CFFF in divers breathing air at 405 kPa (the equivalent of 30 m of seawater (msw)) either inside a hyperbaric chamber or underwater [5–7]. This reduction in CFFF was interpreted as a reduction in cognitive performance due to nitrogen narcosis. Accordingly, it would be expected that CFFF would be further reduced when diving to 608 kPa (50 msw). However, three uncited studies where divers breathed air at 608 kPa (50 msw) inside a hyperbaric chamber or underwater did not show a further reduction in CFFF as one would expect. They found either no change [8] or an increase in CFFF [9,10]. This would indicate that there are possibly other factors influencing the CFFF measurement at 608 kPa, which casts considerable doubt on the suitability of CFFF to measure nitrogen narcosis across the plausible range of air diving exposures. A more elaborative overview of the diving CFFF literature is given elsewhere [8].

Third, in the section about "CFFF and its connection with brainwaves," there seems to be a semantic discrepancy between CFFF, defined as 'critical flicker fusion frequency' and 'flickering light.' The description of the influence of flickering light on the electroencephalogram (EEG) has little or nothing to do with CFFF. It therefore seems out of place in a narrative review about CFFF.

Citation: Vrijdag, X.C.E.; van Waart, H.; Sleigh, J.W.; Mitchell, S.J. Comment on Mankowska et al. Critical Flicker Fusion Frequency: A Narrative Review. *Medicina* 2021, 57, 1096. *Medicina* 2022, 58, 739. https://doi.org/10.3390/medicina58060739

Academic Editor: Enrico Camporesi

Received: 26 April 2022
Accepted: 18 May 2022
Published: 30 May 2022

Publisher's Note: MDPI stays neutral with regard to jurisdictional claims in published maps and institutional affiliations.

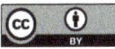

Copyright: © 2022 by the authors. Licensee MDPI, Basel, Switzerland. This article is an open access article distributed under the terms and conditions of the Creative Commons Attribution (CC BY) license (https://creativecommons.org/licenses/by/4.0/).

Author Contributions: Conceptualization, X.C.E.V.; writing—original draft preparation, X.C.E.V.; writing—review and editing, all authors; supervision, H.v.W., J.W.S. and S.J.M. All authors have read and agreed to the published version of the manuscript.

Funding: This study was supported by funding from the Office for Naval Research Global (ONRG), United States Navy (N62909-18-1-2007).

Conflicts of Interest: The authors declare no conflict of interest.

References

1. Mankowska, N.D.; Marcinkowska, A.B.; Waskow, M.; Sharma, R.I.; Kot, J.; Winklewski, P.J. Critical Flicker Fusion Frequency: A Narrative Review. *Medicina* **2021**, *57*, 1096. [CrossRef]
2. Smith, C.R.; Spiess, B.D. The Two Faces of Eve: Gaseous Anaesthesia and Inert Gas Narcosis. *Diving Hyperb. Med.* **2010**, *40*, 68–77. [PubMed]
3. Abraini, J.H.; Kriem, B.; Balon, N.; Rostain, J.C.; Risso, J.J. Gamma-Aminobutyric Acid Neuropharmacological Investigations on Narcosis Produced by Nitrogen, Argon, or Nitrous Oxide. *Anesth. Analg.* **2003**, *96*, 746–749. [CrossRef] [PubMed]
4. Rostain, J.C.; Lavoute, C.; Risso, J.J.; Vallee, N.; Weiss, M. A Review of Recent Neurochemical Data on Inert Gas Narcosis. *Undersea Hyperb. Med.* **2011**, *38*, 49–59. [PubMed]
5. Balestra, C.; Lafère, P.; Germonpré, P. Persistence of Critical Flicker Fusion Frequency Impairment after a 33 Mfw SCUBA Dive: Evidence of Prolonged Nitrogen Narcosis? *Eur. J. Appl. Physiol.* **2012**, *112*, 4063–4068. [CrossRef] [PubMed]
6. Lafère, P.; Balestra, C.; Hemelryck, W.; Guerrero, F.; Germonpré, P. Do Environmental Conditions Contribute to Narcosis Onset and Symptom Severity? *Int. J. Sports Med.* **2016**, *37*, 1124–1128. [CrossRef] [PubMed]
7. Lafère, P.; Hemelryck, W.; Germonpré, P.; Matity, L.; Guerrero, F.; Balestra, C. Early Detection of Diving-Related Cognitive Impairment of Different Nitrogen-Oxygen Gas Mixtures Using Critical Flicker Fusion Frequency. *Diving Hyperb. Med.* **2019**, *49*, 119–126. [CrossRef] [PubMed]
8. Vrijdag, X.C.; van Waart, H.; Sleigh, J.W.; Balestra, C.; Mitchell, S.J. Investigating Critical Flicker Fusion Frequency for Monitoring Gas Narcosis in Divers. *Diving Hyperb. Med.* **2020**, *50*, 377–385. [CrossRef] [PubMed]
9. Tikkinen, J.; Wuorimaa, T.; Siimes, M.A. A Comparison of Simple Reaction Time, Visual Discrimination and Critical Flicker Fusion Frequency in Professional Divers at Elevated Pressure. *Diving Hyperb. Med.* **2016**, *46*, 82–86. [PubMed]
10. Rocco, M.; Pelaia, P.; Di Benedetto, P.; Conte, G.; Maggi, L.; Fiorelli, S.; Mercieri, M.; Balestra, C.; De Blasi, R.A. Inert Gas Narcosis in Scuba Diving, Different Gases Different Reactions. *Eur. J. Appl. Physiol.* **2019**, *119*, 247–255. [CrossRef] [PubMed]

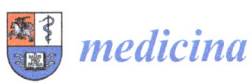

Reply

Reply to Vrijdag et al. Comment on "Mankowska et al. Critical Flicker Fusion Frequency: A Narrative Review. *Medicina* 2021, 57, 1096"

Natalia D. Mankowska [1,*], Anna B. Marcinkowska [1,2,3], Monika Waskow [3], Rita I. Sharma [4,5], Jacek Kot [6] and Pawel J. Winklewski [2,3,4]

1 Applied Cognitive Neuroscience Lab, Department of Human Physiology, Medical University of Gdansk, 80-210 Gdansk, Poland; anna.marcinkowska@gumed.edu.pl
2 2nd Department of Radiology, Medical University of Gdansk, 80-210 Gdansk, Poland; pawelwinklewski@wp.pl
3 Institute of Health Sciences, Pomeranian University in Slupsk, 76-200 Slupsk, Poland; monika.waskow@apsl.edu.pl
4 Department of Human Physiology, Medical University of Gdansk, 80-210 Gdansk, Poland; rita.sharma@gumed.edu.pl
5 Department of Anaesthesiology and Intensive Care, Medical University of Gdansk, 80-210 Gdansk, Poland
6 National Centre for Hyperbaric Medicine, Institute of Maritime and Tropical Medicine in Gdynia, Medical University of Gdansk, 80-210 Gdansk, Poland; jkot@gumed.edu.pl
* Correspondence: natalia.mankowska@gumed.edu.pl; Tel./Fax: +48-58-3491515

Citation: Mankowska, N.D.; Marcinkowska, A.B.; Waskow, M.; Sharma, R.I.; Kot, J.; Winklewski, P.J. Reply to Vrijdag et al. Comment on "Mankowska et al. Critical Flicker Fusion Frequency: A Narrative Review. *Medicina* 2021, 57, 1096". *Medicina* 2022, 58, 765. https://doi.org/10.3390/medicina58060765

Academic Editor: Enrico Camporesi

Received: 27 May 2022
Accepted: 31 May 2022
Published: 6 June 2022

Publisher's Note: MDPI stays neutral with regard to jurisdictional claims in published maps and institutional affiliations.

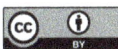

Copyright: © 2022 by the authors. Licensee MDPI, Basel, Switzerland. This article is an open access article distributed under the terms and conditions of the Creative Commons Attribution (CC BY) license (https://creativecommons.org/licenses/by/4.0/).

Thank you very much for your interest and comments [1] on the review by Mankowska et al. [2], aiming at providing an overview of the use of critical flicker fusion frequency (CFFF) to investigate cognitive functions.

We agree with the authors of the Commentary [1] that the $GABA_A$-receptor might be involved in nitrogen narcosis [3,4]. Yet, the precise molecular mechanisms of the adaptation of lipid bilayers to pressure are unknown and require further investigation [5]. The traditional view is that the lipid bilayer of the cellular membrane is the main target for anesthesia and pressure, while newer theories stress the role of transmembrane proteins. It is, however, likely that nitrogen may exert a pluripotent activity, targeting lipids and transmembrane proteins and implicitly affect water molecules at the lipid–solvent interface [5]. Consequently, the membrane theory and the $GABA_A$ theory do not need to exclude each other [5,6]. Most importantly, presenting a discussion of the physiological mechanisms underlying anesthesiologic and pressure effects, although fascinating, was not the aim of the review. Rather, we strived to summarize the existing knowledge regarding the reliability of CFFF in the assessment of cognitive functioning versus other psychometric methods.

We have never implied that a reduction in CFFF while diving should be interpreted as a decline in cognitive performance solely due to nitrogen narcosis. On the contrary, we stressed that it is a multifactorial phenomenon, and, particularly when diving below 50 msw (more than 608 kPa), there might be other variables such as oxygen toxicity. The dose–reaction relations between oxygen and cognitive functions is not clear and actually it is not known whether the increased excitability, and which forms of neuronal excitability, should be considered a part of the learning process or, rather, cellular manifestation of neuronal oxygen poisoning [7]. Consequently, it is not surprising that below 50 msw a further reduction in CFFF is not seen.

Indeed, "critical flicker fusion frequency" is not the same as "flickering light". However, to the best of our knowledge, there are no studies yet that conclusively explain the mechanisms underlying the processing of flickering light, so we do not know how exactly decisions to perceive flicker or light continuity are made, and thus how the CFFF threshold is determined. We believe that it is impossible to understand CFFF without understanding these mechanisms, so describing CFFF in the context of flickering light was intended to suggest the need for further research using neuroimaging (e.g., electroencephalography), which could explain what dependencies and interactions we might expect when using the CFFF test. If we want to use the CFFF test as a measure of an individual's arousal [8–10] or cognitive ability [11–13], including in pathological conditions such as epilepsy [14] or Alzheimer's disease [15,16], we must understand how it interacts with the individual's brain. In diving medicine, the use of electroencephalography to investigate the mechanisms underlying processes measured by CFFF seems particularly interesting in the light of the theory focused on the depth-related "effect on ligand-gated ion-channels in the postsynaptic membrane of excitable neurons".

Author Contributions: Conceptualization, N.D.M., J.K. and P.J.W.; methodology N.D.M.; validation, A.B.M., R.I.S. and M.W.; formal analysis, N.D.M. and A.B.M.; resources, M.W., J.K. and P.J.W.; writing—original draft preparation, N.D.M. and P.J.W.; writing—review and editing, all authors; supervision, A.B.M., J.K. and P.J.W.; project administration, N.D.M. All authors have read and agreed to the published version of the manuscript.

Funding: This research received no external funding.

Conflicts of Interest: The authors declare no conflict of interest.

References

1. Vrijdag, X.C.E.; van Waart, H.; Sleigh, J.W.; Mitchell, S.J. Comment on Mankowska et al. Critical Flicker Fusion Frequency: A Narrative Review. *Medicina* 2021, *57*, 1096. *Medicina* 2022, *58*, 739. [CrossRef]
2. Mankowska, N.D.; Marcinkowska, A.B.; Waskow, M.; Sharma, R.I.; Kot, J.; Winklewski, P.J. Critical Flicker Fusion Frequency: A Narrative Review. *Medicina* 2021, *57*, 1096. [CrossRef] [PubMed]
3. Abraini, J.H.; Kriem, B.; Balon, N.; Rostain, J.C.; Risso, J.J. Gamma-aminobutyric acid neuropharmacological investigations on narcosis produced by nitrogen, argon, or nitrous oxide. *Anesth. Analg.* 2003, *96*, 746–749. [CrossRef] [PubMed]
4. Weir, C.J. The molecular mechanisms of general anaesthesia: Dissecting the GABAA receptor. *Contin. Educ. Anaesth. Crit. Care Pain* 2006, *6*, 49–53. [CrossRef]
5. Moskovitz, Y.; Yang, H. Modelling of noble anaesthetic gases and high hydrostatic pressure effects in lipid bilayers. *Soft Matter* 2015, *11*, 2125–2138. [CrossRef] [PubMed]
6. Rostain, J.C.; Lavoute, C. Neurochemistry of Pressure-Induced Nitrogen and Metabolically Inert Gas Narcosis in the Central Nervous System. *Compr. Physiol.* 2011, *6*, 1579–1590. [CrossRef]
7. Kot, J.; Winklewski, P.J.; Sicko, Z.; Tkachenko, Y. Effect of oxygen on neuronal excitability measured by critical flicker fusion frequency is dose dependent. *J. Clin. Exp. Neuropsychol.* 2015, *37*, 276–284. [CrossRef] [PubMed]
8. Ardestani, S.B.; Balestra, C.; Bouzinova, E.V.; Loennechen, Ø.; Pedersen, M. Evaluation of divers' neuropsychometric effectiveness and high-pressure neurological syndrome via computerized test battery package and questionnaires in operational setting. *Front. Physiol.* 2019, *10*, 1386. [CrossRef] [PubMed]
9. Balestra, C.; Machado, M.-L.L.; Theunissen, S.; Balestra, A.; Cialoni, D.; Clot, C.; Besnard, S.; Kammacher, L.; Delzenne, J.; Germonpré, P.; et al. Critical flicker fusion frequency: A marker of cerebral arousal during modified gravitational conditions related to parabolic flights. *Front. Physiol.* 2018, *9*, 1403. [CrossRef] [PubMed]
10. Lambourne, K.; Audiffren, M.; Tomporowski, P.D. Effects of acute exercise on sensory and executive processing tasks. *Med. Sci. Sports Exerc.* 2010, *42*, 1396–1402. [CrossRef] [PubMed]
11. Dixon, R.; Hughes, A.M.; Nairn, K.; Sellers, M.; Kemp, J.V.; Yates, R.A. Effects of the antimigraine compound zolmitriptan ('Zomig') on psychomotor performance alone and in combination with diazepam in healthy volunteers. *Cephalalgia* 1998, *18*, 468–475. [CrossRef] [PubMed]
12. Skottun, B.C. On using very high temporal frequencies to isolate magnocellular contributions to psychophysical tasks. *Neuropsychologia* 2013, *51*, 1556–1560. [CrossRef] [PubMed]
13. Williams, J.; Ramaswamy, D.; Oulhaj, A. 10 Hz flicker improves recognition memory in older people. *BMC Neurosci.* 2006, *7*, 21. [CrossRef] [PubMed]
14. Achinivu, K.; Staufenberg, E.; Cull, C.; Cavanna, A.E.; Ring, H. Cognitive Function During Vagus Nerve Stimulation for Treatment-Refractory Epilepsy: A Pilot Study Using the Critical Flicker Fusion Test. *J. Neuropsychol.* 2012, *16*, 32–36. [CrossRef]
15. Curran, S.; Wattis, J. Critical flicker fusion threshold: A potentially useful measure for the early detection of Alzheimer's disease. *Hum. Psychopharmacol.* 2000, *15*, 103–112. [CrossRef]
16. Merrill, C.A.; Jonsson, M.A.G.; Minthon, L.; Ejnell, H.; Silander, H.C.S.; Blennow, K.; Karlsson, M.; Nordlund, A.; Rolstad, S.; Warkentin, S.; et al. Vagus nerve stimulation in patients with Alzheimer's disease: Additional follow-up results of a pilot study through 1 year. *J. Clin. Psychiatry* 2006, *67*, 1171–1178. [CrossRef] [PubMed]

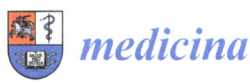

Article

Effect of SCUBA Diving on Ophthalmic Parameters

Laurent Deleu [1,*], Janet Catherine [2], Laurence Postelmans [2] and Costantino Balestra [3,4,*]

1. Cliniques Universitaires de Bruxelles, Department of Ophthalmology, Hôpital Erasme, Université Libre de Bruxelles (ULB), Route de Lennik 808, 1070 Brussels, Belgium
2. CHU Brugmann, Department of Ophthalmology, Université Libre de Bruxelles (ULB), Site Victor Horta Place Arthur Van Gehuchten 4, 1020 Brussels, Belgium; janet.catherine@gmail.com (J.C.); laurencedominique.postelmans@chu-brugmann.be (L.P.)
3. Laboratory of Environmental and Occupational (Integrative) Physiology, Haute Ecole Bruxelles-Brabant, 1160 Brussels, Belgium
4. Physical Activity Teaching Unit, Motor Sciences Department, Université Libre de Bruxelles (ULB), 1050 Brussels, Belgium
* Correspondence: laurent.deleu@gmail.com (L.D.); costantinobalestra@gmail.com (C.B.)

Abstract: *Background and Objective*: Several cases of central serous chorioretinopathy (CSC) in divers have been reported in our medical retina center over the past few years. This study was designed to evaluate possible changes induced by SCUBA diving in ophthalmic parameters and especially subfoveal choroidal thickness (SFCT), since the choroid seems to play a crucial role in physiopathology of CSC. *Materials and Methods*: Intraocular pressure (IOP), SFCT, pachymetry, flow-mediated dilation (FMD), blood pressure, and heart rate were measured in 15 healthy volunteer divers before diving, 30 and 60 min after a standard deep dive of 25 m depth for 25 min in a dedicated diving pool (NEMO 33). *Results*: SFCT reduces significantly to 96.63 ± 13.89% of pre-dive values ($p = 0.016$) 30 min after diving. It recovers after 60 min reaching control values. IOP decreases to 88.05 ± 10.04% of pre-dive value at 30 min, then increases to 91.42 ± 10.35% of its pre-dive value (both $p < 0.0001$). Pachymetry shows a slight variation, but is significantly increased to 101.63 ± 1.01% ($p = 0.0159$) of the pre-dive value, and returns to control level after 60 min. FMD pre-dive was 107 ± 6.7% ($p < 0.0001$), but post-dive showed a diminished increase to 103 ± 6.5% ($p = 0.0132$). The pre-post difference was significant ($p = 0.03$). *Conclusion*: Endothelial dysfunction leading to arterial stiffness after diving may explain the reduced SFCT observed, but SCUBA diving seems to have miscellaneous consequences on eye parameters. Despite this clear influence on SFCT, no clear relationship between CSC and SCUBA diving can be drawn.

Keywords: subfoveal choroidal thickness; intraocular pressure; central corneal thickness; central serous chorioretinopathy; flow-mediated dilation; arterial stiffness; endothelial dysfunction

Citation: Deleu, L.; Catherine, J.; Postelmans, L.; Balestra, C. Effect of SCUBA Diving on Ophthalmic Parameters. *Medicina* 2022, *58*, 408. https://doi.org/10.3390/medicina58030408

Academic Editor: Enrico Camporesi

Received: 6 February 2022
Accepted: 7 March 2022
Published: 9 March 2022

Publisher's Note: MDPI stays neutral with regard to jurisdictional claims in published maps and institutional affiliations.

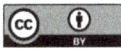

Copyright: © 2022 by the authors. Licensee MDPI, Basel, Switzerland. This article is an open access article distributed under the terms and conditions of the Creative Commons Attribution (CC BY) license (https://creativecommons.org/licenses/by/4.0/).

1. Introduction

Diving is a recreational and professional activity with many potential risks. Effects of SCUBA diving on the eye have been often reported, including retinal complications (ocular barotrauma, decompression sickness syndrome, arterial gas embolism, ultraviolet keratitis, choroidal ischemia, retinal vein occlusion, central serous chorioretinopathy, variation in color/contrast sensibility, etc.) [1–5].

Central serous chorioretinopathy (CSC) is a potentially severe ocular disease of the retina characterized by recurrent and/or persistent subretinal fluid, causing severe retinal pigment epithelial alterations and a variable degree of visual loss. In our medical retina center, we noticed the presence of common history of SCUBA diving among CSC patients representing around 4% of cases during a two-year period. It is known that CSC is commonly associated with choroidal hyperpermeability and increased subfoveal choroidal thickness (SFCT), but its physiopathology is still poorly understood [6,7].

Considering the importance of SFCT in the diagnostic of CSC, we studied the effect of diving on SFCT and other parameters before and after a deep dive.

2. Methods

2.1. Patients and Timing of the Study

For this study, 15 volunteer healthy divers were first interrogated about their medical and diving history, and signed an inform consent. Divers were otherwise healthy Caucasian males between 28 and 72 years old (median 48.93 years). Body mass index 20–25, good general health, nonsmoking (except one), and certified as "advanced divers" with at least 50 logged dives. Of these, three presented treated arterial hypertension, and one with diabetes mellitus without related ophthalmic impairment. Exclusion criteria included previous eye diseases. The study protocol was approved by the Local Ethic Committee Brussels (Academic Bioethical Committee, Brussels, Belgium. Reference Number: B200-2020-088. Date: 10 October 2020), and each subject gave written informed consent before participation. All studies were performed in accordance with the Declaration of Helsinki [8]. The study is part of a series of ongoing field studies on vascular gas emboli (VGE).

All divers received one drop of tropicamide 0.5% (5 mg/mL) in both eyes. Then, 20 min after instillation, they were examined for intraocular pressure (IOP), pachymetry (PACHY), keratometry (KR), subfoveal choroidal thickness (SFCT), and retinal autofluorescence. They were all tested for post-ischemic flow-mediated dilation (FMD), blood pressure (BP), and heart rate (HR). They also underwent transthoracic heart echography (TTE). After pre-dive measures, all divers went for 25 m dive for 25 min in Nemo 33 diving pool in Brussels. Half of the divers underwent measures during the morning, and the other half in the afternoon. All divers respected published decompression tables while coming back to the surface.

Respectively 30 and 60 min after regaining surface, the patients were retested for the same ocular tests. FMD of brachial artery was measured 30 min after regaining surface. BP, HR, and TTE were also controlled after diving looking for post-dive vascular gas emboli (VGE). All divers drank 500 mL water 60 min after the dive.

2.2. Data Acquisition

2.2.1. Ophthalmic Measurements

Nidek Tonoref III (NIDEK Co., Ltd., Tokyo, Japan) was used to measure IOP, PACHY, and KR. Pachymetry is here defined by the central corneal thickness, and keratometry is defined by the corneal curvature of the main corneal meridians. Results were calculated using mean of three values for each eye. IOP was not corrected by pachymetry. Nidek Tonoref III provides accurate and reliable measurements of IOP, compared with Goldmann applanation tonometry, considered as the gold-standard for IOP measurements [9]. Even older devices of air tonometers show low variability ranging from -2 mmHg to $+2$ mmHg, principally due to the cardiac cycle, explaining why three measures should be taken in regular practice [10].

SFCT was measured with enhanced depth imaging (EDI) modality using a Spectral Domain-Optical Coherence Tomography (SD-OCT) (Spectralis, wavelength: 870 nm; Heidelberg Engineering Co. Manufacturer: Heidelberg Engineering GmbH, Heidelberg, Germany). The same device was used for retinal autofluorescence imaging. SD-OCT gives two or three-dimensional images of the retina with near-cellular resolution, allowing ophthalmologists to analyze histologic-like images. SD-OCT uses near-infrared wavelength, and thus does not expose patients to radiation. The procedure for SFCT measurement that we used was previously described by Spaide et al. [11], and is defined as the vertical distance from the hyperreflective line of Bruch's membrane to the hyperreflective line of the inner surface of the sclera. All images were taken by one clinician, and were assessed by three different clinicians. Clinicians were blinded, as they did not know the patient's identification and timing of the measure (pre or post dive). Personal keratometry was encoded in Heidelberg OCT to improve each diver's measurements.

2.2.2. Flow-Mediated Dilation (FMD)

FMD, an established measure of the endothelium-dependent vasodilation mediated by nitric oxide (NO) [12], was used to assess the effect of diving on main conduit arteries. Subjects were at rest for 15-min in a supine position before the measurements were taken. They were asked not to drink caffeinated beverages for the 6 h preceding measurements. Subjects were instructed not to perform strenuous physical exercise 24 h before, or stay in altitude up to 2 weeks before and during the entire study protocol. Brachial artery diameter was measured by means of a 5.0–10.0 MHz linear transducer using a Mindray DP-30 digital diagnostic ultrasound system immediately before and 1-min after a 5-min ischemia induced by inflating a cuff placed on the forearm to 180 mmHg as previously described [13].

All ultrasound assessments were performed by an experienced operator, with more than 100 scans/year, which is recommended to maintain competency with the FMD method [14].

When the images were chosen for analysis, the boundaries for diameter measurement were identified manually with an electronic caliper (provided by the ultrasonography software) in a threefold repetition pattern to calculate the mean value. In our laboratory, the mean intra-observer variability for FMD measurement for the operator (CB) recorded the same day, on the same site, and on the same subject was $1.2 \pm 0.2\%$.

Post-dive values were obtained 20–30 min after surfacing. The divers were given a specific time to enter into the water with their companion (buddy) in order to make it possible to respect the tight timing after the dive for the measurements to be taken. FMD were calculated as the percent increase in arterial diameter from the resting state to maximal dilation.

2.2.3. Post Diving Vascular Gas Emboli (VGE)

Post-dive vascular gas emboli (VGE) (decompression bubbles) were observed using transthoracic echocardiography and a "frame-based" counting method for VGE recently described [15], allowing for continuous values and parametric statistical approaches. Echocardiography was done with a Vivid-I portable echocardiograph (Manufacturer: GE Healthcare, Chalfont Saint Giles, UK) used at the poolside; echocardiography loops were recorded on hard disk for offline analysis by three blinded evaluators. VGE numbers were counted at 30 min and 60 min post dive.

3. Statistical Analysis

The normality of data was performed by means of Shapiro–Wilk or D'Agostino-Pearson tests. When a Gaussian distribution was assumed, they were analyzed with a one-way ANOVA for repeated measures with Dunnett's post-hoc test; when comparisons were limited to two samples, paired or non-paired t-test were applied. If the Gaussian distribution was not assumed, the analysis was performed by means of a non-parametric multiple comparisons using Dunn's test or, if limited to two samples, a Wilcoxon test. Taking the baseline measures as 100%, percentage changes were calculated for each diver, allowing for an appreciation of the magnitude of change rather than the absolute values. All statistical tests were performed using a standard computer statistical package, GraphPad Prism version 5.00 for Windows (GraphPad Software, San Diego, CA, USA). A threshold of $p < 0.05$ was considered statistically significant. All data are presented as mean ± standard deviation (SD). Sample size was calculated setting the power of the study at 95%, and assuming that variables associated to diving would have been affected on a similar extent than that observed in our previous studies [16–18].

4. Results

4.1. Generalities

All results are expressed in a percentage of pre-dive values (relative values) rather than absolute values. Studied parameters and especially SFCT have high interindividual variability. As each diver acts as his/her own control, results were expressed in percentage of pre-dive values so that this proportion could be compared and analyzed with others. As explained in statistical analysis section, taking the baseline measures as 100%, percentage changes were calculated for each diver, allowing an appreciation of the magnitude of change rather than the absolute values.

4.2. Diving Related

FMD comparison between pre/post dive situation and control values is shown in Figure 1. FMD in our divers is increased in pre-dive situation (107.15 ± 6.6% ($p < 0.0001$)). This dilatation is significantly reduced after the dive (103 ± 6.5%, $p = 0.026$). This reduction between the two conditions shows a difference consistent with previously published data and is significant ($p = 0.027$) [19].

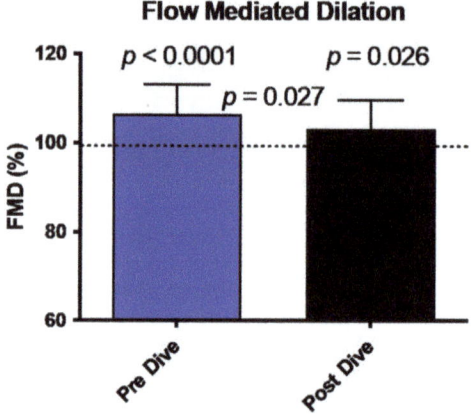

Figure 1. Bar graph illustrating the reduction of FMD 30 min post dive (black bar) compared to predive values (Blue Bar) (mean ± SD). ($N = 15$).

All divers underwent trans-thoracic echocardiography (TTE) 30 min and 60 min after the dive. Figure 2 shows that divers had, on average, eight bubbles per heartbeat (8.0 ± 9.3; mean ± SD) in the right heart (ventricle or atrium) 30 min after the dive. This number is reduced to a mean of 5.25 ± 8.8 Bubbles per HB. The number of circulating decompression bubbles per heartbeat after an hour post the dive was significantly reduced. No participant had symptoms of decompression disease, and the number of VGE found and its decrease is consistent with previously published data [20,21].

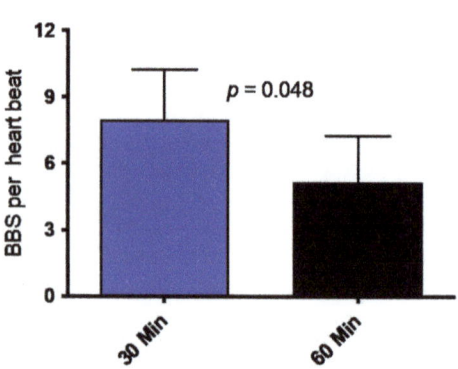

Figure 2. Number of bubbles (BBS = Bubbles) per heartbeat 30 min (blue bar) and 60 min (black bar) after diving. (Mean ± SD).

4.3. Ophthalmological

Comparisons between pre and post-dive values appear in Table 1, and are expressed as a percentage relative to pre-dive values. SFCT and IOP both decrease significantly 30 min after the dive. SFCT recovers pre-dive thickness after 60 min, but IOP is still diminished after an hour. Corneal thickness tends to slightly increase, but the change is no longer significant after 60 min. Table 2 presents mean ± SD of measurements. Ophthalmic data post-dive are significantly altered 30 min post-dive, most of which returned to basal levels 60 min post diving, except IOP, which stayed still reduced 60 min post dive. Figure 3 shows OCT imaging of normal posterior pole of the eye, with color code to distinguish retina from choroid and sclera. This figure helps better understanding of Figure 4, which shows comparison between SFCT before and 30 min after diving in a same eye. High magnification was used to highlight the 11 μm difference in this case.

Table 1. Comparison (in percentage of pre-dive values) of SFCT, IOP, and pachymetry between pre- and post-dive values at 30 min and 60 min post dive.

Mean ± SD	Pre-Dive	30 min Post-Dive	*p*-Value	60 min Post-Dive	*p*-Value
SFCT (%)	100	96.6 (±13.89)	0.016	98.4 (±5.7)	0.21 (ns)
IOP (%)	100	88.05 (±10.03)	<0.0001	91.4 (±10.3)	<0.0001
Pachymetry (%)	100	101.6 (±1.0)	0.015	100.2 (±1.4)	ns

(ns = not significant).

Table 2. Mean measures ± SD of SFCT (expressed in μm), IOP (expressed in mmHg) and pachymetry (expressed in μm).

Mean ± SD	Pre-Dive	30 min Post-Dive	*p*-Value	60 min Post-Dive	*p*-Value
SFCT (μm)	327.1 (±102.0)	318.1 (±109.7)	0.0326	322.2 (±102.1)	0.2434
IOP (mmHg)	16.4 (±2.009)	14.3 (±2.27)	<0.0001	14.98 (±2.67)	<0.0001
Pachymetry (μm)	559.3 (±27.83)	566.5 (±33.53)	0.0120	562.9 (±28.62)	ns

(ns = not significant).

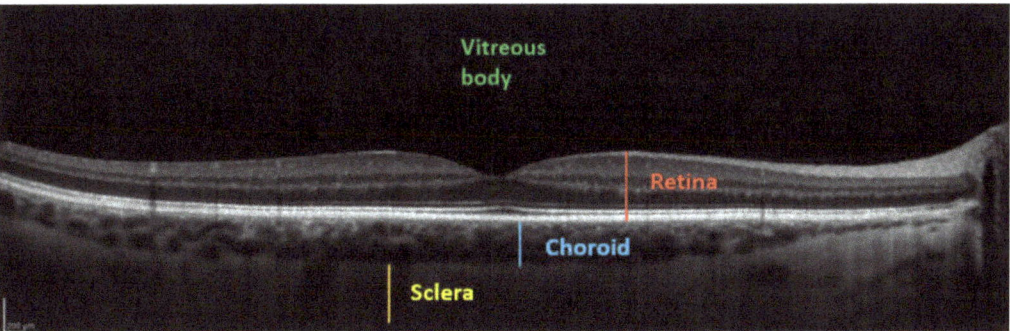

Figure 3. Enhanced depth imaging-optical coherence tomography (EDI-OCT) showing different structures. From anterior to posterior: Vitreous body (green), neurosensory retina and the retinal pigment epithelium (red), choroid (SFCT in blue), and sclera (yellow).

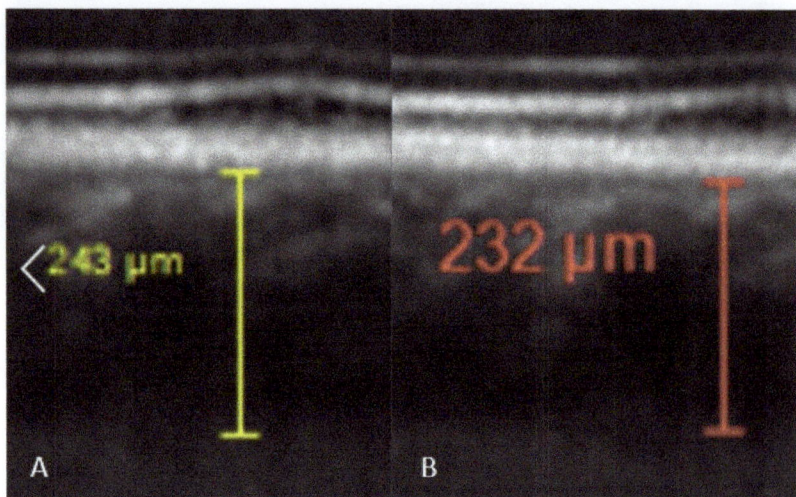

Figure 4. Comparison of SFCT in the same diver before the dive ((**A**), SFCT estimated at 243 μm by one of the investigators), and 30 min after the dive ((**B**), SFCT estimated at 232 μm).

5. Discussion
5.1. Subfoveal Choroidal Thickness

The choroid is a vascular layer situated between the sclera and the retina. It is composed of several layers: the choriocapillaris, 10 μm-thick capillary network; the Sattler's layer, composed of arterioles, small arteries, and veins; Haller's layer, composed of larger blood vessels; the suprachoroid, which is non-vascular, composed of melanocytes, fibroblasts and collagen; and the lamina fusca, separating the choroid from the sclera [22]. It is a highly vascularized space, as the flow per perfused volume is the highest of any other human tissue [23]. While it is well-known that myopic eyes (with greater axial length) tend to have thinner choroid, myopic shift can induce thickening of SFCT in animals, while hyperopic shift induces thinning of SFCT [24]. Mechanisms remain hypothetic, but Wallman et al. observed that, at least in birds, SFCT variation is linked to expansion or compression of lacunae present in the outer choroid [25]. Liquid redistribution seems to be the key of SFCT variation by different suggested mechanisms [24]. However, people with myopic eyes tend to have thinner choroid than emmetropic or hyperopic eyes. These factors make it difficult to know what abnormal SFCT is or not. Studies may give different normal values. Akhtar et al. concluded that subfoveal choroidal thickness was 307 ± 79 μm in an Indian population of any age [26]. Entezari et al. concluded 363 ± 84 μm in an Iranian population [27]. Karapetyan et al. compared SFCT in Caucasians, Africans, and Asians populations, and concluded no significant differences between those ethnics. The mean SFCT in Caucasians was 403.62 ± 37.4 μm. The literature presents sometimes normal SFCT ranges that may be different from ours [28]. Moreover, SFCT seems to decrease over day time [11]. All of these considerations show the importance of measuring variations taking the baseline measures as 100%, for each diver, allowing an appreciation of the magnitude of change rather than the absolute values.

To the best of our knowledge, acute effects of diving on SFCT have never been studied. Our study shows transient and significant SFCT decrease in the 30 first minutes following a deep dive. After 60 min, SFCT returns to its initial thickness. Different hypotheses were investigated to explain those results.

Our preferred hypothesis is that SFCT decreases due to vascular phenomena. As previously said and confirmed by other studies, FMD decreases after a deep dive due to endothelial dysfunction [29,30]. Considering the density of blood vessels in the choroid, reduced dilation of this vascular meshwork could explain by itself the reduction in SFCT.

Moreover, diving involves an increase in oxygen partial pressure leading to oxidative stress by increased free radical concentration in blood. This contributes to endothelial dysfunction and, ultimately, arterial stiffness. It seems likely that vascular smooth muscles also have a role in FMD reduction, but various results are found in studies [29,31]. Implications of smooth-muscle cells might be important, as it has been shown that non-vascular smooth-muscle cells are present in primates in the suprachoroid (just next to lacunae), and in a single layer just beneath Bruch's membrane [32]. It has been suggested that contraction of those smooth-muscle cells oppose the tendency of lacunae to gain fluid [24]. Insufficient relaxation of these cells might prevent swelling of the lacunae, inducing vascular shift from the choroid to general circulation, decreasing SFCT. Thus, both arterial stiffness due to endothelial dysfunction and insufficient relaxation in choroidal smooth-muscle cells reduce the choroidal intravascular fluid and are an explanation to reduced SFCT post diving.

In the literature, SFCT tends to be negatively correlated to IOP [33–38]. As both IOP and SFCT decrease in our study, IOP variation does not explain the SFCT decreases. It is also interesting to notice that pachymetry increases in our study and would be expected to falsely elevate the IOP. We can confidently conclude that changes in IOP and pachymetry are not responsible for the diminution of SFCT after the dive. It is a good argument to suggest that there is an extra-ophthalmological phenomenon explaining SFCT reduction.

Other hypotheses were also considered as being unlikely with our experimental setting:

Effects of physical exercise on SFCT have been reported but results are various and not well established [39–41].

Tropicamide was instilled before pre-dive measures, therefore there was no influence in comparison between pre- and post-dive values. Iovino et al. published in 2020 that there was no significant difference in SFCT before or after mydriatic instillation [42].

SFCT presents diurnal variation and tends to decrease over the day. Some divers underwent measures in the morning, other in the afternoon. Both are periods of decreasing SFCT, so we do not expect any difference between those two cohorts for relative measurements. Moreover, this circadian cycle does not explain the re-increase of SFCT 60 min after the dive. This points out an extra-physiological phenomenon allowing us to exclude this hypothesis.

5.2. Flow-Mediated Dilation (FMD) and Vascular Gas Emboli

A nitric oxide (NO) mediated change in the surface properties of the vascular endothelium favoring the elimination of gas micronuclei has previously been suggested to explain this protection against bubble formation [43]. It was shown that NO synthase activity increases following 45 min of exercise, and that NO administration immediately before a dive reduces VGE [44]. Nevertheless, bubble production is increased by NO blockade in sedentary but not in exercised rats [45], suggesting other biochemical pathways such HSPs, antioxidant defenses or blood rheology.

Vascular gas emboli are probably involved in the post dive reduction of FMD. Nevertheless the available literature refrains us to draw a direct link between FMD reduction and VGE, since micro and macro vascularization react differently [30], and different preconditioning procedures before diving have specific actions independently on FMD and VGE, while others interfere with both [20].

It appears that FMD seems more linked to oxygen partial pressure changes during diving, whereas VGE are more depending on preexisting gas micronuclei population in the tissues and vascular system and coping with inflammatory responses [20,46,47].

FMD is a marker of endothelial function and is reduced in the brachial artery of healthy divers after single or repetitive dives [48,49]. This effect does not seem to be related to the amount of VGE, and was partially reversed by acute and long-term pre-dive supplementation of antioxidants, implicating oxidative stress as an important contributor to post-dive endothelial dysfunction [29]. Decreased nitroglycerin-mediated dilation after diving highlights dysfunction in vascular smooth-muscle cells as possible etiology of those results [29]. Very recent data show that the FMD reduction encountered after a single dive without presence of VGE, is comparable to the reduction encountered with the presence of VGE [19].

Our results about FMD are in tune with what has been previously described in literature on the subject and, with its consequences, is the most likely explanation to decreased SFCT observed in this study.

5.3. Central Serous Chorioretinopathy

CSC is characterized by localized serous retinal detachment associated with focal altered retinal pigment epithelium. Known risk factors are genetics, male gender, cardiovascular diseases and arterial hypertension, increased corticosteroids blood concentration by any income, pregnancy, psychopathology (type A personality), peptic ulcer and Helicobacter Pylori, some drugs (including phosphodiesterase-5 inhibitors), and sleep disturbances. Despite being a common chorioretinal disease, pathophysiology of CSC remains ambiguous. Advances in imaging techniques have shown that CSC is associated with localized areas of delayed choriocapillaris perfusion, congestion of choroidal vessels, choroidal hyperpermeability, and increased SFCT, causing damage to the retinal pigmented epithelium. Imbalance in mineralocorticoid pathway has also been suggested as potential cause. Sympathetic overaction and a decreased parasympathetic tone might also play a role [7,50].

In our department of ophthalmology, there have been several cases of CSC in SCUBA divers in the past years. However, CSC in divers was rarely described in literature [4]. The relationship between hyperbaric environment and CSC could be easily overlooked.

A hypobaric environment might also have influence on SFCT. CSC was reported in at least four air pilots [51–54] and a case during hypobaric chamber exposure [55] together with a small but significant CCT increase was described in high-altitude exposure [56].

Diving has been suspected to cause macular damages since 1988 by the study of Polkinghorne et al. [57]. They highlighted that divers had significantly more retinal pigment epithelial defects, and the prevalence of defects increased with years of diving experience and history of decompression sickness. However, many other studies revealed no significant differences with control groups regarding retinal pigment epithelial alterations [58–60]. A total of three eyes (10%) were found to present retinal epithelium alterations in our study. It is difficult to know if those are the results of diving practice or if it is just incidental finding similar to general population. Decrease in SFCT has been demonstrated in our study, while CSC is typically described with the pachychoroid, which is the opposite.

Regarding those elements, it seems uncertain if SCUBA diving is a risk factor for CSC. Transient decreased SFCT would not explain increased CSC incidence. We did not observe more macular damage, significant retinal pigment alterations nor increased SFCT in our divers compared with general population seen in our daily practice. It seems more likely that cases of CSC in divers reported in our center are just coincidental, as patients had other risk factors of CSC.

5.4. Intraocular Pressure

Our results demonstrated decrease of 88.05% ($p < 0.0001\%$) in IOP 30 min after diving.

Lowered IOP is widely described following physical exercise. However, it still remains a poorly understood phenomenon [61]. A total of three theories of its etiology involve decreased blood pH, elevated blood plasma osmolarity, and elevated blood lactate [62]. Increases in trabecular meshwork thickness, area, and perimeter of Schlemm's canal have also been observed after physical activity, and are thought to be a consequence of sympathetic response to exercise. It was not significantly correlated with the decrease in IOP [63]. Similar observations are expected in SCUBA diving, and it is the most likely hypothesis to explain our results. Other hypotheses were also considered as being unlikely with our experimental setting:

Goenadi et al. suggest that in contrast with swimming goggles, diving masks can induce small decrease of 0.43 mmHg in IOP after diving [64]. All divers wore diving masks (different from swimming goggles), respected mask pressure normalization during diving, and no mask squeeze was observed.

Corneal parameters as central corneal thickness and external curvature radius have influence on IOP measurements [65]. Increased pachymetry is associated with overestimated IOP measures, which also does not explain the results. Intraocular bubbles might block trabecular outflow, increasing IOP.

Fadini et al. interestingly showed that patients without any cardiovascular risk factors but suffering from ocular hypertension and primary open-angle glaucoma (POAG) had both FMD and endothelial progenitor cell (EPC) reduced [66]. It seems likely that chronic reduced FMD and endothelial dysfunction increase IOP. However, it was not demonstrated in transient FMD variation. No other description of decreased IOP after SCUBA diving was found on Pubmed. In contrast to our results, Maverick et al. showed increase IOP post-dive negatively correlated to pachymetry [67].

Instillation of tropicamide was made before pre-dive measures, and so does not explain our results. Effects of tropicamide on IOP vary in literature [68–72].

Our results on IOP are in tune with previous papers studying influence of sports on IOP [61]. Also, as IOP is negatively correlated to SFCT, we can formally exclude the role of IOP in the diminution of SFCT after the dive. It is a good argument to suggest that there is an extra-ophthalmological phenomenon explaining SFCT reduction.

5.5. Pachymetry

This study shows increase in pachymetry 30 min after diving ($101.6 \pm 1.0\%$; $p = 0.015$). Results are not significant anymore at 60 min.

Maverick et al. described no significant change of pachymetry in 24 eyes after diving from 34 to 100 feet of depth [67]. However, in a major review, Butler et al. explained how the use of diving mask may, if the divers do compensate air compression in the mask exhaling gas through the nose into the mask, cause a negative pressure around the eye [1]. In severe cases, this can lead to ocular barotrauma. We can easily imagine that this negative pressure may be responsible for increased pachymetry after the dive.

Increased pachymetry also does not explain the SCFT decrease nor IOP decrease.

6. Conclusions

SCUBA diving appears to have miscellaneous consequences on ophthalmic parameters. We postulate that SFCT is transiently reduced as a consequence of vascular changes, involving increased arterial stiffness and insufficient relaxation in vascular smooth-cells due to oxidative stress and endothelial dysfunction. IOP showed transient decrease until 60 min after the dive, and was not correlated with changes of SFCT or pachymetry. It is a strong argument to point out an extra-ophthalmic phenomenon to explain our results. The results brought us no argument to conclude in a relationship between CSC and SCUBA diving.

Author Contributions: All authors listed have made a substantial, direct and intellectual contribution to the work, and approved it for publication Conceptualization, C.B., J.C. and L.P.; writing, L.D. and C.B.; review and editing, C.B., J.C. and L.P. All authors have read and agreed to the published version of the manuscript.

Funding: This submission received no external funding.

Institutional Review Board Statement: The study was conducted in accordance with the Declaration of Helsinki and received ethical approval from Local Ethic Committee Brussels (Academic Bioethical Committee, Brussels, Belgium. Reference Number: B200-2020-088). Date: 10 October 2020.

Informed Consent Statement: Informed consent was obtained from all subjects involved in the study.

Data Availability Statement: Data are available at request from the authors.

Acknowledgments: Authors are grateful to volunteer participants and John Beernaerts, owner of NEMO 33 (https://www.nemo33.com/en/ accessed on 8 March 2022), for letting us use their facilities.

Conflicts of Interest: The authors declare no conflict of interest.

Abbreviations

BP	Blood pressure
CSC	Central Serous Chorioretinopathy
FMD	Flow-mediated dilation
HR	Heart rate
IOP	Intraocular pressure
KR:	Keratometry
NO	Nitric Oxide
PACHY	Pachymetry
SD-OCT	Spectral-Domain
SFCT	Subfoveal choroidal thickness
TTE	Transthoracic echocardiography
VGE	Vascular gas emboli

References

1. Butler, F.K. Diving and hyperbaric ophthalmology. *Surv. Ophthalmol.* **1995**, *39*, 347–366. [CrossRef]
2. Merle, H.; Drault, J.N.; Gerard, M.; Alliot, E.; Mehdaoui, H.; Elisabeth, L. Retinal vein occlusion and deep-sea diving. *J. Français d'Ophtalmol.* **1997**, *20*, 456–460.
3. Iordanidou, V.; Gendron, G.; Khammari, C.; Rodallec, T.; Baudouin, C. Choroidal Ischemia Secondary to a Diving Injury. *Retin. Cases Brief Rep.* **2010**, *4*, 262–265. [CrossRef] [PubMed]
4. Cochard, G.; Lacour, J.; Egreteau, J. A Propos d'un accident Oculaire de Plongée Sous-Marine. 1996. Available online: https://www.semanticscholar.org/paper/A-propos-d\T1\textquoterightun-accident-oculaire-de-plong%C3%A9e-Cochard-Lacour/8b891aa6732b66070eb6c2ce519014522ef55755#citing-papers (accessed on 5 August 2021).
5. Macarez, R.; Dordain, Y.; Hugon, M.; Kovalski, J.-L.; Guigon, B.; Bazin, S.; May, F.; Colin, J. Retentissement à long terme de la plongée sous-marine sur le champ visuel, la vision des couleurs et la sensibilité au contraste du plongeur professionnel. *J. Français d'Ophtalmol.* **2005**, *28*, 825–831. [CrossRef]
6. Chung, Y.-R.; Kim, J.W.; Choi, S.-Y.; Park, S.W.; Kim, J.H.; Lee, K. subfoveal Choroidal Thickness and Vascular Diameter in Active and Resolved Central Serous Chorioretinopathy. *Retina* **2018**, *38*, 102–107. [CrossRef]
7. Semeraro, F.; Morescalchi, F.; Russo, A.; Gambicorti, E.; Pilotto, A.; Parmeggiani, F.; Bartollino, S.; Costagliola, C. Central Serous Chorioretinopathy: Pathogenesis and Management. *Clin. Ophthalmol.* **2019**, *13*, 2341–2352. [CrossRef]
8. World Medical Association. World Medical Association Declaration of Helsinki: Ethical principles for medical research involving human subjects. *JAMA* **2013**, *310*, 2191–2194. [CrossRef]
9. Lazari, K.C.; Karpathaki, M.N.; Linardakis, M.; Christodoulakis, E.V. Evaluation of differences in Intraocular Pressure (IOP) measurement between Tonoref III and Goldmann Applanation Tonometry (GAT). *Investig. Ophthalmol. Vis. Sci.* **2019**, *60*, 2420.
10. Myers, K.J.; Scott, C.A. The non-contact ("air puff") tonometer: Variability and corneal staining. *Am. J. Optom. Physiol. Opt.* **1975**, *52*, 36–46. [CrossRef]
11. Margolis, R.; Spaide, R.F. A Pilot Study of Enhanced Depth Imaging Optical Coherence Tomography of the Choroid in Normal Eyes. *Am. J. Ophthalmol.* **2009**, *147*, 811–815. [CrossRef]
12. Pyke, K.E.; Tschakovsky, M.E.; Bandi, E.; Bernareggi, A.; Grandolfo, M.; Mozzetta, C.; Augusti-Tocco, G.; Ruzzier, F.; Lorenzon, P. The relationship between shear stress and flow-mediated dilatation: Implications for the assessment of endothelial function. *J. Physiol.* **2005**, *568*, 357–369. [CrossRef]
13. Corretti, M.C.; Anderson, T.J.; Benjamin, E.; Celermajer, D.; Charbonneau, F.; Creager, M.A.; Deanfield, J.; Drexler, H.; Gerhard-Herman, M.; Herrington, D.; et al. Guidelines for the ultrasound assessment of endothelial-dependent flow-mediated vasodilation of the brachial artery: A report of the International Brachial Artery Reactivity Task Force. *J. Am. Coll. Cardiol.* **2002**, *39*, 257–265. [CrossRef]
14. Areas, G.P.T.; Mazzuco, A.; Caruso, F.R.; Jaenisch, R.B.; Cabiddu, R.; Phillips, S.A.; Arena, R.; Borghi-Silva, A. Flow-mediated dilation and heart failure: A review with implications to physical rehabilitation. *Heart Fail. Rev.* **2019**, *24*, 69–80. [CrossRef]
15. Germonpré, P.; Papadopoulou, V.; Hemelryck, W.; Obeid, G.; Lafère, P.; Eckersley, R.J.; Tang, M.-X.; Balestra, C. The use of portable 2D echocardiography and 'frame-based' bubble counting as a tool to evaluate diving decompression stress. *Diving Hyperb. Med. J.* **2014**, *44*, 5–13.
16. Theunissen, S.; Schumacker, J.; Guerrero, F.; Tillmans, F.; Boutros, A.; Lambrechts, K.; Mazur, A.; Pieri, M.; Germonpré, P.; Balestra, C. Dark chocolate reduces endothelial dysfunction after successive breath-hold dives in cool water. *Eur. J. Appl. Physiol.* **2013**, *113*, 2967–2975. [CrossRef]
17. Theunissen, S.; Balestra, C.; Boutros, A.; De Bels, D.; Guerrero, F.; Germonpré, P. The effect of pre-dive ingestion of dark chocolate on endothelial function after a scuba dive. *Diving Hyperb. Med. J.* **2015**, *45*, 4–9.

18. Theunissen, S.; Guerrero, F.; Sponsiello, N.; Cialoni, D.; Pieri, M.; Germonpré, P.; Obeid, G.; Tillmans, F.; Papadopoulou, V.; Hemelryck, W.; et al. Nitric oxide-related endothelial changes in breath-hold and scuba divers. *Undersea Hyperb. Med.* **2013**, *40*, 135–144.
19. Levenez, M.; Lambrechts, K.; Mrakic-Sposta, S.; Vezzoli, A.; Germonpré, P.; Pique, H.; Virgili, F.; Bosco, G.; Lafère, P.; Balestra, C. Full-Face Mask Use during SCUBA Diving Counters Related Oxidative Stress and Endothelial Dysfunction. *Int. J. Environ. Res. Public Health* **2022**, *19*, 965. [CrossRef]
20. Germonpré, P.; Balestra, C. Preconditioning to Reduce Decompression Stress in Scuba Divers. *Aerosp. Med. Hum. Perform.* **2017**, *88*, 114–120. [CrossRef]
21. Balestra, C.; Theunissen, S.; Papadopoulou, V.; Le Mener, C.; Germonpré, P.; Guerrero, F.; Lafère, P. Pre-dive Whole-Whole Body Vibration Better Reduces Decompression Induced Vascular Gas Emboli than Oxygenation or a Combination of Both. In *Physiology in Extreme Conditions: Adaptation and Unexpected Reactions*; Electronic Edition; Trivella, M.G., Capobianco, E., L'Abbate, A., Eds.; Frontiers Media: Lausnne, Switzerland, 2017.
22. Ferrara, M.; Lugano, G.; Sandinha, M.T.; Kearns, V.R.; Geraghty, B.; Steel, D.H.W. Biomechanical properties of retina and choroid: A comprehensive review of techniques and translational relevance. *Eye* **2021**, *35*, 1818–1832. [CrossRef]
23. Ethier, C.R.; Johnson, M.; Ruberti, J. Ocular Biomechanics and Biotransport. *Annu. Rev. Biomed. Eng.* **2004**, *6*, 249–273. [CrossRef]
24. Nickla, D.L.; Wallman, J. The multifunctional choroid. *Prog. Retin. Eye Res.* **2010**, *29*, 144–168. [CrossRef]
25. Wallman, J.; Wildsoet, C.; Xu, A.; Gottlieb, M.D.; Nickla, D.L.; Marran, L.; Krebs, W.; Christensen, A.M. Moving the retina: Choroidal modulation of refractive state. *Vis. Res.* **1995**, *35*, 37–50. [CrossRef]
26. Akhtar, Z.; Rishi, P.; Srikanth, R.; Rishi, E.; Bhende, M.; Raman, R. Choroidal thickness in normal Indian subjects using Swept source optical coherence tomography. *PLoS ONE* **2018**, *13*, e0197457. [CrossRef]
27. Karimi, S.; Entezari, M.; Ramezani, A.; Nikkhah, H.; Fekri, Y.; Kheiri, B. Choroidal thickness in healthy subjects. *J. Ophthalmic Vis. Res.* **2018**, *13*, 39–43. [CrossRef]
28. Tan, C.; Ouyang, Y.; Ruiz, H.; Sadda, S.R. Diurnal Variation of Choroidal Thickness in Normal, Healthy Subjects Measured by Spectral Domain Optical Coherence Tomography. *Investig. Opthalmol. Vis. Sci.* **2012**, *53*, 261–266. [CrossRef]
29. Lambrechts, K.; Pontier, J.-M.; Balestra, C.; Mazur, A.; Wang, Q.; Buzzacott, P.; Theron, M.; Mansourati, J.; Guerrero, F. Effect of a single, open-sea, air scuba dive on human micro- and macrovascular function. *Eur. J. Appl. Physiol.* **2013**, *113*, 2637–2645. [CrossRef]
30. Lambrechts, K.; Balestra, C.; Theron, M.; Henckes, A.; Galinat, H.; Mignant, F.; Belhomme, M.; Pontier, J.-M.; Guerrero, F. Venous gas emboli are involved in post-dive macro, but not microvascular dysfunction. *Eur. J. Appl. Physiol.* **2017**, *117*, 335–344. [CrossRef]
31. Obad, A.; Valic, Z.; Palada, I.; Brubakk, A.O.; Modun, D.; Dujić, Z. Antioxidant pretreatment and reduced arterial endothelial dysfunction after diving. *Aviat. Space Environ. Med.* **2007**, *78*, 1114–1120. [CrossRef]
32. Poukens, V.; Glasgow, B.J.; Demer, J.L. Nonvascular contractile cells in sclera and choroid of humans and monkeys. *Investig. Ophthalmol. Vis. Sci.* **1998**, *39*, 1765–1774.
33. Akahori, T.; Iwase, T.; Yamamoto, K.; Ra, E.; Terasaki, H. Changes in Choroidal Blood Flow and Morphology in Response to Increase in Intraocular Pressure. *Investig. Opthalmol. Vis. Sci.* **2017**, *58*, 5076–5085. [CrossRef] [PubMed]
34. Zhang, X.; Cole, E.; Pillar, A.; Lane, M.; Waheed, N.; Adhi, M.; Magder, L.; Quigley, H.; Saeedi, O. The Effect of Change in Intraocular Pressure on Choroidal Structure in Glaucomatous Eyes. *Investig. Opthalmol. Vis. Sci.* **2017**, *58*, 3278–3285. [CrossRef] [PubMed]
35. Kara, N.; Baz, O.; Altan, C.; Satana, B.; Kurt, T.; Demirok, A. Changes in choroidal thickness, axial length, and ocular perfusion pressure accompanying successful glaucoma filtration surgery. *Eye* **2013**, *27*, 940–945. [CrossRef] [PubMed]
36. Silva, D.; Lopes, A.S.; Henriques, S.; Lisboa, M.; Pinto, S.; Vaz, F.T.; Prieto, I. Changes in choroidal thickness following trabeculectomy and its correlation with the decline in intraocular pressure. *Int. Ophthalmol.* **2018**, *39*, 1097–1104. [CrossRef] [PubMed]
37. Bouillot, A.; Pierru, A.; Blumen-Ohana, E.; Brasnu, E.; Baudouin, C.; Labbé, A. Changes in choroidal thickness and optic nerve head morphology after filtering surgery: Nonpenetrating deep sclerectomy versus trabeculectomy. *BMC Ophthalmol.* **2019**, *19*, 24. [CrossRef] [PubMed]
38. Wang, Y.X.; Jiang, R.; Ren, X.L.; Chen, J.D.; Shi, H.L.; Xu, L.; Bin Wei, W.; Jonas, J.B. Intraocular pressure elevation and choroidal thinning. *Br. J. Ophthalmol.* **2016**, *100*, 1676–1681. [CrossRef] [PubMed]
39. Mauget-Faÿsse, M.; Arej, N.; Paternoster, M.; Zuber, K.; Derrien, S.; Thevenin, S.; Alonso, A.-S.; Salviat, F.; Lafolie, J.; Vasseur, V. Retinal and choroidal blood flow variations after an endurance exercise: A real-life pilot study at the Paris Marathon. *J. Sci. Med. Sport* **2021**, *24*, 1100–1104. [CrossRef]
40. Sayin, N.; Kara, N.; Pekel, G.; Altinkaynak, H. Choroidal thickness changes after dynamic exercise as measured by spectral-domain optical coherence tomography. *Indian J. Ophthalmol.* **2015**, *63*, 445–450. [CrossRef]
41. Hong, J.; Zhang, H.; Kuo, D.S.; Wang, H.; Huo, Y.; Yang, D.; Wang, N. The Short-Term Effects of Exercise on Intraocular Pressure, Choroidal Thickness and Axial Length. *PLoS ONE* **2014**, *9*, e104294. [CrossRef]
42. Iovino, C.; Chhablani, J.; Rasheed, M.A.; Tatti, F.; Bernabei, F.; Pellegrini, M.; Giannaccare, G.; Peiretti, E. Effects of different mydriatics on the choroidal vascularity in healthy subjects. *Eye* **2021**, *35*, 913–918. [CrossRef]

43. Dujić, Ž.; Palada, I.; Valic, Z.; Duplančić, D.; Obad, A.; Wisløff, U.; Brubakk, A.O. Exogenous Nitric Oxide and Bubble Formation in Divers. *Med. Sci. Sports Exerc.* **2006**, *38*, 1432–1435. [CrossRef]
44. Wisløff, U.; Richardson, R.S.; Brubakk, A.O. Exercise and nitric oxide prevent bubble formation: A novel approach to the prevention of decompression sickness? *J. Physiol.* **2004**, *555*, 825–829. [CrossRef]
45. Wisløff, U.; Richardson, R.S.; Brubakk, A.O. Nos inhibition increases bubble formation and reduces survival in sedentary but not exercised rats. *J. Physiol.* **2003**, *546*, 577–582. [CrossRef]
46. Lautridou, J.; Dugrenot, E.; Amérand, A.; Guernec, A.; Pichavant-Rafini, K.; Goanvec, C.; Inizan, M.; Albacete, G.; Belhomme, M.; Galinat, H.; et al. Physiological characteristics associated with increased resistance to decompression sickness in male and female rats. *J. Appl. Physiol.* **2020**, *129*, 612–625. [CrossRef]
47. Imbert, J.-P.; Egi, S.M.; Germonpré, P.; Balestra, C. Static Metabolic Bubbles as Precursors of Vascular Gas Emboli During Divers' Decompression: A Hypothesis Explaining Bubbling Variability. *Front. Physiol.* **2019**, *10*, 807. [CrossRef]
48. Marinovic, J.; Ljubkovic, M.; Breskovic, T.; Gunjaca, G.; Obad, A.; Modun, D.; Bilopavlovic, N.; Tsikas, D.; Dujic, Z. Effects of successive air and nitrox dives on human vascular function. *Eur. J. Appl. Physiol.* **2011**, *112*, 2131–2137. [CrossRef]
49. Brubakk, A.O.; Duplancic, D.; Valic, Z.; Palada, I.; Obad, A.; Bakovic, D.; Wisløff, U.; Dujic, Z. A single air dive reduces arterial endothelial function in man. *J. Physiol.* **2005**, *566*, 901–906. [CrossRef]
50. Daruich, A.; Matet, A.; Dirani, A.; Bousquet, E.; Zhao, M.; Farman, N.; Jaisser, F.; Behar-Cohen, F. Central serous chorioretinopathy: Recent findings and new physiopathology hypothesis. *Prog. Retin. Eye Res.* **2015**, *48*, 82–118. [CrossRef]
51. Dietrich, K.C. Fighter Pilot with Recurrent Central Serous Chorioretinopathy. *Aerosp. Med. Hum. Perform.* **2016**, *87*, 901–905. [CrossRef]
52. Gross, M.; Froom, P.; Tendler, Y.; Mishori, M.; Ribak, J. Central serous retinopathy (choroidopathy) in pilots. *Aviat. Space Environ. Med.* **1986**, *57*, 457–458.
53. Newman, D.G. Central serous retinopathy with permanent visual deficit in a commercial air transport pilot: A case report. *Aviat. Space Environ. Med.* **2002**, *73*, 1122–1126.
54. Richmond, M.R.R.; Rings, M.M. Recurrent Central Serous Retinopathy with Permanent Visual Loss in a U.S. Naval Fighter Pilot. *Mil. Med.* **2018**, *183*, e671–e675. [CrossRef]
55. Ide Central Serous Chorioretinopathy Following Hypobaric Chamber Exposure. *Aviat. Space Environ. Med.* **2014**, *85*, 1053–1055. [CrossRef]
56. Fischer, M.D.; Schatz, A.; Seitz, I.P.; Schommer, K.; Bartz-Schmidt, K.U.; Gekeler, F.; Willmann, G. Reversible Increase of Central Choroidal Thickness During High-Altitude Exposure. *Investig. Opthalmol. Vis. Sci.* **2015**, *56*, 4499–4503. [CrossRef]
57. Polkinghorne, P.; Cross, M.; Sehmi, K.; Minassian, D.; Bird, A. Ocular Fundus Lesions in Divers. *Lancet* **1988**, *332*, 1381–1383. [CrossRef]
58. Holden, R.; Morsman, C.D.; Lane, C.M. Ocular fundus lesions in sports divers using safe diving practices. *Br. J. Sports Med.* **1992**, *26*, 90–92. [CrossRef]
59. Peyraud-Gilly, V.M.; Daubas, P.; Joly, T.; Filliard, G.; Monroux-Rousseau, S. Macular functions in professional divers. *J. Français d'Ophtalmol.* **2000**, *23*, 472–474.
60. Murrison, A.W.; Pethybridge, R.J.; Rintoul, A.J.; Jeffrey, M.N.; Sehmi, K.; Bird, A.C. Retinal angiography in divers. *Occup. Environ. Med.* **1996**, *53*, 339–342. [CrossRef]
61. McMonnies, C.W. Intraocular pressure and glaucoma: Is physical exercise beneficial or a risk? *J. Optom.* **2016**, *9*, 139–147. [CrossRef]
62. Risner, D.; Ehrlich, R.; Kheradiya, N.S.; Siesky, B.; McCranor, L.; Harris, A. Effects of exercise on intraocular pressure and ocular blood flow: A review. *J. Glaucoma* **2009**, *18*, 429–436. [CrossRef]
63. Yan, X.; Li, M.; Song, Y.; Guo, J.; Zhao, Y.; Chen, W.; Zhang, H. Influence of Exercise on Intraocular Pressure, Schlemm's Canal, and the Trabecular Meshwork. *Investig. Opthalmol. Vis. Sci.* **2016**, *57*, 4733–4739. [CrossRef] [PubMed]
64. Goenadi, C.J.; Law, D.Z.; Lee, J.W.; Ong, E.L.; Chee, W.K.; Cheng, J. The Effect of a Diving Mask on Intraocular Pressure in a Healthy Population. *Case Rep. Ophthalmol.* **2016**, *7*, 328–332. [CrossRef] [PubMed]
65. Guzmán, A.F.; Castilla, A.A.; Guarnieri, F.A.; Rodríguez, F.R. Intraocular pressure: Goldmann tonometry, computational model, and calibration equation. *J. Glaucoma* **2013**, *22*, 10–14. [CrossRef] [PubMed]
66. Fadini, G.P.; Pagano, C.; Baesso, I.; Kotsafti, O.; Doro, D.; De Kreutzenberg, S.V.; Avogaro, A.; Agostini, C.; Dorigo, M.T. Reduced endothelial progenitor cells and brachial artery flow-mediated dilation as evidence of endothelial dysfunction in ocular hypertension and primary open-angle glaucoma. *Acta Ophthalmol.* **2010**, *88*, 135–141. [CrossRef]
67. Maverick, K.J.; Conners, M.S. Corneal Thickness and Intraocular Pressure Changes Associated with Scuba Diving. *Investig. Ophthalmol. Vis. Sci.* **2003**, *44*, 2571.
68. Pukrushpan, P.; Tulvatana, W.; Kulvichit, K. Intraocular pressure change following application of 1% tropicamide for diagnostic mydriasis. *Acta Ophthalmol. Scand.* **2005**, *84*, 268–270. [CrossRef]
69. Marchini, G.; Babighian, S.; Tosi, R.; Perfetti, S.; Bonomi, L. Comparative Study of the Effects of 2% Ibopamine, 10% Phenylephrine, and 1% Tropicamide on the Anterior Segment. *Investig. Opthalmol. Vis. Sci.* **2003**, *44*, 281–289. [CrossRef]
70. Oltulu, R.; Satirtav, G.; Altunkaya, O.; Bitirgen, G.; Okka, M. Effect of mydriasis induced by topical 0.5% tropicamide instillation on the corneal biomechanical properties in healthy individuals measured by ocular response analyzer. *Cutan. Ocul. Toxicol.* **2014**, *34*, 35–37. [CrossRef]

71. Qian, C.X.-Y.; Duperré, J.; Hassanaly, S.; Harissi-Dagher, M. Pre- versus post-dilation changes in intraocular pressure: Their clinical significance. *Can. J. Ophthalmol.* **2012**, *47*, 448–452. [CrossRef]
72. Atalay, E.; Tamçelik, N.; Arici, C.; Özkök, A.; Dastan, M.; Arıcı, C. The change in intraocular pressure after pupillary dilation in eyes with pseudoexfoliation glaucoma, primary open angle glaucoma, and eyes of normal subjects. *Int. Ophthalmol.* **2014**, *35*, 215–219. [CrossRef]

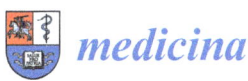

Article

Pulmonary Effects of One Week of Repeated Recreational Closed-Circuit Rebreather Dives in Cold Water

Emmanuel Gouin [1,2,†], Costantino Balestra [3,4,5,6,†], Jeremy Orsat [2], Emmanuel Dugrenot [1,7] and Erwan L'Her [8,9,*]

1. TEK Diving SAS, 29200 Brest, France
2. Laboratoire ORPHY, EA 4324, Université de Bretagne Occidentale, 29200 Brest, France
3. Environmental, Occupational, Aging (Integrative) Physiology Laboratory, Haute Ecole Bruxelles-Brabant (HE2B), 1050 Brussels, Belgium
4. Anatomical Research and Clinical Studies (ARCS), Vrije Universiteit Brussels (VUB), 1090 Brussels, Belgium
5. DAN Europe Research Division (Roseto-Brussels), 1020 Brussels, Belgium
6. Physical Activity Teaching Unit, Motor Sciences Department, Université Libre de Bruxelles (ULB), 1050 Brussels, Belgium
7. Divers Alert Network, Durham, NC 27605, USA
8. Médecine Intensive et Réanimation, CHRU de la Cavale Blanche, 29200 Brest, France
9. LaTIM INSERM UMR 1101, Université de Bretagne Occidentale, 29200 Brest, France
* Correspondence: erwan.lher@chu-brest.fr; Tel.: +33-2-92-34-71-81
† These authors contributed equally to this work.

Abstract: *Background and Objectives*: The use of closed-circuit rebreathers (CCRs) in recreational diving is gaining interest. However, data regarding its physiological effects are still scarce. Immersion, cold water, hyperoxia, exercise or the equipment itself could challenge the cardiopulmonary system. The purpose of this study was to examine the impact of CCR diving on lung function and autonomous cardiac activity after a series of CCR dives in cold water. *Materials and Methods*: Eight CCR divers performed a diving trip (one week) in the Baltic Sea. Spirometry parameters, SpO_2, and the lung ultrasonography score (LUS) associated with hydration monitoring by bioelectrical impedance were assessed at the end of the week. Heart rate variability (HRV) was recorded during the dives. *Results*: No diver declared pulmonary symptoms. The LUS increased after dives combined with a slight non-pathological decrease in SpO_2. Spirometry was not altered, and all body water compartments were increased. Global HRV decreased during diving with a predominant increase in sympathetic tone while the parasympathetic tone decreased. All parameters returned to baseline 24 h after the last dive. *Conclusions*: The lung aeration disorders observed seem to be transient and not associated with functional spirometry alteration. The HRV dynamics highlighted physiological constraints during the dive as well as environmental-stress-related stimulation that may influence pulmonary changes. The impact of these impairments is unknown but should be taken into account, especially when considering long and repetitive CCR dives.

Keywords: adverse effects; autonomic nervous system; decompression; lung ultrasound; mixed gas diving; pulmonary function; technical diving

Citation: Gouin, E.; Balestra, C.; Orsat, J.; Dugrenot, E.; L'Her, E. Pulmonary Effects of One Week of Repeated Recreational Closed-Circuit Rebreather Dives in Cold Water. *Medicina* 2023, 59, 81. https://doi.org/10.3390/medicina59010081

Academic Editor: Enrico Mario Camporesi

Received: 23 November 2022
Revised: 21 December 2022
Accepted: 28 December 2022
Published: 30 December 2022

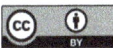

Copyright: © 2022 by the authors. Licensee MDPI, Basel, Switzerland. This article is an open access article distributed under the terms and conditions of the Creative Commons Attribution (CC BY) license (https://creativecommons.org/licenses/by/4.0/).

1. Introduction

The use of closed-circuit rebreathers (CCRs) has become increasingly common in the recreational scuba diving community over the past two decades. Their use allows longer and deeper dives than classical open-circuit (OC) scuba equipment. CCRs bring major advantages in terms of gas consumption, an optimal oxygen mix, and warm humidified breathing gas [1]. Conversely, since the breathing system is much more complicated to use, it exposes the diver to technical failures or specific emergencies [2].

During a dive, the cardio-pulmonary system is challenged by various combinations of stressors and adaptive mechanisms such as blood shift, thermal strain, exercise, gas density, hypercapnia, narcosis and hyperoxia [3–5]. In addition, the breathing apparatus by itself may add to the respiratory workload (work of breathing) that could be increased by the negative transpulmonary pressure gradient in the prone position with back-mounted counterlungs on the CCR used [6]. A number of studies have investigated pulmonary function following OC diving under varying conditions, but the results remain contradictory [4]. Many did not show any spirometric alteration after a single OC dive for a maximum depth of 65 m [7,8]. However, changes in pulmonary function have been found to be associated with depth, cold temperatures, oxidative or decompression stress and duration. These post-dive obstructive pattern changes appeared to be limited and transient [9,10]. Exposure to pure oxygen, even at shallow depths (5 msw), leads to a lung diffusing capacity alteration [11]. CCR diving exposes to high, and potentially prolonged, PpO_2 and specific mechanical constraints [1,6]. There is a lack of data about cardio-pulmonary effects during CCR diving. A CCR deep diving study has shown an almost 30% decrease in forced vital capacity (FVC) after bounce dives at 100 msw [12]. Conversely, CCR use did not affect the spirometry despite the long duration at a maximum depth of 20 msw [13,14]. The impact of CCR repeated dives has not been evaluated in cold conditions (<10 °C) and no data are available about the evolution of such abnormalities over time. More recently, asymptomatic lung aeration defects were assessed by ultrasound with B-line detection after dives. These artefacts may suggest extravascular lung water accumulation [15,16]. Most studies have shown an accumulation of B-lines with incomplete resolution between each in repetitive deep OC dives to 60–80 msw, which is not observed at a 33 msw depth [3,8,17]. With CCR, a lung aeration loss was detected, even in shallow water, between 1 and 10 msw, and was substantially amplified by exercise and negative-pressure breathing. The right-to-left heart imbalance and increase in pulmonary vasoconstriction seem to be related to these impairments [5,6]. This phenomenon was already described during breath-hold diving and was related to diaphragmatic spasms with a closed glottis adding to the negative pressure gradient explanation [18].

All immersion constraints, such as blood centralization, pulmonary workload, or hyperoxia, also modulate the autonomic nervous system (ANS). Heart rate variability (HRV) reflects the constant fluctuation of the interaction between pulmonary ventilation, blood pressure, and cardiac output to maintain homeostasis [19]. It can be used to indirectly study changes in parasympathetic (PNS) and sympathetic (SNS) nervous system activity, which express the level of intensity in physiological adaptation. There are marked changes in autonomic cardiac activity during and after scuba diving with a predominance of PNS activity [20,21]. There are complex and sometimes conflicting additional ANS modulations, and CCR diving seems to provoke a different HRV response in divers as compared to OC diving [22].

We hypothesize that in-water breathing constraints may have a negative impact on the lung after CCR dives, especially in case of repetitive exposures. Better knowledge of the physiological impacts of CCR appears essential given the growing diving community and technical developments. Data regarding the cardio-pulmonary effects of repetitive CCR diving are still needed for different depths and environments. The aim of this study was to examine the impact of CCR diving on lung function together with autonomous cardiac activity in asymptomatic healthy volunteers after a recurrent diving exposure in cold water.

2. Methods

2.1. Diving Sites

The "Vräk diving expedition" took place in the Stockholm archipelago (Sweden) in September 2022. This study was approved by the Bio-Ethical Committee for Research and Higher Education, Brussels (No B200-2020-088), and adhered to the principles of the Declaration of Helsinki [23].

2.2. Study Population

This observational study was an intrasubject experimental design with repeated measures. A total of eight male divers were included. Table 1 summarizes the anthropometric data. None were smokers and none were taking medication. All of the subjects were at least recreational rebreather mixed-gas divers. The median CCR experience was 4.5 (2.9–8.3) years. Two divers (25%) have DCS history (one musculoskeletal and one lymphatic manifestations). All divers were fit to dive and had a valid medical certificate for diving. None dived in the previous week. They were all informed about the physiological study and its implications. All participants gave written consent prior to the program.

Table 1. Participants' anthropometric parameters (n = 8).

	Median (1st–3rd Quartile)
Age (years)	40.5 [36.25; 47]
Weight (kg)	80 [75; 103]
Height (cm)	178 [175; 187]
BMI (kg.cm^{-2})	25.7 [23; 30.3]

BMI, body mass index.

2.3. Diving Procedures

The dives were performed in accordance with usual CCR dive planning and were not modified for the study requirements. All dives were performed from a rigid inflatable boat. The dive sites were 30 min to 2 h away from the harbor. One to two dives were performed daily, depending on the maximal planned depth. A surface interval of 2 to 3 h between the first and second dive was met. Helium mixed-gases were used for dives below 40 m. Day 2 was taken off. The surface and bottom temperatures were 16.5 (16–17) and 8.5 (6–15.5) °C, respectively, with a thermocline at approximately 15 m. The dive parameters are shown in Table 2. Five divers performed five more comparable consecutive diving days in a second week.

Table 2. Diving description during the monitoring week. The third dive on the first day were performed by 5 divers to test equipment. Cumulative central nervous system oxygen toxicity (CNS) represents the time spent at a given oxygen partial pressure (PpO$_2$) and dividing by the NOAA time limit for that PpO$_2$ (corresponding to the cumulative oxygen exposition).

	D1 (2 or 3 Dives) Air Diluent	D3 (2 Dives) Air Diluent	D4 (2 Dives) Air Diluent	D5 (1 Dive) Trimix 15/40	D6 (1 Dive) Trimix 10/50
Maximal depth (msw)	19.7 [13; 20.9]	29.3 [28.6; 33.8]	32.9 [28.6; 37.8]	44.8 [41.6; 44.9]	64.7 [46.1; 70.1]
Mean depth (msw)	14.3 [9.3; 16.0]	22.3 [20.8; 23.3]	22.0 [21; 22.3]	24.2 [23; 24.5]	24.1 [23.6; 24.3]
Each dive time (min)	54 [41; 63]	66 [55; 94]	64 [58; 73]	99 [83; 99]	90 [88; 92]
Total dive time (min)	147 [98; 172]	136 [93; 168]	126 [109; 141]	99 [83; 99]	90 [88; 92]
Cumulative CNS (%)	38 [22; 48]	47 [39; 58]	43 [34; 50]	52 [46; 53]	49 [45; 52]

Divers used back-mounted counter lung electronic controlled rebreathers (rEvo™ Rebreathers, Brugge, Belgium; n = 5 or JJ-CCR DiveCAN®, Presto, Denmark; n = 3). Decompression (Buhlmann ZHL-16C algorithm) was conducted using a connected Petrel 2 computer (Shearwater, Richmond, BC, Canada). The gradient factors were set to 30% (low) and 70% (high) for all dives. The oxygen partial pressure (PpO$_2$) was maintained at 130 kPa during the entire dive. Subjects each wore a dry-suit with dry-gloves and an active heating system [24].

2.4. Measurements

Divers were monitored prior to the first dive, after the dive during the first five diving days, and 24 h after their last dive (i.e., after five diving days for three divers and ten days for five divers) in a dry and heated room (temperature 18–20 °C). The study flowchart is shown in Figure 1.

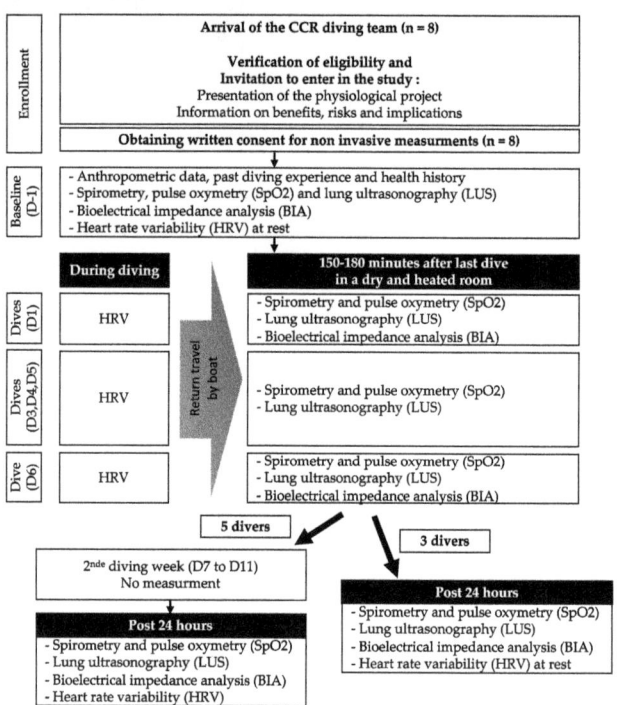

Figure 1. Experimental flowchart.

2.4.1. Functional and Anatomical Pulmonary Monitoring

Measurement of pulmonary parameters was performed daily, 150 to 180 min after the dive. All measurements were performed in the sitting position and at rest. Pulse oxygen saturation (SpO_2) and heart rate (HR) were recorded for 30 s, using a dedicated oximetry module connected to the spirometer (Spirobank II Smart; MIR Medical International Research Srl, Rome, Italy). The mean value for SpO_2 and HR was considered. Spirometric parameters were collected including the forced vital capacity (FVC), forced expiratory volume in one second (FEV1), FEV1/FVC ratio, peak expiratory flow (PEF), and forced expiratory flow (FEF25-75) following GLI (Global Lung Initiative) 2017 for Caucasian adults [25]. The device used for measurements meets the ISO26782:2009 international standards technical characteristics and is CE marked [26]. Flow data were recorded in real time in a dedicated computer, using the manufacturer WinspiroPRO v8.1.0 software. Three repeated loops were performed to assess the reproducibility under the investigator's supervision. The highest FVC and FEV1 values observed over the measurement series were reported [26].

The anatomical pulmonary aeration was evaluated by lung ultrasonography with a 1.1–4.7 MHz phased array probe (Venue Go™, General Electric Healthcare, Buc, France). Six areas were longitudinally scanned on each hemithorax (anterosuperior, anteroinferior, laterosuperior, lateroinferior, posterosuperior and posteroinferior) to count the total number of B-lines [27]. The exam was performed simultaneously by two trained operators to assess consistent scoring after comparison. A B-line is defined as an echogenic, coherent, wedge-shaped signal with a narrow origin arising from the hyperechogenic pleural line and extending to the far edge of the viewing area [15]. The amount of lung aeration loss was calculated in a semi-quantitative approach using the validated lung ultrasound score (LUS). For each explored region, the worst finding was reported according to the following rating: normal: 0; well-separated B-lines: 1; coalescent B-lines: 2; and consolidation: 3 [27]. The LUS corresponded to the sum of each scanning site score (range 0 to 36). An increase in score indicates a decrease in lung aeration without necessarily reaching pathology levels [28].

2.4.2. Hydration Status

All divers had unrestricted access to drinking water. Bioelectrical impedance analysis (BIA) is a safe and fast method to evaluate the body composition or hydration status [29–31]. These changes were estimated by a multifrequency tetrapolar impedancemetry Biody XPert^{ZM} (Aminogram, La Ciotat, France) in order to evaluate the total body hydration status and its related changes after diving. It is presented as a hand–foot analyzer and the measuring time is within the minute. Data were measured according to the manufacturer's instructions in a seated position before the first dive, 150 to 180 min after the first-day dive and at the end of the fifth-day dive, and 24 h after the last-day dive. The data were directly transferred via Bluetooth using the proprietary Aminogram Biodymanager app for Android. The device is accredited to the ISO13485:2016 standard and is CE marked. The response of different body tissues to the application of a weak alternating current at five different frequencies (range 5 to 200 KHz) determines the resistant indices (IRs) and the phase angle at 50 kHz (PA°). It allows an estimate of the total body (TBW), intracellular (ICW) and extracellular (ECW) water. The phase angle expresses both changes in the amount as well as the quality of soft tissue mass (i.e., cell membrane permeability and soft tissue hydration) [32,33].

2.4.3. Heart Rate Variability

Heart rate variability (HRV) is a non-invasive assessment of the variation in time between consecutive inter-beat intervals (R–R intervals) that results in a dynamic relationship between PNS and SNS [19]. It represents the ability of the heart to respond to a variety of physiological and environmental stimuli. Each diver wore a chest elastic belt sensor Polar H10 connected to the Polar Unite watch (Polar Electro Oy, Kempele, Finland) to record the R-to-R interval at a 1000 Hz sampling frequency. The validity of this device for HRV measurement has already been demonstrated in several studies [22,34]. The resting baseline was recorded in a sitting position, after ten minutes at rest, before the first dive and 24 h after the last day for ten minutes. During diving, the Polar watches were placed on the shoulder strap of the undergarment inside the dry suit after starting recording. Full data were extracted daily and analyzed using the Kubios HRV Premium Analysis Software 3.5.0 (UKU, Kuopio, Finland). The automatic artifact correction function of the program was used to correct data corruption for each subject before analysis. Time–domain results with mean HR, standard deviation of normal-to-normal R waves (SDNN), root mean square of the successive difference (RMSSD) of the R–R intervals, and integral of the density of the R–R interval histogram divided by the maximum of its weight (RR triangular index) were calculated. RMSSD mainly reflects the parasympathetic tone while the SDNN and triangular index are indicators of the overall ANS activity frequency-domain measures including the very-low-frequency (VLF), low-frequency (LF), and high-frequency (HF) spectral absolute power and LF/HF ratio. These estimate the distribution of absolute or relative power in different frequency bands [35]. Quantitative analyses of Poincare plot features (SD1, SD2, and SD2/SD1 ratio), Shannon entropy (ShanEn), and Multi-scale entropy (MSE) were computed. This non-linear approach is less dependent on the respiratory sinusal arrythmia variations in the R–R intervals [22]. Furthermore, two composite indexes were calculated. These indexes are based on known HRV parameters that reflect PNS and SNS activity. PNS and SNS indexes were based on the mean R-to-R interval, RMSSD and

SD1, and the mean HR interval, the stress index, and SD2, respectively [36]. An index value of zero reflected that the PNS or SNS activity is equal to the normal population average [37].

3. Statistical Analysis

Statistical analysis was performed with GraphPad Prism v9.0.2 (GraphPad Software Inc., San Diego, CA, USA). All data are presented as the median (first and third quartile). The normality of distribution was assessed by Shapiro–Wilk test. ANOVA for repeated measures was used to analyze more than two related groups followed by multiple comparison Tukey's post hoc test. A two-way ANOVA for repeated measures was used to assess the effects of the dive day and chest site on the LUS. If non-normality was found, a non-parametric Friedman test was used followed by multiple comparison Dunn test. Statistical significance was set at a p-value < 0.05.

The sample size was calculated setting the power of the study at 95% and assuming that variables associated with diving would have been affected to a similar extent as observed in our previous studies where our sample reached 98% [12,30].

4. Results

4.1. Respiratory and Pulmonary Parameters

Divers performed the repetitive diving program without any pulmonary symptoms or any other disturbance. No modification of spirometry parameters was observed (Table 3). The mean SpO_2 significantly decreased during all diving days by −1.4 [−2.6; −0.8] % (F = 5.02, p = 0.02). Few B-lines were observed on the baseline for several divers, with a median LUS at 1.5 [0.3; 2.8] and a basal predominance.

Table 3. Spirometry parameters. Data were assessed at baseline and 150–180 min after each day dive. FCV, forced vital capacity; FEV1, forced expiratory volume in one second; PEF, peak expiratory flow; FEF2575, forced expiratory flow; SpO_2, pulse oxygen saturation; HR, heart rate. Data are expressed in absolute value and the percentage of expected values according to the GLI (% pred). p-value for the ANOVA. Tukey's multiple comparisons test is expressed versus baseline with * p < 0.05. Differences versus post-24 h are expressed with † p < 0.05 and †† p < 0.01.

	Baseline	D1	D3	D4	D5	D6	Post 24 h	p-Value
FVC (l)	5.6 [4.8; 6]	5.8 [5.1; 6.5]	6.0 [5.9; 6.6]	5.9 [5.4; 6.5]	6.2 [4.9; 6.5]	6.2 [5.4; 6.4]	6.1 [5.2; 6.4]	0.2
(% pred)	106 [101; 111]	112 [100; 117]	115 [108; 123]	112 [106; 118]	107 [101; 115]	112 [102; 119]	107 [104; 117]	
FEV1 (l)	4.4 [4.0; 4.5]	4.5 [4.2; 4.7]	4.5 [4.1; 4.7]	4.6 [4.3; 4.7]	4.6 [4.0; 4.8]	4.5 [4.2; 4.8]	4.5 [4.3; 4.6]	0.5
(% pred)	101 [96; 111]	104 [98; 117]	107 [94; 113]	103 [95; 116]	100 [93; 113]	101 [91; 114]	105 [95; 113]	
FEV1/FVC (%)	78 [72; 84]	78 [71; 81]	74 [70; 78]	78 [72; 79]	77 [72; 81]	77 [72; 78]	77 [71; 82]	0.4
(% pred)	96 [89; 105]	97 [88; 101]	91 [88; 97]	97 [89; 99]	95 [89; 102]	94 [89; 97]	96 [88; 102]	
PEF (l.s^{-1})	11.6 [11.1; 12.2]	12.3 [10.9; 13.0]	11.7 [10.7; 12.4]	12.0 [10.9; 12.5]	11.6 [10.4; 12.6]	11.7 [10.6; 13.2]	11.5 [10.6; 13.6]	0.4
(% pred)	125 [117; 134]	133 [115; 138]	122 [115; 136]	132 [121; 134]	120 [110; 129]	123 [108; 132]	125 [113; 147]	
FEF2575 (l.s^{-1})	3.8 [3.1; 4.7]	3.7 [3.0; 4.9]	3.3 [3.1; 3.6]	3.4 [3.3; 4.0]	3.8 [3.2; 4.4]	3.4 [3.0; 4.2]	3.5 [3.2; 4.5]	0.8
(% pred)	95 [74; 120]	97 [75; 116]	82 [70; 97]	92 [71; 113]	86 [74; 115]	97 [67; 100]	91 [72; 119]	
SpO_2 (%)	97.8 [97.4; 98.4]	96.2 [95.7; 97.2] *	96.6 [95.5; 97.3] *	96.5 [96.3; 97.1]	96.6 [95.5; 97.1]	96.2 [95; 96.7] *	97.4 [96.7; 97.7]	0.02
HR (bpm)	78 [67; 86]	98 [97; 104] *,††	94 [87; 103] *,†	94 [84; 99] †	98 [96; 104] *,†	91 [80; 97]	80 [71; 83]	<0.0001

There was significative B-line accumulation after diving days 3, 4, 5 and 6 for all participants (Figure 2, F = 8.50, p = 0.003) with a return to baseline 24 h after the last dive (p > 0.99). There was no difference in chest site repartition (F = 1.02, p = 0.4) between lung territories or interaction with the day effect (F = 0.67, p = 0.9).

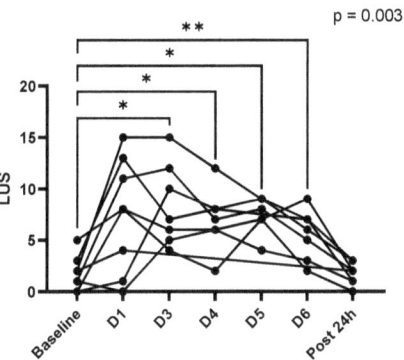

Figure 2. Evolution of individual lung ultrasound score (LUS) throughout repetition of day dives. All divers developed B-lines after several dive days and a return to baseline 24 h after the last one. *p*-value for the ANOVA. Tukey's multiple comparisons test is expressed versus baseline with * $p < 0.05$, ** $p < 0.01$.

4.2. Impedancemetry

All body water compartments and TBW increased after dives. Figure 3 depicts variation as compared to the baseline. No significative variation was found 24 h after dives in each compartment. A trend towards an IR (impedance ratio) decrease between baseline and after dives was observed at D1 and D6 (-1.5 [-2.3; -0.2] % and -1.85 [-3.4; -0.6] % F = 4.35, $p = 0.06$, respectively). There was no change in the angle phase (F = 0.20, $p = 0.8$).

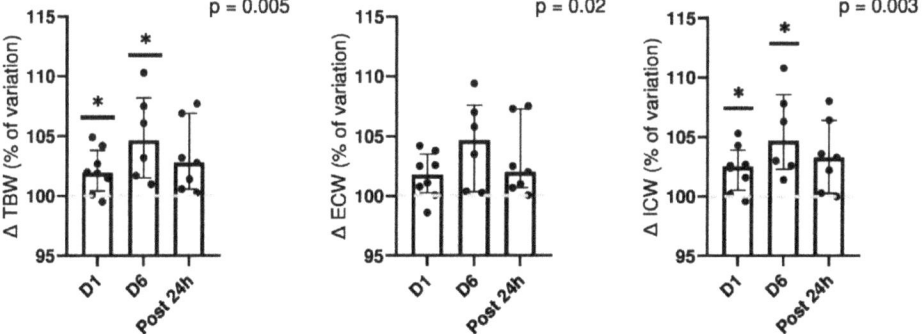

Figure 3. Evolution of hydration status measured by impedancemetry. Results are expressed in percentage of baseline variation. TBW, total body water; ECW, extra-cellular water; ICW, intra-cellular water. The *p*-value for the ANOVA. Tukey's multiple comparisons test is expressed versus baseline with * $p < 0.05$.

4.3. Heart Rate Variability

Only 23 measurements of HRV were accurately recorded during dives due to methodological issues. HRV data are shown in Table 4. No change was observed between baseline and 24 h post-dive. RMSSD and HF were significatively lower in dive versus rest measurements. Similarly, the global activity showed a decrease in variability with lower triangular index, SD2/SD1 and LF/HF ratios. The SDNN decrease was not significative (F = 5.83, $p = 0.05$).

At baseline, the PNS index was -1.92 [-2.17; -0.69] and decreased to -3.26 [-2.17; -2.8] on immersion ($p < 0.001$). Conversely, the SNS index varied to 5.570 [4.97; 6.62] at 13.5 [9.38; 19.72] ($p = 0.02$). The PNS index decreased on immersion (F = 35.83, $p < 0.0001$) while the SNS increased (F = 23.74, $p < 0.0001$), as shown in Figure 4.

Table 4. HRV parameters. Data were recorded at rest, in sitting position at baseline and 24 h after last day dive. Dive measurements were recorded in immersion during the diving program (*n* = 23). HR, heart rate; SDNN, standard deviation of normal-to-normal R waves; RMSSD, root mean square of the successive difference; RR triangular index, R–R intervals, and integral of the density of the R–R interval histogram divided by the maximum of its weight; VLF, very low-frequency; LF, low frequency; HF, high frequency; SD1, beat-to-beat HR variability; SD2, global HR variability; ShanEn, Shannon entropy; MSE, multi-scale entropy. *p*-value for the Friedman test. Dunn's multiple comparisons test is expressed versus dive with * $p < 0.05$, ** $p < 0.01$, *** $p < 0.001$ and **** $p < 0.0001$. Differences versus baseline are expressed with † $p < 0.05$ and †† $p < 0.01$.

	Baseline (Rest)	Dive	Post 24 h (Rest)	*p*-Value
Time domain				
Mean HR (bpm)	90 [65; 92] ***	118 [108; 135]	75 [74; 82] ****	<0.0001
SDNN (ms)	54.6 [51.4; 95]	35.7 [28.2; 65.3]	53.9 [53; 81.8]	0.05
RMSSD (ms)	24.2 [20.3; 26.6] **	6.1 [3.3; 9.1]	20.4 [19.8; 38.9] ****	<0.0001
RR triangular index	14.47 [13.21; 18.25] *	9.71 [7.99; 15.12]	14.41 [11.07; 22.05]	0.02
Frequency domain				
VLF (ms2)	1302 [947; 2683]	802 [467; 1908]	1843 [1780; 1932]	0.1
LF (ms2)	1259 [1000; 2445] ****	69 [28; 210]	775 [773; 2885] **	<0.0001
HF (ms2)	117 [92; 253] **	10 [3; 50]	134 [97; 629] ****	<0.0001
LF/HF ratio	11.35 [4.936; 13.68] *	5.764 [3.629; 9.095]	5.75 [4.585; 7.504] †	0.01
Non-linear results				
SD1 (ms)	17.1 [14.4; 18.8] ***	4.3 [2.3; 6.4]	14.4 [14; 27.5] ***	<0.0001
SD2 (ms)	74.8 [71.3; 133.2]	50.1 [39.8; 78.3]]	74.9 [73.4; 112.4]	0.05
SD2/SD1 ratio	4.965 [3.976; 5.553] ****	12.59 [7.818; 18.04]	5.187 [4.087; 5.249] ****	<0.0001
ShanEn	3.37 [2.946; 3.47] ****	4.238 [3.934; 4.553]	3.463 [3.102; 3.578] ***	<0.0001
MSE min	0.758 [0.711; 0.892]	0.658 [0.447; 0.797]	1.044 [0.914; 1.124] ****, ††	<0.0001
MSE max	2.787 [2.224; 2.902] ****	1.544 [1.358; 1.79]	2.485 [2.208; 2.65] ***	<0.0001

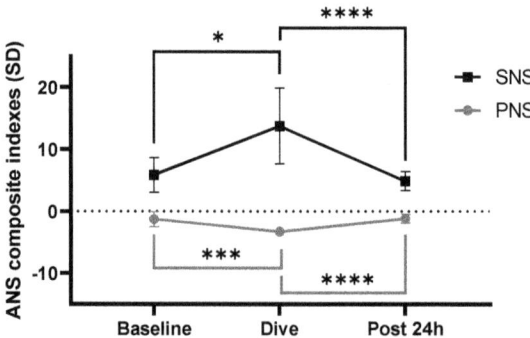

Figure 4. Autonomic nervous system (ANS) composite index measured by HRV. HRV parameters were performed at rest, in sitting position at baseline and 24 h after last day dive. Dive measurements were recorded in immersion during the diving program (*n* = 23). PNS, in parasympathetic nervous system; SNS, sympathetic nervous system; SD, standard deviation of measurement to the normal population average. Dunn's multiple comparisons test is expressed versus dive with * $p < 0.05$, *** $p < 0.001$ and **** $p < 0.0001$.

5. Discussion

The present study depicts that lung aeration disorders are observed during repeated CCR dives. However, these abnormalities, associated with a slight but significant SpO_2 decrease, may be transient and not associated with lung spirometry modifications.

A long-term FVC increase has already been reported in the experienced diving community, in relation to the chest muscular workload at depth. This change suggests a distension of the alveoli wall that may cause narrowing of small airways [4]. It could explain the moderate but not significant basal FEF 25–75 alteration observed in our study. However, the absence of any significant spirometric alteration after such shallow dives is similar to previous studies on CCR diving. There is a general consensus in pulmonary medicine and anesthesiology that breathing oxygen at an oxygen partial pressure (PpO_2) higher than 50 kPa causes acute pulmonary injury, which can result in atelectasis, interstitial oedema, and inflammation [38]. In such diving conditions, there was no significant clinically relevant impairment of clinical airway physiology. After breathing PpO_2 at 140 kPa for 20 min at 15 msw, an increase in oxidative stress urinary markers has been described but was not considered sufficient to affect the spirometry [14]. The pulmonary function also remained unchanged either after a prolonged 3- and 12 h exposure at 5 msw and 20 msw, respectively, with a PpO_2 of 150 kPa or after repeated dives (20 dives within 11 days) at an average depth of 69 msw during 112 min with a PpO_2 set at 130–140 kPa. It should be noted that the recommended maximal repetition excursion oxygen exposure (REPEX) threshold was approached in these studies [11,13,39]. In contrast, for deeper dives (90–120 msw) with a duration of 2 or 3 h, we previously found a gradual FVC decrease from 109 to 73% of the predicted value after a second dive, without returning to baseline between dives. No alteration of pulmonary resistance was observed, which might suggest other physiological mechanisms than hyperoxia. Considering all these arguments, one might consider that the alteration of spirometry data seems more likely to result from the effects of prolonged and deeper immersion at depth than from oxygen toxicity by itself [12].

A loss of lung aeration was observed after dives, as shown by the accumulation of B-lines without the alteration of spirometry. B-lines are an index of extravascular congestive lung fluid, which has been previously validated with high sensitivity and intra-patient reliability, allowing good interrater consistency of pulmonary fluid assessment using radiographic imaging [16,28]. Some authors have reported up to 75% of divers showing extravascular lung water detected as B-line accumulation. Many factors seem to be associated with asymptomatic changes in cardiovascular and pulmonary physiology in diving, therefore linked to the development of extravascular lung water [40]. However, B-lines are not specific, and their occurrence may also reflect any interstitial disorder or ventilation impairment. Some studies indicate a good correlation between their number and the intensity of damages [41]. An aeronautic study has shown that hyperoxia and hypergravity are independent risk factors of pulmonary atelectasis formation in healthy humans after a long arm centrifuge session. The increase in B-lines has been reported to reflect the onset of hyperoxic atelectasis [42]. Our study does not enable us to distinguish extravascular lung water or atelectasis contribution. It is interesting to note, while not significant, that a higher LUS number was observed during the first two days. Dives were shallower but the total immersion time and oxygen exposure were longer. Moreover, helium mixed gases were used for the deepest following dives, thus inducing a lesser gas density and a decrease in breathing workload. Two or three hours after surfacing from a deep Trimix dive, the B-lines were already largely resolved, similar to what has been reported by a previous Croatian study with similar dives [8]. Our results suggested that most of the pulmonary changes including loss of aeration lasted only for a short time after dives with a return to baseline 24 h post-dive.

A reduction in pulmonary diffusing capacity was shown only after a wet shallow oxygen dive as compared to a dry similar dive that suggested the implication of cardiopulmonary changes in immersion [11]. This impairment was inconsistent and was not correlated with the presence of B-lines [8]. In our study, SpO_2 slightly decreased after dives but remained within physiological values considered to be normal [43]. This oxygenation decrease may be related to the lung aeration loss and a potential alteration of alveolo-capillary gas exchange, even though it persists while LUS values have decreased and/or returned to baseline values. Atelectasis could lead to a pulmonary ventilation/perfusion mismatch and shunt opening [42]. Although non-pathological, this may interfere with gas elimination and decompression. Similar results were found after CCR dives at 10 msw [5] but not after deep dives despite spirometric alteration [12]. This SpO_2 decrease might be compensated by a prolonged high PpO_2 up to 150 kPa during long decompression stop after deep dives. Several artefacts can interfere with SpO_2 monitoring. However, data were always recorded after rewarming, in dry conditions, and after hydration in order to reduce these methodological artefacts [43].

It is well known that immersion induces hyperdiuresis, which in turn alters the hydration status with a loss of body weight of up to 3% and a potential impact on the cardio-pulmonary system [12,44]. Conversely, our results showed an increase in body water after diving. Considering that dehydration plays a role in decompression stress and that water intake could provide a decrease in the risk of decompression sickness (DCS), no specific instruction was given to fluid management for the team [45,46]. Technical divers were aware of this problem, and they probably rehydrated themself effectively during hours prior to measurements. There is no direct evidence within the literature that immersion pulmonary oedema is related to hydration in healthy divers [47,48]. In our study, there is no clear evidence that the observed state of hyperhydration could have contributed to lung ultrasound abnormalities.

HRV monitoring during scuba diving is only available from a limited number of studies, and CCR diving seems to induce a different HRV response than OC diving [22,49]. Immersion stimulates both the PNS and SNS branches. A predominant PNS is usually observed during descent and bottom stay, in accordance with human diving responses [49]. After emersion and continuation of atmospheric air breathing, the SNS takes over the PNS. A PNS tone increase in dive, related to dive length and depth, has been demonstrated [50]. Nitrox diving seems to induce a higher PNS activation [51] but also to be the principal dynamic component of SNS [50]. Short-term HRV is in fact influenced by many other factors, including PNS/SNS balance, as well as respiration via the respiratory sinus arrhythmia, heart and vascular tone via baroreceptor and cardiac stretch receptor activity, the central nervous system (CNS), the endocrine system, and chemoreceptors [21]. The PNS activity is a major contributor to the HF component (which reflects the power of vagally modulated respiratory sinus arrhythmia) [19]. Non-linear analysis revealed complexity in heart-rate patterns, which could not be perceived from time–domain [52]. Compared to OC diving, no variation in HF power or SDNN at depth was found in CCR diving, while the non-linear analysis increased. This suggests a lower PNS dynamic and variability in CCR dives [22]. In CCR cold diving (2 to 4 °C), the PNS index significatively decreased at submersion and increased gradually throughout the dive. At the same time, the SNS index sharply increased during immersion and then slowly declined back to the pre-dive rest levels [21]. Our results demonstrate a similar PNS dynamic. However, the SNS index appeared mostly predominant while global HRV activity and PNS decreased, which is contradictory to previous observations during OC diving. The SNS activity can be stimulated by many factors including physical activity or psychologically stressful situations [53]. The divers wore heavy equipment and were not necessarily previously familiar with the diving conditions that they experienced in this dynamic. Our HRV analysis has some limitations as we were only able to record 23 measurements due to interference between the heating system and the sensor. Moreover, the dive profiles varied over time, and we are not able to compare the responses at these different depths.

6. Limitations

The findings of this study have to be viewed with caution due to the small number of subjects and lack of daily pre-dive measurements due to logistical constraints. All measurements are compared to the first-day dive baseline, which reduces the accuracy in the assessment of physiological variations throughout the program. That may have particularly affected our impedancemetry analyses. In addition, the lack of monitoring fluid intake makes the interpretation difficult.

The mandatory boat travel-back time led to many hours of delay before measurements. Thus, we are aware of the risk of missing potential transient changes in the measured parameters. Our study was not conducted in controlled laboratory-like conditions. Essential parameters that could interfere with our results such as temperature, visibility, current, depth, or dive duration could not be controlled. Unfortunately, due to the small number of dives, the effect of the dive profile and breathing mixture cannot be evaluated.

7. Conclusions

The present observation represents the first original data regarding the pulmonary effects of repetitive CCR dives, combining spirometry, oxygenation evaluation and lung ultrasound imaging. Despite no detectable change in pulmonary function, we observed a significative loss of lung aeration. The impact of these impairments is unknown but should be taken into account, especially when considering long and repetitive dives. The marked changes that were also observed in autonomic cardiac activity highlight the important physiological and environmental constraints in CCR diving. All cardiac and pulmonary function changes were, however, transient, without the negative effect of dive repetition, and returned to baseline within 24 h after the last dive. Further research on this topic is encouraged to gain better knowledge about cardiopulmonary constraints during CCR diving.

Author Contributions: All authors listed have made a substantial, direct and intellectual contribution to the work, and approved it for publication. Conceptualization, E.G., C.B., J.O., E.D. and E.L.; methodology, C.B., E.D. and E.L.; validation, C.B. and E.L.; formal analysis, E.G., C.B. and E.L.; investigation, E.G., E.D. and E.L.; resources, E.G., C.B., J.O., E.D. and E.L.; data curation, E.G., E.D. and E.L.; writing—original draft preparation, E.G.; writing—review and editing, E.G., C.B. and E.L.; visualization, E.G.; supervision, C.B. and E.L.; funding acquisition, C.B. and E.L. All authors have read and agreed to the published version of the manuscript.

Funding: This research was funded by the Divers Alert Network (DAN), (Grant 10-25-2022) and Brest University Foundation.

Institutional Review Board Statement: The study was conducted in accordance with the Declaration of Helsinki, and approved by the Bio-Ethical Committee for Research and Higher Education, Brussels (No B200-2020-088, Date: 22 August 2020).

Informed Consent Statement: Informed written consent was obtained from all subjects involved in the study.

Data Availability Statement: Data are available on request from the authors.

Acknowledgments: The authors wish to thank General Electric Healthcare France and Sweden for their technical support. We acknowledge all divers and film crew for their kind collaboration and taking for a genuine interest in the research with special mention to Emmy Ahlén and Björn Lindoff from Vrakdykarpensionatet (Dalarö) for their logistical support and warm hospitality.

Conflicts of Interest: The authors declare no conflict of interest.

Abbreviations

ANOVA	analysis of variance	MSE	multi-scale entropy
ANS	autonomic nervous system	msw	meters of sea water
CCR	closed-circuit rebreather	OC	open circuit
DCS	decompression sickness	PEF	peak expiratory flow
ECW	extracellular body water	PNS	parasympathetic nervous system
FEF	forced expiratory flow	PpO_2	oxygen partial pressure
FEV1	forced expiratory volume in one second	RMSSD	root mean square of the successive difference
FVC	forced vital capacity	SDNN	standard deviation of normal-to-normal R waves
HF	high frequency	ShanEn	Shannon entropy
HR	heart rate	SNS	sympathetic nervous system
HRV	heart-rate variability	SpO_2	pulse oxygen saturation
ICW	intracellular body water	TBW	total body water
LF	low frequency	VLF	very low frequency
LUS	lung ultrasound score		

References

1. Mitchell, S.J.; Doolette, D.J. Recreational Technical Diving Part 1: An Introduction to Technical Diving Methods and Activities. *Diving Hyperb. Med.* **2013**, *43*, 86–93. [PubMed]
2. Gempp, E.; Louge, P.; Blatteau, J.-E.; Hugon, M. Descriptive Epidemiology of 153 Diving Injuries With Rebreathers Among French Military Divers From 1979 to 2009. *Mil. Med.* **2011**, *176*, 446–450. [CrossRef] [PubMed]
3. Marinovic, J.; Ljubkovic, M.; Obad, A.; Breskovic, T.; Salamunic, I.; Denoble, P.J.; Dujic, Z. Assessment of Extravascular Lung Water and Cardiac Function in Trimix SCUBA Diving. *Med. Sci. Sports Exerc.* **2010**, *42*, 1054–1061. [CrossRef] [PubMed]
4. Tetzlaff, K.; Thomas, P.S. Short- and Long-Term Effects of Diving on Pulmonary Function. *Eur. Respir. Rev.* **2017**, *26*, 160097. [CrossRef]
5. Martinez-Villar, M.; Tello-Montoliu, A.; Olea, A.; Pujante, Á.; Saura, D.; Martín, S.; Venero, N.; Carneiro-Mosquera, A.; Ruiz de Pascual, N.; Valero, N.; et al. Global Longitudinal Strain Assessment of Cardiac Function and Extravascular Lung Water Formation after Diving Using Semi-Closed Circuit Rebreather. *Eur. J. Appl. Physiol.* **2022**, *122*, 945–954. [CrossRef] [PubMed]
6. Castagna, O.; Regnard, J.; Gempp, E.; Louge, P.; Brocq, F.X.; Schmid, B.; Desruelle, A.-V.; Crunel, V.; Maurin, A.; Chopard, R.; et al. The Key Roles of Negative Pressure Breathing and Exercise in the Development of Interstitial Pulmonary Edema in Professional Male SCUBA Divers. *Sports Med.-Open* **2018**, *4*, 1. [CrossRef]
7. Dujic, Z.; Bakovic, D.; Marinovic-Terzic, I.; Eterovic, D. Acute Effects of a Single Open Sea Air Dive and Post-Dive Posture on Cardiac Output and Pulmonary Gas Exchange in Recreational Divers. *Br. J. Sports Med.* **2005**, *39*, e24. [CrossRef]
8. Ljubkovic, M.; Gaustad, S.E.; Marinovic, J.; Obad, A.; Ivancev, V.; Bilopavlovic, N.; Breskovic, T.; Wisloff, U.; Brubakk, A.; Dujic, Z. Ultrasonic Evidence of Acute Interstitial Lung Edema after SCUBA Diving Is Resolved within 2–3 h. *Respir. Physiol. Neurobiol.* **2010**, *171*, 165–170. [CrossRef]
9. Skogstad, M.; Thorsen, E.; Haldorsen, T.; Melbostad, E.; Tynes, T.; Westrum, B. Divers' Pulmonary Function after Open-Sea Bounce Dives to 10 and 50 Meters. *Undersea Hyperb. Med. J. Undersea Hyperb. Med. Soc. Inc.* **1996**, *23*, 71–75.
10. Tetzlaff, K.; Friege, L.; Koch, A.; Heine, L.; Neubauer, B.; Struck, N.; Mutzbauer, T.S. Effects of Ambient Cold and Depth on Lung Function in Humans after a Single Scuba Dive. *Eur. J. Appl. Physiol.* **2001**, *85*, 125–129. [CrossRef]
11. Van Ooij, P.J.A.M.; Van Hulst, R.A.; Houtkooper, A.; Sterk, P.J. Differences in Spirometry and Diffusing Capacity after a 3-h Wet or Dry Oxygen Dive with a PO2 of 150 KPa: Spirometry and Diffusing Capacity after a 3-h Oxygen Dive. *Clin. Physiol. Funct. Imaging* **2011**, *31*, 405–410. [CrossRef] [PubMed]
12. Dugrenot, E.; Balestra, C.; Gouin, E.; L'Her, E.; Guerrero, F. Physiological Effects of Mixed-Gas Deep Sea Dives Using a Closed-Circuit Rebreather: A Field Pilot Study. *Eur. J. Appl. Physiol.* **2021**, *121*, 3323–3331. [CrossRef] [PubMed]
13. Castagna, O.; Bergmann, C.; Blatteau, J.E. Is a 12-h Nitrox Dive Hazardous for Pulmonary Function? *Eur. J. Appl. Physiol.* **2019**, *119*, 2723–2731. [CrossRef] [PubMed]
14. Bosco, G.; Rizzato, A.; Quartesan, S.; Camporesi, E.; Mrakic-Sposta, S.; Moretti, S.; Balestra, C.; Rubini, A. Spirometry and Oxidative Stress after Rebreather Diving in Warm Water. *Undersea Hyperb. Med.* **2018**, *45*, 191–198. [CrossRef] [PubMed]
15. Lichtenstein, D.; Mézière, G.; Biderman, P.; Gepner, A.; Barré, O. The Comet-Tail Artifact. An Ultrasound Sign of Alveolar-Interstitial Syndrome. *Am. J. Respir. Crit. Care Med.* **1997**, *156*, 1640–1646. [CrossRef] [PubMed]
16. Picano, E.; Pellikka, P.A. Ultrasound Assessment of Extravascular Lung Water: A New Standard for Pulmonary Congestion. *Eur. Heart J.* **2016**, *37*, 2097–2104. [CrossRef] [PubMed]
17. Dujic, Z.; Marinovic, J.; Obad, A.; Ivancev, V.; Breskovic, T.; Jovovic, P.; Ljubkovic, M. A No-Decompression Air Dive and Ultrasound Lung Comets. *Aviat. Space Environ. Med.* **2011**, *82*, 40–43. [CrossRef]

18. Lambrechts, K.; Germonpré, P.; Charbel, B.; Cialoni, D.; Musimu, P.; Sponsiello, N.; Marroni, A.; Pastouret, F.; Balestra, C. Ultrasound Lung "Comets" Increase after Breath-Hold Diving. *Eur. J. Appl. Physiol.* **2011**, *111*, 707–713. [CrossRef]
19. Shaffer, F.; Ginsberg, J.P. An Overview of Heart Rate Variability Metrics and Norms. *Front. Public Health* **2017**, *5*, 258. [CrossRef]
20. Chouchou, F.; Pichot, V.; Garet, M.; Barthélémy, J.-C.; Roche, F. Dominance in Cardiac Parasympathetic Activity during Real Recreational SCUBA Diving. *Eur. J. Appl. Physiol.* **2009**, *106*, 345–352. [CrossRef]
21. Lundell, R.V.; Tuominen, L.; Ojanen, T.; Parkkola, K.; Räisänen-Sokolowski, A. Diving Responses in Experienced Rebreather Divers: Short-Term Heart Rate Variability in Cold Water Diving. *Front. Physiol.* **2021**, *12*, 649319. [CrossRef] [PubMed]
22. Lafère, P.; Lambrechts, K.; Germonpré, P.; Balestra, A.; Germonpré, F.L.; Marroni, A.; Cialoni, D.; Bosco, G.; Balestra, C. Heart Rate Variability During a Standard Dive: A Role for Inspired Oxygen Pressure? *Front. Physiol.* **2021**, *12*, 635132. [CrossRef] [PubMed]
23. World Medical Association. World Medical Association Declaration of Helsinki: Ethical Principles for Medical Research Involving Human Subjects. *JAMA* **2013**, *310*, 2191. [CrossRef] [PubMed]
24. Lafère, P.; Guerrero, F.; Germonpré, P.; Balestra, C. Comparison of Insulation Provided by Dry or Wetsuits among Recreational Divers during Cold Water Immersion (<5 °C). *Int. Marit. Health* **2021**, *72*, 217–222. [CrossRef]
25. Quanjer, P.H.; Stanojevic, S.; Cole, T.J.; Baur, X.; Hall, G.L.; Culver, B.H.; Enright, P.L.; Hankinson, J.L.; Ip, M.S.M.; Zheng, J.; et al. Multi-Ethnic Reference Values for Spirometry for the 3–95-Yr Age Range: The Global Lung Function 2012 Equations. *Eur. Respir. J.* **2012**, *40*, 1324–1343. [CrossRef]
26. Graham, B.L.; Steenbruggen, I.; Miller, M.R.; Barjaktarevic, I.Z.; Cooper, B.G.; Hall, G.L.; Hallstrand, T.S.; Kaminsky, D.A.; McCarthy, K.; McCormack, M.C.; et al. Standardization of Spirometry 2019 Update. An Official American Thoracic Society and European Respiratory Society Technical Statement. *Am. J. Respir. Crit. Care Med.* **2019**, *200*, e70–e88. [CrossRef]
27. Bouhemad, B.; Mongodi, S.; Via, G.; Rouquette, I. Ultrasound for "Lung Monitoring" of Ventilated Patients. *Anesthesiology* **2015**, *122*, 437–447. [CrossRef]
28. Mongodi, S.; De Luca, D.; Colombo, A.; Stella, A.; Santangelo, E.; Corradi, F.; Gargani, L.; Rovida, S.; Volpicelli, G.; Bouhemad, B.; et al. Quantitative Lung Ultrasound: Technical Aspects and Clinical Applications. *Anesthesiology* **2021**, *134*, 949–965. [CrossRef]
29. Marini, E.; Campa, F.; Buffa, R.; Stagi, S.; Matias, C.N.; Toselli, S.; Sardinha, L.B.; Silva, A.M. Phase Angle and Bioelectrical Impedance Vector Analysis in the Evaluation of Body Composition in Athletes. *Clin. Nutr.* **2020**, *39*, 447–454. [CrossRef]
30. Balestra, C.; Guerrero, F.; Theunissen, S.; Germonpré, P.; Lafère, P. Physiology of Repeated Mixed Gas 100-m Wreck Dives Using a Closed-Circuit Rebreather: A Field Bubble Study. *Eur. J. Appl. Physiol.* **2022**, *122*, 515–522. [CrossRef]
31. Wekre, S.L.; Landsverk, H.D.; Lautridou, J.; Hjelde, A.; Imbert, J.P.; Balestra, C.; Eftedal, I. Hydration Status during Commercial Saturation Diving Measured by Bioimpedance and Urine Specific Gravity. *Front. Physiol.* **2022**, *13*, 971757. [CrossRef] [PubMed]
32. Kyle, U. Bioelectrical Impedance Analysis?Part I: Review of Principles and Methods. *Clin. Nutr.* **2004**, *23*, 1226–1243. [CrossRef] [PubMed]
33. Bosy-Westphal, A.; Danielzik, S.; Dörhöfer, R.-P.; Later, W.; Wiese, S.; Müller, M.J. Phase Angle From Bioelectrical Impedance Analysis: Population Reference Values by Age, Sex, and Body Mass Index. *J. Parenter. Enter. Nutr.* **2006**, *30*, 309–316. [CrossRef] [PubMed]
34. Plews, D.J.; Scott, B.; Altini, M.; Wood, M.; Kilding, A.E.; Laursen, P.B. Comparison of Heart-Rate-Variability Recording With Smartphone Photoplethysmography, Polar H7 Chest Strap, and Electrocardiography. *Int. J. Sports Physiol. Perform.* **2017**, *12*, 1324–1328. [CrossRef]
35. Malik, M. Heart Rate Variability: Standards of Measurement, Physiological Interpretation, and Clinical Use. *Circulation* **1996**, *93*, 1043–1065. [CrossRef]
36. Tarvainen, M.P.; Niskanen, J.-P.; Lipponen, J.A.; Ranta-aho, P.O.; Karjalainen, P.A. Kubios HRV–Heart Rate Variability Analysis Software. *Comput. Methods Programs Biomed.* **2014**, *113*, 210–220. [CrossRef]
37. Nunan, D.; Sandercock, G.R.H.; Brodie, D.A. A Quantitative Systematic Review of Normal Values for Short-Term Heart Rate Variability in Healthy Adults: Review of Short-Term HRV Values. *Pacing Clin. Electrophysiol.* **2010**, *33*, 1407–1417. [CrossRef]
38. Clark, J.M.; Lambertsen, C.J. Pulmonary Oxygen Toxicity: A Review. *Pharmacol. Rev.* **1971**, *23*, 37–133.
39. Fock, A.; Harris, R.; Slade, M. Oxygen Exposure and Toxicity in Recreational Technical Divers. *Diving Hyperb. Med.* **2013**, *43*, 67–71.
40. Castagna, O.; Gempp, E.; Poyet, R.; Schmid, B.; Desruelle, A.-V.; Crunel, V.; Maurin, A.; Choppard, R.; MacIver, D.H. Cardiovascular Mechanisms of Extravascular Lung Water Accumulation in Divers. *Am. J. Cardiol.* **2017**, *119*, 929–932. [CrossRef]
41. Soldati, G.; Demi, M.; Smargiassi, A.; Inchingolo, R.; Demi, L. The Role of Ultrasound Lung Artifacts in the Diagnosis of Respiratory Diseases. *Expert Rev. Respir. Med.* **2019**, *13*, 163–172. [CrossRef] [PubMed]
42. Dussault, C.; Gontier, E.; Verret, C.; Soret, M.; Boussuges, A.; Hedenstierna, G.; Montmerle-Borgdorff, S. Hyperoxia and Hypergravity Are Independent Risk Factors of Atelectasis in Healthy Sitting Humans: A Pulmonary Ultrasound and SPECT/CT Study. *J. Appl. Physiol.* **2016**, *121*, 66–77. [CrossRef] [PubMed]
43. Jubran, A. Pulse Oximetry. *Crit. Care* **2015**, *19*, 272. [CrossRef] [PubMed]
44. Castagna, O.; Desruelle, A.; Blatteau, J.-E.; Schmid, B.; Dumoulin, G.; Regnard, J. Alterations in Body Fluid Balance During Fin Swimming in 29 °C Water in a Population of Special Forces Divers. *Int. J. Sports Med.* **2015**, *36*, 1125–1133. [CrossRef] [PubMed]
45. Gempp, E.; Blatteau, J.E.; Pontier, J.-M.; Balestra, C.; Louge, P. Preventive Effect of Pre-Dive Hydration on Bubble Formation in Divers. *Br. J. Sports Med.* **2009**, *43*, 224–228. [CrossRef]

46. Han, K.-H.; Hyun, G.-S.; Jee, Y.-S.; Park, J.-M. Effect of Water Amount Intake before Scuba Diving on the Risk of Decompression Sickness. *Int. J. Environ. Res. Public Health* **2021**, *18*, 7601. [CrossRef]
47. Henckes, A.; Cochard, G.; Gatineau, F.; Louge, P.; Gempp, E.; Demaistre, S.; Nowak, E.; Ozier, Y. Risk Factors for Immersion Pulmonary Edema in Recreational Scuba Divers: A Case-Control Study. *Undersea Hyperb. Med. J. Undersea Hyperb. Med. Soc. Inc.* **2019**, *46*, 611–618. [CrossRef]
48. Weiler-Ravell, D.; Shupak, A.; Goldenberg, I.; Halpern, P.; Shoshani, O.; Hirschhorn, G.; Margulis, A. Pulmonary Oedema and Haemoptysis Induced by Strenuous Swimming. *BMJ* **1995**, *311*, 361–362. [CrossRef]
49. Ackermann, S.P.; Raab, M.; Backschat, S.; Smith, D.J.C.; Javelle, F.; Laborde, S. The Diving Response and Cardiac Vagal Activity: A Systematic Review and Meta-analysis. *Psychophysiology* **2022**, *00*, e14183. [CrossRef]
50. Noh, Y.; Posada-Quintero, H.F.; Bai, Y.; White, J.; Florian, J.P.; Brink, P.R.; Chon, K.H. Effect of Shallow and Deep SCUBA Dives on Heart Rate Variability. *Front. Physiol.* **2018**, *9*, 110. [CrossRef]
51. Zenske, A.; Kähler, W.; Koch, A.; Oellrich, K.; Pepper, C.; Muth, T.; Schipke, J.D. Does Oxygen-Enriched Air Better than Normal Air Improve Sympathovagal Balance in Recreational Divers?An Open-Water Study. *Res. Sports Med.* **2020**, *28*, 397–412. [CrossRef] [PubMed]
52. Stein, P.K.; Reddy, A. Non-Linear Heart Rate Variability and Risk Stratification in Cardiovascular Disease. *Indian Pacing Electrophysiol. J.* **2005**, *5*, 210–220. [PubMed]
53. Kim, H.-G.; Cheon, E.-J.; Bai, D.-S.; Lee, Y.H.; Koo, B.-H. Stress and Heart Rate Variability: A Meta-Analysis and Review of the Literature. *Psychiatry Investig.* **2018**, *15*, 235–245. [CrossRef] [PubMed]

Disclaimer/Publisher's Note: The statements, opinions and data contained in all publications are solely those of the individual author(s) and contributor(s) and not of MDPI and/or the editor(s). MDPI and/or the editor(s) disclaim responsibility for any injury to people or property resulting from any ideas, methods, instructions or products referred to in the content.

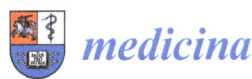

Article

Vascular Function Recovery Following Saturation Diving

Jean-Pierre Imbert [1,2], Salih-Murat Egi [1,3] and Costantino Balestra [1,4,5,6,*]

[1] Environmental, Occupational, Aging (Integrative) Physiology Laboratory, Haute Ecole Bruxelles-Brabant (HE2B), 1090 Brussels, Belgium
[2] Divetech, 1543 Chemin des Vignasses, 06410 Biot, France
[3] Computer Engineering Department, Galatasaray University, Istanbul 34349, Turkey
[4] Anatomical Research and Clinical Studies (ARCS), Vrije Universiteit Brussels (VUB), 1090 Brussels, Belgium
[5] DAN Europe Research Division, 64026 Roseto, Italy
[6] Physical Activity Teaching Unit, Motor Sciences Department, Université Libre de Bruxelles (ULB), 1050 Brussels, Belgium
* Correspondence: costantinobalestra@gmail.com

Abstract: *Background and Objectives*: Saturation diving is a technique used in commercial diving. Decompression sickness (DCS) was the main concern of saturation safety, but procedures have evolved over the last 50 years and DCS has become a rare event. New needs have evolved to evaluate the diving and decompression stress to improve the flexibility of the operations (minimum interval between dives, optimal oxygen levels, etc.). We monitored this stress in saturation divers during actual operations. *Materials and Methods*: The monitoring included the detection of vascular gas emboli (VGE) and the changes in the vascular function measured by flow mediated dilatation (FMD) after final decompression to surface. Monitoring was performed onboard a diving support vessel operating in the North Sea at typical storage depths of 120 and 136 msw. A total of 49 divers signed an informed consent form and participated to the study. Data were collected on divers at surface, before the saturation and during the 9 h following the end of the final decompression. *Results*: VGE were detected in three divers at very low levels (insignificant), confirming the improvements achieved on saturation decompression procedures. As expected, the FMD showed an impairment of vascular function immediately at the end of the saturation in all divers but the divers fully recovered from these vascular changes in the next 9 following hours, regardless of the initial decompression starting depth. *Conclusion*: These changes suggest an oxidative/inflammatory dimension to the diving/decompression stress during saturation that will require further monitoring investigations even if the vascular impairment is found to recover fast.

Keywords: flow-mediated dilation; FMD; decompression; arterial stiffness; endothelial dysfunction; underwater; hyperbaric; commercial diver; off-shore energy operation; human

Citation: Imbert, J.-P.; Egi, S.-M.; Balestra, C. Vascular Function Recovery Following Saturation Diving. *Medicina* 2022, 58, 1476. https://doi.org/10.3390/medicina58101476

Academic Editor: Marcus Daniel Lancé

Received: 29 September 2022
Accepted: 13 October 2022
Published: 17 October 2022

Publisher's Note: MDPI stays neutral with regard to jurisdictional claims in published maps and institutional affiliations.

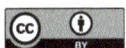

Copyright: © 2022 by the authors. Licensee MDPI, Basel, Switzerland. This article is an open access article distributed under the terms and conditions of the Creative Commons Attribution (CC BY) license (https://creativecommons.org/licenses/by/4.0/).

1. Introduction

Saturation diving is a standard technique of divers' intervention in the North Sea because of its depth (average 100 to 150 msw). Saturation is conducted from large diving support vessel that employs around 80 divers in multiple rotations during a working season. The contractors have developed saturation procedures empirically over the last 40 years and reached a mature level of technology and safety. On the other hand, the need for evaluating the diving and decompression stress to improve flexibility of the operations (minimum interval between dives, optimal oxygen levels, etc.) arose.

An increasing number of research reports have been published to document procedures, diver's subjective evaluations [1], hematological changes [2], high pressure nervous syndrome [3], divers hydration status [4] or oxidative stress [5]. Saturation permits divers to live under pressure in chambers onboard of a vessel and to be deployed directly to the seabed by a diving bell. Historically, commercial saturation diving was developed during the 1970s for the North Sea oil platform installations. At the time, the concern was decompression sickness (DCS) that was associated with bubbles in the divers' blood. During these "early days" when diving in such a harsh environment was not as safe, and still difficult today, alarming reports were available:

"Records show that since 1966 seventy-seven diving personnel tragically have lost their lives in the quest for, depending on your perspective "Black Gold" or "Devil's excrement" in the North Sea Basin. By nationality: 53 British/Commonwealth subjects, 9 American, 7 Norwegian, 4 Dutch, 3 French, and 1 Italian. Prior to 1971/1974, applicable laws & regulations (if any) required no accurate fatal accident statistics. One can conclude that the actual combined number of deaths is higher. However, it is known that several divers received severe injuries from which they never recovered."

(https://the-norwegian.com/north-sea-diving-fatalities (accessed on 20 September 2022))

Fifty years later, saturation procedures have improved a lot and decompression sickness has become a rare event. Official safety records published in Norway on the Website of the PSA (Petroleum safety Authority) indicate an incidence of less than one case per 2000 exposure over the last 10 years (https://www.ptil.no/en/technical-competence/explore-technical-subjects (accessed on 20 September 2022)). As a result, the diving companies have the duty to evaluate the performances of their procedures such as the minimal permitted interval between two saturations. This minimum interval has been arbitrarily defined for a long time by industry guidelines or diving regulations but the divers' recovery between saturations has never been studied scientifically. This recovery period remains important for companies to optimize their crew changes and divers to manage their professional career.

Saturation diving is obviously associated with multiple stressors that may be organized along three dimensions for simplicity. The first dimension is characterized by the diving work and includes stresses such as the physical, mental, or thermal.

The second dimension is associated with the vascular gas emboli (VGE) produced during decompression. Although there is no clear relation between the number of VGE measured and the risk of DCS, it is recognized that the smaller the number of VGE detected, the safer is the decompression [6]. The number of circulating VGE was therefore taken as the principal measurement of the decompression stress.

The third dimension covers several biological processes recently identified in the literature [7]. New insight demonstrate that bubbles tear the vessel inner layer away and create microparticles of endothelial debris when detaching from the endothelium during decompression [8–10]. Bubbles and oxygen partial pressure increase trigger defense mechanisms like platelets and neutrophil activation that will also elicit some microparticles [11,12]. In this study, the vascular function assessed by means of Flow Mediated Dilation (FMD) was considered as the third dimension representing the oxidative and or inflammatory stress [10,13,14].

The objective of the study was to define a monitoring package and use it on board a vessel to monitor saturation divers at surface, before the saturation and after exiting saturation (after decompression), in order to evaluate their recovery during the 9 h following the end of their final decompression.

2. Methods

2.1. Worksites

A leading diving company provided access to one of their diving support vessels (DSV) operating in the North Sea for this study. Two monitoring sessions were conducted onboard the DSV Deep Arctic (The vessel DEEP ARCTIC is an Offshore Support Vessel built in 2009 with particulars of Gross Tonnage 18,640 t; Summer Deadweight 13,000 t; Length Overall 157 m; Beam 31 m.) in April and October 2016, during two different projects, one in the Norwegian sector at 121 m of sea water (msw) and the other in the UK sector at 155 msw working depth. The two projects, performed on the same vessel, corresponded to a well intervention on the seabed; the divers used the same breathing gasses, the same diving equipment and performed the same tasks (see Figure 1).

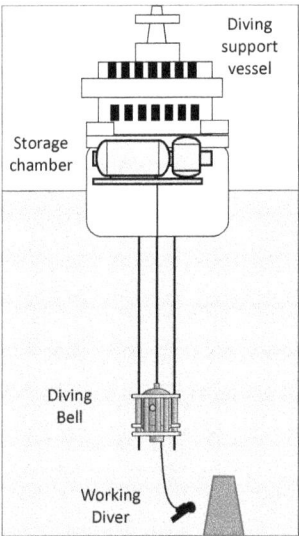

Figure 1. A typical saturation worksite. The divers are deployed from the diving support vessel inside a diving bell. Once on site, the bell's door opens, and the divers lock out in the water using an umbilical attached to the bell to breathe and being supplied with hot water in their suit for thermal comfort. The working depth corresponds to the maximum depth reached by the divers. The working depth defines the chamber storage depth from excursion tables prepared in the company diving manual. The bell depth is usually set at 5 msw deeper than the storage depth to clear from subsea structures when opened. The "storage" and the "bell" are almost at the same pressure allowing for getting back to storage after work without decompression needed. The excursion of the diver out of the diving bell is limited to some meters not to add additional decompression time. The breathing gas is Heliox (Helium-Oxygen) to limit the density of the breathed gas (significant at such pressures) to reduce the work of breathing as well as Oxygen toxicity and Nitrogen narcosis.

2.2. Saturation Procedures

The two projects were conducted with saturations according to the Company procedures defined in their diving manuals. However, specific requirements are defined in the Norwegian diving regulations that introduced slight variations.

The chambers were initially compressed to 10 msw in 10 min for a 20 min leaks check. Compression then proceeded to the "storage" depth at 1 msw/min.

The chamber PO_2 at storage depth was controlled at 40 hPa. The storage depth was selected from the working depth using the standard excursion tables (110 msw storage depth for 121 msw working depth in the Norwegian sector, 136 msw storage depth for 155 msw working depth in the UK sector). During the bottom phase, divers performed one bell dive of 8 h per day but may sometime skip a dive due to weather conditions or vessel transit. During the dives, the divers' breathing mixture was Heliox with a PO_2 ranging from 60 to 80 hPa.

The final decompression can only start after an 8 h period following the last excursion dive.

The decompression is performed in two phases. It starts with constant chamber PO_2 (50 hPa in the UK, 48 hPa in Norway) until 15 msw and finishes with a chamber oxygen percentage maintained between 23.1 and 23% to limit the fire hazard and optimize inert gas exhalation.

Despite the difference between sectors, the total decompression durations were very similar (5 days 5 h in the UK sector and 5 days 11 h in the Norwegian sector, a difference of less than 3%).

The divers were organized in three men teams (two divers and the bellman). Teams worked in shifts (12:00 p.m. to midnight and midnight to 12:00 p.m.). Each team was involved in one bell excursion dive per day during their shift. The divers' in-water time was limited to 6 h with a mandatory break at mid-excursion.

2.3. Participant Eligibility and Enrollment

The study group consisted of volunteer, male, certified commercial saturation divers. These divers were declared fit for the saturation by the vessel hyperbaric nurse after a mandatory pre-dive medical examination.

All experimental procedures were conducted in accordance with the Declaration of Helsinki [8] and were approved by the Academic Ethical Committee of Brussels (B200-2009-039). The methods and potential risks were explained in detail to the participants. Each subject gave written informed consent before participation.

A total of 49 divers accepted to participate to the study.

The group anthropometric parameters were obtained after a confidential interview in the vessel hospital. (See Table 1).

Table 1. Participants anthropometric parameters (n = 49).

	Mean ± SD
Age	45.7 ± 7.32
Height	180.4 ± 7.2 cm
Weight	86.4 ± 11.5 kg
BMI	26.5 ± 2.4

As expected from saturation divers, all were very experienced divers with a long diving career. (See Table 2).

Table 2. Participants diving experience (commercial experience includes Saturation experience).

	Mean ± SD
Experience as a commercial air diver	21.3 ± 8.3 years
Experience as a saturation diver	14.7 ± 8.1 years

Part of the group freely took of antioxidant supplements (commercially available products containing as vitamin C, D, or E) before and during the saturation. (See Table 3).

Table 3. Group antioxidant supplement intake (free administration).

Antioxidant Supplements	Yes	No	Sometimes
During normal surface life	58%	38%	4%
During saturation	59%	29%	12%

Saturation divers generally spend a lot of time maintaining a high level of physical fitness and are involved in all sorts of sports. Every diver in the group except one had a daily or at least weekly physical activity when at home. (See Table 4).

Table 4. Participants' usual physical activities.

Type of Physical Activity	Percentage
Outdoor, intense like running, surfing, cycling, climbing, biking, kitesurf	72.9%
Outdoor, moderate like golf, hiking	6.8%
Indoor, intense: swimming, hockey, boxing, gym	13.6%
Moderate, or no sport	5%
Unclassified (i.e., working as a farmer)	1.7%

The participants were divided as follows: 37 divers in saturation in the Norwegian project (75%) and 12 divers in saturation in the UK project (25%). The saturation duration depended on the sector regulations. It is 14 days maximum bottom time in Norway and 28 days total saturation time in the UK. The mean saturation duration was 19.70 ± 6.5 days (minimum 10 days, maximum 28 days) (see Figure 2).

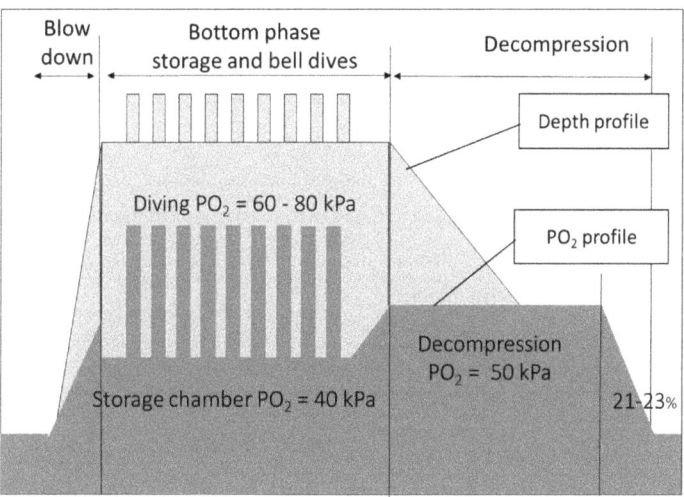

Figure 2. Description of the saturation in the UK sector: depth profile (compression, storage depth, bell dives, decompression) and associated PO_2 profile.

2.4. Organizational Constraints

The voluntary divers were first involved in the study in the few hours after arriving onboard, after their pre-saturation medical examination, just before entering the saturation chambers. Baseline (control) measurements (FMD and Questionnaires) were recorded. The group of divers were then monitored during the next 12 h following the end of the decompression to surface.

The questionnaires and measurements were run in the vessel hospital room that warranted confidentiality.

It is admitted that after the decompression, due to operational constraints, it was difficult to "catch" the divers at regular times and some subjects (30%) only performed one or two sessions of the four initially planned (see Figure 3).

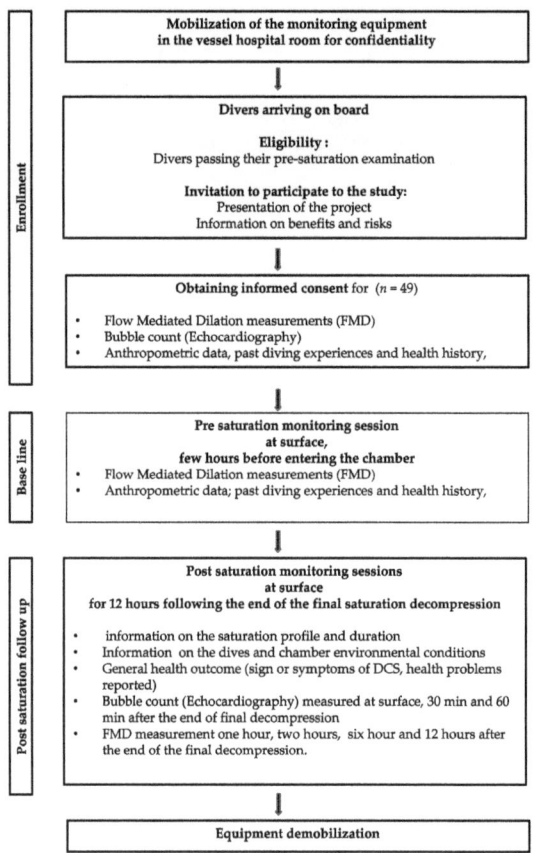

Figure 3. Experimental flowchart.

2.5. Data Acquisition

2.5.1. Flow-Mediated Dilation (FMD)

FMD, an established measure of the endothelium-dependent vasodilation mediated by nitric oxide (NO) [15], was used to assess the effect of diving on main conduit arteries. Subjects were at rest for 15-min in a supine position before the measurements were taken. Brachial artery diameter was measured by means of a 5.0–10.0 MHz linear transducer M-Turbo portable echocardiograph (Sonosite M-Turbo, FUJIFILM Sonosite Inc., Amsterdam, The Netherlands) immediately before and 1-min after a 5-min ischemia (induced by inflating a sphygmomanometer cuff placed on the forearm to 180 mmHg as previously described [16].

All ultrasound assessments were performed by an experienced operator, with more than 100 scans/year, which is recommended to maintain competency with the FMD method [17].

When the images were chosen for analysis, the boundaries for diameter measurement were identified manually with an electronic caliper (provided by the ultrasonography proprietary software) in a threefold repetition pattern to calculate the mean value. In our laboratory, the mean intra observer variability for FMD measurement for the operator recorded the same day, on the same site and on the same subject was $1.2 \pm 0.2\%$.

FMD were calculated as the percent increase in arterial diameter from the resting state to maximal dilation.

2.5.2. Post Saturation Diving Decompression Vascular Gas Emboli (VGE)

The echocardiographic VGE signals over the 1 min recording were evaluated by frame-based bubble counting as described by Germonpré et al. [18], but also scored according to the Eftedal-Brubakk categorical score [19].

Echocardiography was performed with a M-Turbo portable echocardiograph (Sonosite M-Turbo, FUJIFILM Sonosite Inc, Amsterdam, The Netherlands) used in a medical clinic included in the vessel while the patient was comfortably lying in a medical bed (Left Lateral Decubitus); four chamber view echocardiography loops were recorded on hard disk for offline analysis by three blinded evaluators. VGE numbers were counted at 30 min and 60 min post saturation decompression.

Evaluation of decompression stress and of the potential benefit of preventive measures has been done historically based on the presence or absence of clinical symptoms of DCS. However, for obvious ethical reasons, this is not acceptable in the field of recreational or professional diving [20]. Although imperfect, it is now accepted that research projects can use VGE data as a surrogate endpoint [6,21]. Different methods of detection of VGE are possible, such as Doppler ultrasonic bubble detectors or 2D cardiac echography [22]. During field studies, bubbles are usually detected in the right atrium, ventricle (right heart), and pulmonary artery. Then, the amount of detected VGE is graded according to different systems, either, categorical [19], semi-quantitatively [18] or continuous [21,22].

3. Statistical Analysis

The normality of data was performed by means of Shapiro–Wilk or D'Agostino-Pearson tests.

When a Gaussian distribution was assumed, and when comparisons were limited to two samples, paired or non-paired t-test were applied. If the Gaussian distribution was not assumed, the analysis was performed by means of a non-parametric Mann-Whitney U test or, a Wilcoxon paired test. Taking the baseline measures as 100%, percentage changes were calculated for each diver, allowing for an appreciation of the magnitude of change rather than the absolute values (one sample t-test). All statistical tests were performed using a standard computer statistical package, GraphPad Prism version 5.00 for Windows (GraphPad Software, San Diego, CA, USA).

A threshold of $p < 0.05$ was considered statistically significant. All data are presented as mean $\pm$ standard deviation (SD).

Sample size was calculated setting the power of the study at 95%, and assuming that variables associated with diving would have been affected to a similar extent as that observed in our previous studies [16–18] our sample reached 99%.

The linear regression line was performed using the least squares method and the lateral bands represented are in the 95% predictivity range.

4. Results

4.1. Vascular Gas Emboli

A very low number of bubbles were found in the participants after their decompression during their "bend-watch" period (the first 9 h).

Among all divers ($n = 49$), only three showed circulating gas emboli according to the EB scale that represented 0.2 ± 0.05 (mean $\pm$ SD) bubbles per heartbeat, which represents less than grade 1 on the EB grading scale in three divers. This is extremely low and doesn't allow statistical analysis. To allow the reader to compare with other diving situations this grading is 10 times lower than an average number of bubbles after a simple dive of 25 min at 25 m considered within safety limits [23].

4.2. Flow Mediated Dilation

FMD comparison between pre/post dive situation and control values is shown in Figure 4. Flow Mediated Dilation is calculated as the percentage increase of arterial diameter after an occlusion period (5 min); this post occlusion dilation was normal in our divers in pre-dive situations (107.15 ± 6.6%). After vascular occlusion, the dilation provoked by the imposed shear stress was around 7–10%. Taking the individual FMD of each diver as the baseline, the percentual mean reduction reaches 94.7 ± 0.9 % ($p < 0.0001$) during the first two hours after decompression and quickly recovers reaching 98.75 ± 0.91 ($p < 0.0001$) in the last two hours (6–8 h after decompression) (see Figure 4).

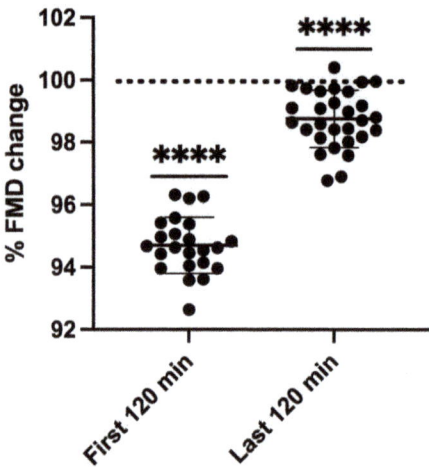

Figure 4. Bar graph illustrating FMD changes during the first 2 h (First 120 min.) ($n = 23$) and last 2 h ($n = 29$) (7–9 h) after saturation decompression (**** = $p < 0.0001$) (One sample t-test). (FMD Changes are presented compared to predive values represented by the dotted line at 100%).

Our data suggest that total vascular function recovery has not yet reached 8 h after the end of decompression. We then computed a best fit equation to extrapolate the time needed to achieve recovery. The linear regression line and the equation are shown in Figure 5.

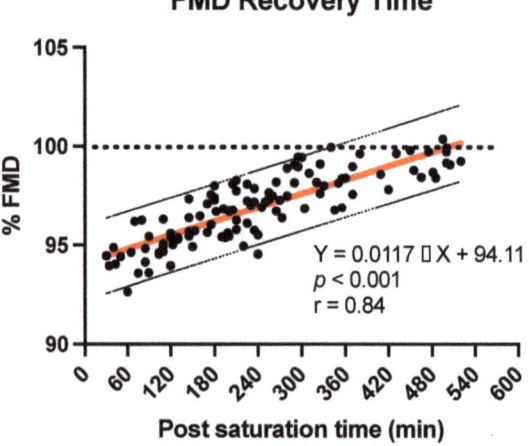

Figure 5. FMD evolution after exiting saturation the linear solution has been selected as the best fit approach, and the dotted lateral bands represent the 95% prediction bands.

5. Discussion

Few scientific studies have been performed in real commercial saturation conditions during the last ten years. These studies are difficult because of the offshore constraints and project planning that do not allow much time for scientific testin—not to mention the cost of accommodating the scientific team onboard. Available studies are related to the subjective evaluation of saturation operations by the divers themselves [1]. More advanced studies such as evolution of plasma or blood derived measurements have been conducted [2,24]. Given the difficulties to achieve blood sampling, other studies are conducted based on salivary, urine, epithelial, or other minimally invasive sampling techniques [24–27].

Our goal in this experiment was to document vascular recovery post saturation diving (after decompression). Vascular gas emboli are probably involved in the post dive reduction of FMD. Nevertheless, the available literature refrains us to draw a direct link between FMD reduction and VGE, since micro and macro vascularization react differently [28], and different preconditioning procedures before diving have specific actions independently on FMD and VGE, while others interfere with both [29].

In a recent experiment, a similar reduction in FMD was found in a setting excluding bubble formation, but a significant change in FMD was demonstrated depending on the oxygen partial pressure of the breathed gas [30].

Moreover, in this experimental setting, we only saw minimal levels of bubbles allowing for neglecting this stressor in such saturation decompression procedures. Decompression bubbles are very likely not to be found post decompression after saturation diving. Further investigations are needed to monitor bubbles production after excursions while being in saturation or during the decompression phase.

A nitric oxide (NO) mediated change in the surface properties of the vascular endothelium favoring the elimination of gas micronuclei has previously been suggested to explain this protection against bubble formation [31]. It was shown that NO synthase activity increases following 45 min of exercise, and, if done before a dive, it reduces VGE [32]. In saturation, although work can be considered as an exercise, it should be considered that the divers are otherwise sedentary.

It appears that FMD seems more linked to oxygen partial pressure changes during diving, whereas VGE are more depending on preexisting gas micronuclei population [33,34] in the tissues and vascular system and coping with inflammatory responses [29,35].

FMD is a marker of endothelial function and is reduced in the brachial artery of healthy divers after single or repetitive dives [29,35]. This effect does not seem to be related to the amount of VGE and was partially reversed by acute and long-term pre-dive supplementation of antioxidants, implicating oxidative stress as an important contributor to post-dive endothelial dysfunction [36,37].

Decreased nitroglycerin-mediated dilation after diving highlights dysfunction in vascular smooth-muscle cells as possible etiology of those results [37].

Very recent data show that the FMD reduction encountered after a single dive without the presence of VGE, is comparable to the reduction found with the presence of VGE [30].

The divers that volunteered in our saturation experiment were taking some antioxidant "medication" (see Table 3) as a protective measure, the trend of our data doesn't show a clear inflexion for some participants that could be explained by antioxidants intake, although 60% of the divers declared doing so.

A recent manuscript [25] shows very interesting results allowing for following the oxidative defenses status post saturation. Although the depth and duration differ from our setting, the recovery time for NOx is around 24 h.

Our data are in tune with the NOx returning to baseline, since FMD is closely related to the availability of nitric oxide (NO), and we can see from our results that FMD almost fully recovers after 8 h. If we apply the formula extracted from our data the mean time needed to reach 100% recovery would be around 540 min (9 h) and in the least predictive range (−95%) around 600 min (10 h) would be needed to fully recover, which is confirmed by Mrakic-Sposta et al. (2020) results. In fact, their results show that 24 h post saturation, the ROS

(Reactive Oxygen Species) are still significantly higher than baseline, but concomitantly TAC (Total Antioxidant Capacity) is also still high. From our results we can consider that the vascular dysfunction has already recovered and that the balance between antioxydants and prooxydants is clearly efficient and therefore fostering recovery. Another parameter measured by Mrakic-Sposta et al. [25] was IL-6 (Interleukin-6), this citokine reflects pro/anti-inflammatory response, and was increased during saturation but it was not significantly different than baseline 24 h post saturation.

6. Limitations

Strengths:
- This study builds on established modern methods of evaluation of decompression stress including vascular function and current theories of VGE generation.
- As there is possible large inter-individual variation for VGE and FMD effects after diving, the subjects served as their own controls.
- The measured effects are consistent with the theoretical rationale and do not require complicated new hypotheses.
- The equipment used for these experiments is readily available and reliable, inviting other research groups to repeat the study.
- The study was performed in real operational activities.
- A large number of divers volunteered for the study (never a saturation diving study addressed so many participants).

Weaknesses:
- The subjects were not homogenous or necessarily similar in body composition (age, weight, fat/lean mass distribution, sex).
- Operational constraints sometimes altered the planning of the measurements.
- Gender balance was impossible to reach.

7. Conclusions

This monitoring session has no equivalent in the commercial diving industry because of its duration (6 month), conditions (a working diving support vessel) and the large number of divers who volunteered for the study. It was the first time that the possibility for assessing onsite the vascular function of divers was offered during actual saturation diving operations. The study not only confirmed the role of inflammation and oxidative stress in saturation diving but it also permitted to obtain an estimation of the recovery time needed.

The lessons learnt from this experiment were that (1) scientific studies are possible even on a diving support vessel during operations under extreme environmental conditions. (2) Both national safety rules seem to provide health of the divers. (3) The equipment selected for the study was too heavy to be easily mobilized, and it could only work at ambient pressure and required a specific expertise. The future monitoring sessions, if any, should aim at using simpler equipment, which could be operated by the divers themselves inside the chamber, under pressure. Future experiments should include pressure resistance bubble measuring devices such as the O'Dive system tool to ascertain a minimal bubble number in the sub-clavian vein during excursion dives and during decompression [38].

Author Contributions: All authors listed have made a substantial, direct and intellectual contribution to the work, and approved it for publication. Conceptualization, J.-P.I., S.-M.E. and C.B. Onboard monitoring J.-P.I.; Writing, J.-P.I., S.-M.E. and C.B.; Review and editing, J.-P.I., S.-M.E. and C.B. All authors have read and agreed to the published version of the manuscript.

Funding: Technip FMC, generously hosted the study and the research team on one of their diving support vessels which is a major contribution. The work is also supported with a grant by The Scientific and Technological Research Council of Turkey (TUBITAK) (for S.-M.E.) The sponsors had no role in the design and conduct of the study; collection, management, analysis, and interpretation of the data; preparation, review, or approval of the manuscript; and the decision to submit the manuscript for publication.

Institutional Review Board Statement: The study was conducted in accordance with the Declaration of Helsinki and received ethical approval from Local Ethic Committee Brussels (Academic Bioethical Committee, Brussels, Belgium. Reference Number: B200-2009-039). Date: 10 October 2015.

Informed Consent Statement: Informed consent was obtained from all subjects involved in the study.

Data Availability Statement: Data are available at request from the authors.

Acknowledgments: The authors are grateful to Technip FMC that supported the study and, in particular to Andy Butler, Diving Technical Authority & Lead; Technip FMC who actively promoted the study within the Company and organized the venue of the team onboard the Deep Arctic DSV. We also want to express special acknowledgements to the divers who volunteered to participate to study and all the surface operational personnel who made the monitoring sessions possible.

Conflicts of Interest: The authors declare no conflict of interest.

Abbreviations

NO	Nitric Oxide
TAC	Total Antioxidant Capacity
FMD	Flow-Mediated Dilation
HR	Heart Rate
ROS	Reactive Oxygen Species
NOx	Nitric Oxide Metabolites
NO	Nitric Oxide
DSV	Diving Support Vessel
EB	Eftedal – Brubakk Score
hPa	Hecto-Pascal
msw	Meters of sea water
VGE	Vascular Gas Emboli
IL-6	Interleukin-6

References

1. Imbert, J.P.; Balestra, C.; Kiboub, F.Z.; Loennechen, O.; Eftedal, I. Commercial Divers' Subjective Evaluation of Saturation. *Front. Psychol.* **2018**, *9*, 2774. [CrossRef] [PubMed]
2. Kiboub, F.Z.; Balestra, C.; Loennechen, O.; Eftedal, I. Hemoglobin and Erythropoietin after Commercial Saturation Diving. *Front. Physiol.* **2018**, *9*, 1176. [CrossRef] [PubMed]
3. Berenji Ardestani, S.; Balestra, C.; Bouzinova, E.V.; Loennechen, O.; Pedersen, M. Evaluation of Divers' Neuropsychometric Effectiveness and High-Pressure Neurological Syndrome via Computerized Test Battery Package and Questionnaires in Operational Setting. *Front. Physiol.* **2019**, *10*, 1386. [CrossRef] [PubMed]
4. Wekre, S.L.; Landsverk, H.D.; Lautridou, J.; Hjelde, A.; Imbert, J.P.; Balestra, C.; Eftedal, I. Hydration status during commercial saturation diving measured by bioimpedance and urine specific gravity. *Front. Physiol.* **2022**, *13*, 971757. [CrossRef]
5. Mrakic-Sposta, S.; Gussoni, M.; Vezzoli, A.; Dellanoce, C.; Comassi, M.; Giardini, G.; Bruno, R.M.; Montorsi, M.; Corciu, A.; Greco, F.; et al. Acute Effects of Triathlon Race on Oxidative Stress Biomarkers. *Oxid. Med. Cell. Longev.* **2020**, *2020*, 3062807. [CrossRef]
6. Balestra, C.; Germonpre, P.; Rocco, M.; Biancofiore, G.; Kot, J. Diving physiopathology: The end of certainties? Food for thought. *Minerva Anestesiol.* **2019**, *85*, 1129–1137. [CrossRef]
7. Thom, S.R.; Milovanova, T.N.; Bogush, M.; Bhopale, V.M.; Yang, M.; Bushmann, K.; Pollock, N.W.; Ljubkovic, M.; Denoble, P.; Dujic, Z. Microparticle production, neutrophil activation, and intravascular bubbles following open-water SCUBA diving. *J. Appl. Physiol.* **2012**, *112*, 1268–1278. [CrossRef]
8. Arieli, R. Nanobubbles Form at Active Hydrophobic Spots on the Luminal Aspect of Blood Vessels: Consequences for Decompression Illness in Diving and Possible Implications for Autoimmune Disease-An Overview. *Front. Physiol.* **2017**, *8*, 591. [CrossRef]
9. Thom, S.R.; Milovanova, T.N.; Bogush, M.; Yang, M.; Bhopale, V.M.; Pollock, N.W.; Ljubkovic, M.; Denoble, P.; Madden, D.; Lozo, M.; et al. Bubbles, microparticles, and neutrophil activation: Changes with exercise level and breathing gas during open-water SCUBA diving. *J. Appl. Physiol.* **2013**, *114*, 1396–1405. [CrossRef]
10. Tremblay, J.C.; Thom, S.R.; Yang, M.; Ainslie, P.N. Oscillatory shear stress, flow-mediated dilatation, and circulating microparticles at sea level and high altitude. *Atherosclerosis* **2017**, *256*, 115–122. [CrossRef]
11. Balestra, C.; Arya, A.K.; Leveque, C.; Virgili, F.; Germonpré, P.; Lambrechts, K.; Lafère, P.; Thom, S.R. Varying Oxygen Partial Pressure Elicits Blood-Borne Microparticles Expressing Different Cell-Specific Proteins—Toward a Targeted Use of Oxygen? *Int. J. Mol. Sci.* **2022**, *23*, 7888. [CrossRef]

12. Thom, S.R.; Bhopale, V.M.; Yu, K.; Huang, W.; Kane, M.A.; Margolis, D.J. Neutrophil microparticle production and inflammasome activation by hyperglycemia due to cytoskeletal instability. *J. Biol. Chem.* **2017**, *292*, 18312–18324. [CrossRef]
13. Thom, S.R.; Yang, M.; Bhopale, V.M.; Huang, S.; Milovanova, T.N. Microparticles initiate decompression-induced neutrophil activation and subsequent vascular injuries. *J. Appl. Physiol.* **2011**, *110*, 340–351. [CrossRef]
14. Mause, S.F.; Ritzel, E.; Liehn, E.A.; Hristov, M.; Bidzhekov, K.; Müller-Newen, G.; Soehnlein, O.; Weber, C. Platelet microparticles enhance the vasoregenerative potential of angiogenic early outgrowth cells after vascular injury. *Circulation* **2010**, *122*, 495–506. [CrossRef]
15. Pyke, K.E.; Tschakovsky, M.E. The relationship between shear stress and flow-mediated dilatation: Implications for the assessment of endothelial function. *J. Physiol.* **2005**, *568*, 357–369. [CrossRef]
16. Corretti, M.C.; Anderson, T.J.; Benjamin, E.J.; Celermajer, D.; Charbonneau, F.; Creager, M.A.; Deanfield, J.; Drexler, H.; Gerhard-Herman, M.; Herrington, D.; et al. Guidelines for the ultrasound assessment of endothelial-dependent flow-mediated vasodilation of the brachial artery: A report of the International Brachial Artery Reactivity Task Force. *J. Am. Coll. Cardiol.* **2002**, *39*, 257–265. [CrossRef]
17. Areas, G.P.T.; Mazzuco, A.; Caruso, F.R.; Jaenisch, R.B.; Cabiddu, R.; Phillips, S.A.; Arena, R.; Borghi-Silva, A. Flow-mediated dilation and heart failure: A review with implications to physical rehabilitation. *Heart Fail. Rev.* **2019**, *24*, 69–80. [CrossRef]
18. Germonpre, P.; Papadopoulou, V.; Hemelryck, W.; Obeid, G.; Lafere, P.; Eckersley, R.J.; Tang, M.X.; Balestra, C. The use of portable 2D echocardiography and 'frame-based' bubble counting as a tool to evaluate diving decompression stress. *Diving Hyperb. Med.* **2014**, *44*, 5–13.
19. Eftedal, O.; Brubakk, A.O. Agreement between trained and untrained observers in grading intravascular bubble signals in ultrasonic images. *Undersea Hyperb. Med.* **1997**, *24*, 293–299.
20. Ozyigit, T.; Yavuz, C.; Egi, S.M.; Pieri, M.; Balestra, C.; Marroni, A. Clustering of recreational divers by their health conditions in a database of a citizen science project. *Undersea Hyperb. Med.* **2019**, *46*, 171–183. [CrossRef]
21. Doolette, D.J. Venous gas emboli detected by two-dimensional echocardiography are an imperfect surrogate endpoint for decompression sickness. *Diving Hyperb. Med.* **2016**, *46*, 4–10. [PubMed]
22. Møllerløkken, A.; Blogg, S.L.; Doolette, D.J.; Nishi, R.Y.; Pollock, N.W. Consensus guidelines for the use of ultrasound for diving research. *Diving Hyperb. Med.* **2016**, *46*, 26–32. [PubMed]
23. Lambrechts, K.; Germonpré, P.; Vandenheede, J.; Delorme, M.; Lafère, P.; Balestra, C. Mini Trampoline, a New and Promising Way of SCUBA Diving Preconditioning to Reduce Vascular Gas Emboli? *Int. J. Environ. Res. Public Health* **2022**, *19*, 5410. [CrossRef] [PubMed]
24. Łuczyński, D.; Lautridou, J.; Hjelde, A.; Monnoyer, R.; Eftedal, I. Hemoglobin during and following a 4-Week Commercial Saturation Dive to 200 m. *Front. Physiol.* **2019**, *10*, 1494. [CrossRef]
25. Mrakic-Sposta, S.; Vezzoli, A.; D'Alessandro, F.; Paganini, M.; Dellanoce, C.; Cialoni, D.; Bosco, G. Change in Oxidative Stress Biomarkers during 30 Days in Saturation Dive: A Pilot Study. *Int. J. Environ. Res. Public Health* **2020**, *17*, 7118. [CrossRef]
26. Monnoyer, R.; Haugum, K.; Lautridou, J.; Flatberg, A.; Hjelde, A.; Eftedal, I. Shifts in the Oral Microbiota during a Four-Week Commercial Saturation Dive to 200 Meters. *Front. Physiol.* **2021**, *12*, 669355. [CrossRef]
27. Monnoyer, R.; Lautridou, J.; Deb, S.; Hjelde, A.; Eftedal, I. Using Salivary Biomarkers for Stress Assessment in Offshore Saturation Diving: A Pilot Study. *Front. Physiol.* **2021**, *12*, 791525. [CrossRef]
28. Lambrechts, K.; Balestra, C.; Theron, M.; Henckes, A.; Galinat, H.; Mignant, F.; Belhomme, M.; Pontier, J.M.; Guerrero, F. Venous gas emboli are involved in post-dive macro, but not microvascular dysfunction. *Eur. J. Appl. Physiol.* **2017**, *117*, 335–344. [CrossRef]
29. Germonpre, P.; Balestra, C. Preconditioning to Reduce Decompression Stress in Scuba Divers. *Aerosp. Med. Hum. Perform.* **2017**, *88*, 114–120. [CrossRef]
30. Levenez, M.; Lambrechts, K.; Mrakic-Sposta, S.; Vezzoli, A.; Germonpré, P.; Pique, H.; Virgili, F.; Bosco, G.; Lafère, P.; Balestra, C. Full-Face Mask Use during SCUBA Diving Counters Related Oxidative Stress and Endothelial Dysfunction. *Int. J. Environ. Res. Public Health* **2022**, *19*, 965. [CrossRef]
31. Arieli, R. Gas micronuclei underlying decompression bubbles may explain the influence of oxygen enriched gases during decompression on bubble formation and endothelial function in self-contained underwater breathing apparatus diving. *Croat. Med. J.* **2019**, *60*, 388. [CrossRef]
32. Blatteau, J.E.; Boussuges, A.; Gempp, E.; Pontier, J.M.; Castagna, O.; Robinet, C.; Galland, F.M.; Bourdon, L. Haemodynamic changes induced by submaximal exercise before a dive and its consequences on bubble formation. *Br. J. Sport. Med.* **2007**, *41*, 375–379. [CrossRef]
33. Arieli, Y.; Katsenelson, K.; Arieli, R. Bubble reduction after decompression in the prawn Palaemon elegans by pretreatment with hyperbaric oxygen. *Undersea Hyperb. Med.* **2007**, *34*, 369–378.
34. Blatteau, J.E.; Souraud, J.B.; Gempp, E.; Boussuges, A. Gas nuclei, their origin, and their role in bubble formation. *Aviat. Space Environ. Med.* **2006**, *77*, 1068–1076.
35. Gempp, E.; Blatteau, J.E. Preconditioning methods and mechanisms for preventing the risk of decompression sickness in scuba divers: A review. *Res. Sport. Med.* **2010**, *18*, 205–218. [CrossRef]

36. Wang, Q.; Mazur, A.; Guerrero, F.; Lambrechts, K.; Buzzacott, P.; Belhomme, M.; Theron, M. Antioxidants, endothelial dysfunction, and DCS: In vitro and in vivo study. *J. Appl. Physiol.* **2015**, *119*, 1355–1362. [CrossRef]
37. Lambrechts, K.; Pontier, J.M.; Balestra, C.; Mazur, A.; Wang, Q.; Buzzacott, P.; Theron, M.; Mansourati, J.; Guerrero, F. Effect of a single, open-sea, air scuba dive on human micro- and macrovascular function. *Eur. J. Appl. Physiol.* **2013**, *113*, 2637–2645. [CrossRef]
38. Germonpre, P.; Van der Eecken, P.; Van Renterghem, E.; Germonpre, F.L.; Balestra, C. First impressions: Use of the Azoth Systems O'Dive subclavian bubble monitor on a liveaboard dive vessel. *Diving Hyperb. Med.* **2020**, *50*, 405–412. [CrossRef]

MDPI
St. Alban-Anlage 66
4052 Basel
Switzerland
Tel. +41 61 683 77 34
Fax +41 61 302 89 18
www.mdpi.com

Medicina Editorial Office
E-mail: medicina@mdpi.com
www.mdpi.com/journal/medicina

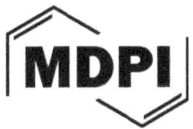

www.ingramcontent.com/pod-product-compliance
Lightning Source LLC
LaVergne TN
LVHW070617100526
838202LV00012B/668